Oral Health and Systemic Diseases

Oral Health and Systemic Diseases

Editor: Theresa Martino

AMERICAN
MEDICAL PUBLISHERS
www.americanmedicalpublishers.com

AMERICAN
MEDICAL PUBLISHERS
www.americanmedicalpublishers.com

Cataloging-in-Publication Data

Oral health and systemic diseases / edited by Theresa Martino.
p. cm.
Includes bibliographical references and index.
ISBN 978-1-63927-771-1
1. Oral manifestations of general diseases. 2. Mouth--Diseases--Complications.
3. Mouth--Infections--Complications. 4. Mouth--Care and hygiene. 5. Dental hygiene.
6. Oral medicine. I. Martino, Theresa.
RK61 .O73 2023
617.522--dc23

American Medical Publishers,
41 Flatbush Avenue,
1st Floor, New York,
NY 11217, USA

ISBN 978-1-63927-771-1 (Hardback)

Contents

Preface

Oral health is essential for maintaining systematic health. A good oral health can decrease the risk of various systemic diseases, such as rheumatoid arthritis, cardiovascular disease and diabetes. Oral diseases are linked to other diseases of the body due to the natural reaction of the human body towards harmful stimuli, which is known as inflammatory response. It is the body's warning response towards viruses and infections. The common symptoms of inflammation include pain, swelling, redness, heat and limited function. Rheumatoid arthritis, cardiovascular disease, gum diseases and diabetes all have similar type of inflammatory response. Severe gum disease can increase systemic inflammation, which develops in the background and may turn into severe systemic diseases. Oral bacteria trigger the formation of C-reactive proteins (CRPs), which cause inflammation resulting in the formation of clots in the arteries, thereby increasing the risk of stroke and heart diseases. The topics included in this book on oral health and systemic diseases are of utmost significance and bound to provide incredible insights to readers. It will serve as a valuable source of reference for graduate and post graduate students.

The information shared in this book is based on empirical researches made by veterans in this field of study. The elaborative information provided in this book will help the readers further their scope of knowledge leading to advancements in this field.

Finally, I would like to thank my fellow researchers who gave constructive feedback and my family members who supported me at every step of my research.

Editor

1

Defining Metaniches in the Oral Cavity According to their Microbial Composition and Cytokine Profile

Corinna L. Seidel [1,*], Roman G. Gerlach [2], Patrick Wiedemann [1], Matthias Weider [1], Gabriele Rodrian [1], Michael Hader [3], Benjamin Frey [3,4], Udo S. Gaipl [3,4], Aline Bozec [4,5], Fabian Cieplik [6], Christian Kirschneck [7], Christian Bogdan [2,4] and Lina Gölz [1]

1 Department of Orthodontics and Orofacial Orthopedics, Universitätsklinikum Erlangen and Friedrich-Alexander Universität (FAU) Erlangen-Nürnberg, Glückstr. 11, 91054 Erlangen, Germany; patrick.wiedemann@fau.de (P.W.); matthias.weider@uk-erlangen.de (M.W.); gabriele.rodrian@uk-erlangen.de (G.R.); lina.goelz@uk-erlangen.de (L.G.)

2 Mikrobiologisches Institut-Klinische Mikrobiologie, Immunologie und Hygiene, Universitätsklinikum Erlangen and Friedrich-Alexander-Universität (FAU) Erlangen-Nürnberg, Wasserturmstraße 3/5, 91054 Erlangen, Germany; roman.gerlach@uk-erlangen.de (R.G.G.); christian.bogdan@uk-erlangen.de (C.B.)

3 Department of Radiation Oncology, Universitätsklinikum Erlangen and Friedrich-Alexander-Universität (FAU) Erlangen-Nürnberg, Universitätsstr. 27, 91054 Erlangen, Germany; michael.hader@uk-erlangen.de (M.H.); benjamin.frey@uk-erlangen.de (B.F.); udo.gaipl@uk-erlangen.de (U.S.G.)

4 Medical Immunology Campus Erlangen, FAU Erlangen-Nürnberg, 91054 Erlangen, Germany

5 Department of Medicine 3, Rheumatology and Immunology, Universitätsklinikum Erlangen and Friedrich-Alexander-Universität (FAU) Erlangen-Nürnberg, Glückstr. 6, 91054 Erlangen, Germany; aline.bozec@uk-erlangen.de

6 Department of Conservative Dentistry and Periodontology, University Hospital Regensburg, Franz-Josef-Strauß-Allee 11, 93053 Regensburg, Germany; fabian.cieplik@ukr.de

7 Department of Orthodontics, University Hospital Regensburg, Franz-Josef-Strauß-Allee 11, 93053 Regensburg, Germany; christian.kirschneck@ukr.de

* Correspondence: corinna.seidel@uk-erlangen.de;

Abstract: The human oral microbiota consists of over 700 widespread taxa colonizing the oral cavity in several anatomically diverse oral niches. Lately, sequencing of the 16S rRNA genes has become an acknowledged, culture-independent method to characterize the oral microbiota. However, only a small amount of data are available concerning microbial differences between oral niches in periodontal health and disease. In the context of periodontitis, the cytokine expression in the gingival crevicular fluid has been studied in detail, whereas little is known about the cytokine profile in hard and soft tissue biofilms. In order to characterize oral niches in periodontal health, the oral microbiota and cytokine pattern were analyzed at seven different sites (plaque (P), gingival crevicular fluid (GCF), saliva (S), tongue (T), hard palate (HP), cheek (C) and sublingual area (U)) of 20 young adults using next-generation sequencing and multiplex immunoassays. Site-specific microbial compositions were detected, which clustered into three distinct metaniches ("P-GCF", "S-T-HP" and "C-U") and were associated with niche-/metaniche-specific cytokine profiles. Our findings allow the definition of distinct metaniches according to their microbial composition, partly reflected by their cytokine profile, and provide new insights into microenvironmental similarities between anatomical diverse oral niches.

Keywords: oral microbiota; oral niches; metaniches; cytokine profile; oral biofilms and fluids; next-generation sequencing; multiplex immunoassay

1. Introduction

The oral cavity serves as the first part of the digestive system and the respiratory tract showing complex environmental conditions and anatomically diverse oral niches, such as supra- and subgingival plaque on teeth, gingival sulcus and gingival crevicular fluid (GCF), keratinized gingiva and bucca mucosa, tongue, sublingual area, hard/soft palate, lips, tonsils and saliva [1].

In 2015, Hajishengallis et al. [2] introduced a new explanatory model in the etiology of periodontal disease: periodontal health was defined as a state of "symbiosis" between the resident, eubiotic microorganisms and the immune cells of the host. Instead, periodontitis was defined as a "dysbiotic inflammatory disease", in which exogenous factors (e.g., plaque accumulation, smoking, malnourishment, stress) can lead to an imbalance between pathogenic and protective bacteria causing dysregulation of the immune response, an excessive inflammatory reaction and the development of periodontal disease [2]. Therefore, the investigation of both the oral microbiota and the cytokine profile is crucial when studying periodontal health and periodontitis.

The oral cavity shows the second-largest microbiota in the human body after the gut microbiota [1,3,4]. Recently, sequencing of the 16S rRNA genes has become an acknowledged, culture-independent method to characterize the oral microbiota, as most of the oral bacteria cannot be cultivated [1]. 775 taxa have been detected up to now, while only 57% are cultivable and named, 30% are uncultivable phylotypes, and 13% are cultivable but unnamed [5,6]. As the intrauterine surrounding is sterile, the development of the neonatal microbiota begins during and after birth, which is an ongoing process during childhood towards an "adult oral microbiota". This process seems to be influenced by the cross-talk between the oral and gut microbiota as well as by exogenous factors, such as the microbiota of family members or the type of diet. The oral-gut microbiota axis also seems to be crucial for the maturation of our immune system, especially during the first year of life [3,7–12]. Regarding bacterial composition in patients with periodontitis and periodontal health, most studies have focused on the characterization of the whole microbiota or investigation of supra- or subgingival plaque [1,13], while only a few elucidated microbial similarities or dissimilarities between distinct oral niches with varying—and at times contradictory—results [4,14–18]. Moreover, there is a lack of a clear definition and differentiation of "symbiosis" and "dysbiosis", complicating the usage of this definition [2] for diagnosis and research purposes.

The immune response against bacterial pathogens in the oral cavity is triggered by several immune cells and humoral mediators like cytokines and chemokines [19]. Inflammation in periodontal disease has been studied intensively by analysis of the cytokine expression in GCF [20,21]. Thereby an increase of pro-inflammatory cytokines such as interleukin (IL)-1β, -2, -6, -8, tumour-necrosis-factor (TNF), and interferon-gamma (IFN-γ) was seen in periodontitis, while a decrease of inflammation was detected after periodontal treatment [19–24]. Moreover, several studies focused on salivary cytokine biomarkers and detected higher levels of pro-inflammatory cytokines not only in periodontitis [25] but also in the saliva of smokers [26] and patients with oral squamous cell carcinoma [27]. However, to our knowledge, so far no correlation analysis of cytokine and chemokine expression with differences in the oral microbiome in periodontal health has been performed. Furthermore, the complex cytokine network and their pathways in the activation of immune cells in oral diseases are crucial [28] and further studies are necessary to gain knowledge about cytokine composition in other oral niches like dental biofilm or the salivary pellicle on different soft tissue surfaces.

Therefore, this study aimed to analyse the microbial composition and the cytokine expression in different oral niches of young adults maintaining periodontal health and excellent oral hygiene (Approximal-Plaque-Index <25%, Bleeding-on-Probing-Index <3%, study population consisting of dental students and dentists with an excellent daily oral hygiene and regular prophylaxis) and to investigate possible similarities or discrepancies in the oral cavity. Defining oral sites in perfect periodontal health is crucial for future studies analysing changes in the composition of the oral microbiota or immune response associated with treatment or oral diseases.

2. Results

Oral microbiota composition and cytokine profiles were studied in 280 samples collected from 7 different oral niches (2 samples per niche) of 20 study participants. To this aim, unstimulated saliva samples (S) were obtained by the spitting method and soft tissue samples were collected from the middle part of the hard palate (HP), the middle and anterior part of the tongue (T), the middle part of the sublingual area (U) and the molar region of the right cheek (C) using sterile swabs. Moreover, hard tissue samples of supragingival plaque (P) were taken by sterile curettes and samples of gingival crevicular fluid (GCF) were collected from 6 periodontal pockets using sterile paper strips.

2.1. *Microbial Composition*

Oral microbiota analyses of 140 samples from 7 different oral niches (P, GCF, S, T, HP, C, U) showed 9 different microbial phyla, 14 classes, 30 orders, 44 families, and 75 genera derived from 300 operational taxonomic units (OTU).

In summary, the oral microbiota of healthy young adults is dominated by *Actinobacteriota, Bacteroidota, Firmicutes* and *Proteobacteria* on phylum level, *Actinobacteria, Bacilli, Bacteroidia, Fusobacteria* and *Gammaproteobacteria* on class level, *Actinomycetales, Bacteroidales, Flavobacteriales, Fusobacteriales, Lactobacillales, Pasteurellales* and *Veillonellales* on order level; *Actinomycetaceae, Camplyobacteriae, Carnobacteriacae, Flavobacteriacae, Fusobacteriaceae, Gemellaceae, Lachnospraceae, Leptotrichiaceae, Micrococcaceae, Porphyromonadacea, Prevotellaceae, Streptococcaceae* and *Veillonellaceae* on family level, and *Actinobacillus, Actinomyces, Alloprevotella, Campylobacter, Capnocytophaga, Corynebacterium, Fusobacterium, Gemella, Granulicatella, Haemophilus, Lautropia, Leptotrichia, Neisseria, Porphyromonas, Prevotella, Rothia* and *Veillonella* on genus level (Figure S1).

2.1.1. Distribution of Microbial Genera in Different Oral Niches and Definition of Metaniches

Regarding the microbial composition of all seven niches for each healthy individual, no clustering was detectable for individual oral microbiotas. However, three distinct clusters were observed in a dendrogram based on generalized UniFrac distances, roughly correlating with groups of sampling sites (Figure 1). The first branch showed clustering of plaque (P) and gingival crevicular fluid (GCF), the second branch for saliva (S), tongue (T), and hard palate (HP), and the last branch showed clusters for cheek (C) and sublingual area (U) with some inter-individual variabilities. According to these branches, the frequencies of microbial genera showed specific patterns for P-GCF, S-T-HP, and C-U (Figure 1). Therefore, we could define three specific microbial "metaniches" according to the given data:

(1) supragingival plaque and gingival crevicular fluid (P-GCF);
(2) saliva-tongue-hard palate (S-T-HP);
(3) cheek and sublingual area (C-U).

Most samples of metaniche P-GCF showed relatively higher proportions of the following genera compared to metaniches S-T-HP and C-U: *Actinomyes, Aggregatibacter, Fusobacterium, Leptotrichia, Capnocytophaga, Corynebacterium, Lautropia, Campylobacter* and *Tannerella*.

Compared to metaniches P-GCF and C-U, samples from branch S-T-HP showed higher proportions of the subsequent genera: *Prevotella, Neisseria, Veillonella, Porphyromonas, Granulicatella,* and *Alloprevotella*.

Regarding metaniche C-U compared to P-GCF and S-T-HP noticeably higher frequencies were seen for the following genera: *Haemophilus, Streptococcus, Gemella* and *Actinobacillus*.

Despite the recognizable differences between the three branches seen in the dendrogram (Figure 1), some genera showed similar amounts in all sites like *Rothia*.

According to the Shannon diversity index, samples of metaniche P-GCF showed a significantly higher alpha diversity compared to metaniche S-T-HP and C-U (3.64 ± 0.07 vs. 3.20 ± 0.05 vs. 2.58 ± 0.13, $p < 0.0001$), while metaniche C-U showed the lowest diversity (Figure 1, right side).

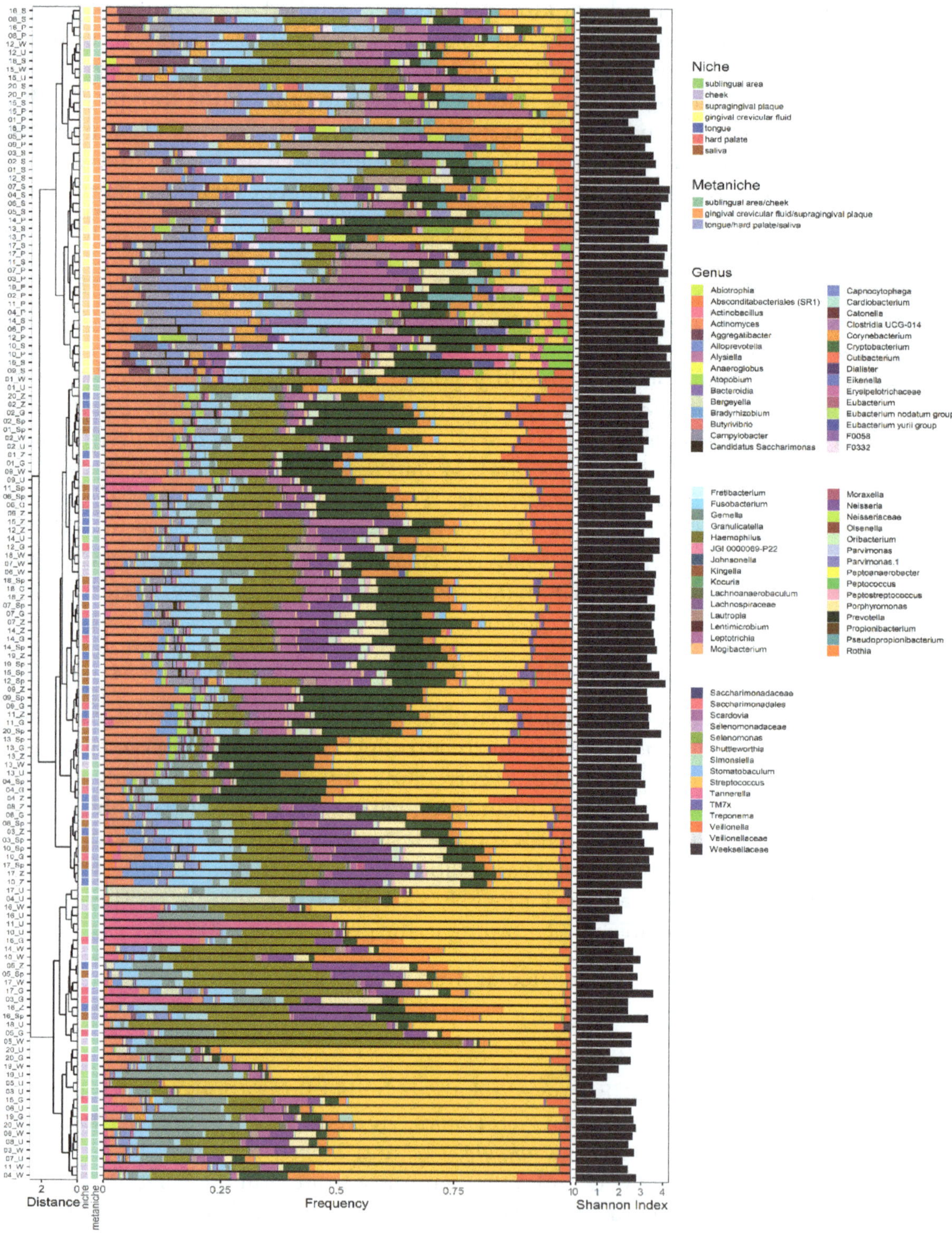

Figure 1. Dendrogram, genus frequencies plot, and Shannon index representing the genera detected in different oral niches and metaniches. A dendrogram based on generalized UniFrac distances is given for all oral niches (sublingual area, cheek, supragingival plaque, gingival crevicular fluid, tongue, hard palate, saliva) and metaniches (sublingual area/cheek; gingival crevicular fluid/supragingival plaque; tongue/hard palate/saliva) for each individual subject and sample (colour key is given on the right side). Genus frequencies found in the individual microbiotas are given with a colour key for the different genera, which are sorted alphabetically and presented horizontally from the left to the right side. The Shannon diversity index is given on the right side.

The grouping of niches into metaniches was confirmed by analysing beta diversity using multidimensional scaling (MDS) plots. We found the ellipse centres of plaque and gingival crevicular fluid, of cheek and sublingual area, and of saliva, tongue and hard palate, each in close proximity to each other (Figure 2a). While showing hardly any overlap to the other groups, the microbial profiles of P-GCF were in closest proximity to saliva (Figure 2a). In contrast, saliva, tongue, hard palate, cheek and sublingual area exhibited overlapping microbial profiles. This would make saliva to be the "connecting part" between all oral niches (Figure 2a). When grouped according to the identified clusters, the multidimensional scaling (MDS) plot underlined the presence of distinct metaniches in the oral cavity (Figure 2b).

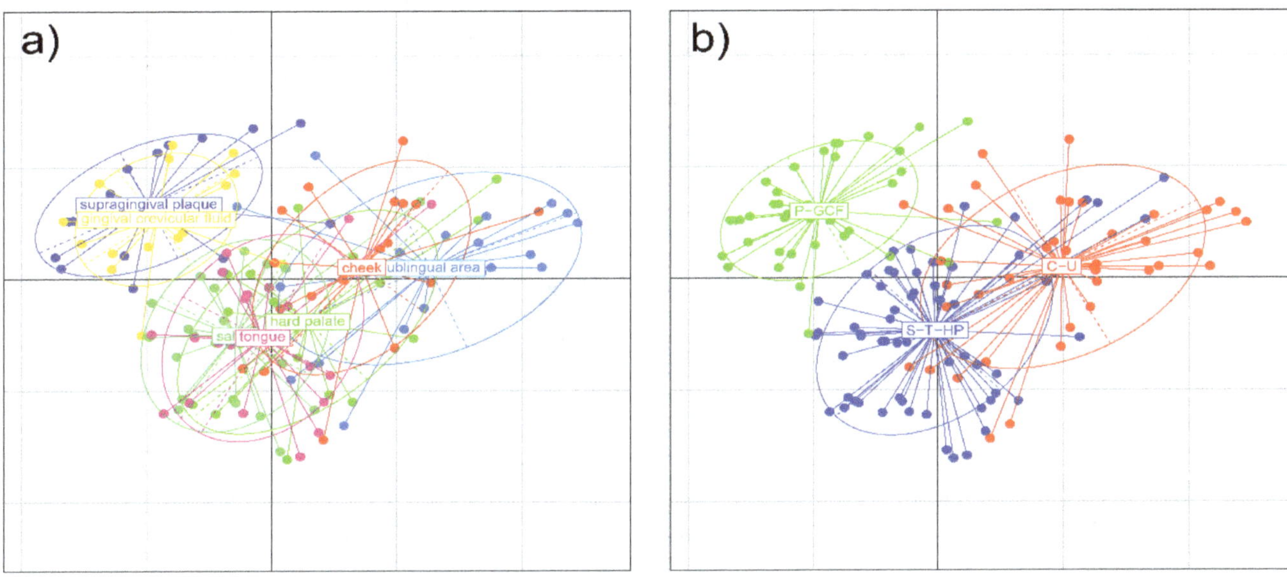

Figure 2. MDS plots of microbial profiles are given. (**a**) MDS plot for microbial profiles for all oral niches (plaque, gingival crevicular fluid, saliva, tongue, palate, cheek, sublingual) are displayed; (**b**) MDS plot of microbial profiles for defined metaniches (P-GCF = plaque/gingival crevicular fluid, S-T-HP = saliva/tongue/palate, C-U = cheek/sublingual) are displayed.

To summarize, we could define three specific microbial metaniches according to the given data "P-GCF", "S-T-HP" and "C-U".

2.1.2. Characteristic Species for Defined Metaniches

Characteristic microbial patterns for defined metaniches were not only seen on the genus level, but also on the OTU/species level. Analysis of statistically significant enrichment or depletion depending on the oral metaniche identified 24 OTUs (Figure 3).

Metaniche "P-GCF" demonstrated clearly higher values of the following OTUs compared to metaniche "C-U" and "S-T-HP": **OTU_14** (*Rothia* sp.); **OTU_16** (*Campylobacter gracilis*); **OTU_20** (*Streptococcus sanguinis*); **OTU_24** (*Fusobacterium nucleatum*); **OTU_92** (*Capnocytophaga* sp.); **OTU_40028** (*Streptococcus* sp.); **OTU_108** (*Prevotella oris*); **OTU_147** (*Leptotrichia buccalis*) and **OTU_231** (*Fusobacterium* sp.).

In **metaniche "S-T-HP"**, various OTUs were much more prevalent compared to metaniche "P-GCF" and "C-U": **OTU_1** (*Streptococcus salivarius*); **OTU_2** (*Fusobacterium (pseudo)periodonticum*); **OTU_4** (*Prevotella melanogenica*); **OTU_6** (*Neisseria* sp.); **OTU_12** (*Granulicatella adiacens*); **OTU_15** (*Veillonella dispar*); **OTU_21** (*Actinomyces* sp.); **OTU_22** (*Streptococcus* sp.); **OTU_29** (*Porphyromonas* sp.); **OTU_39** (*Saccharimonadaceae*) and **OTU_45** (*Campylobacter* sp.).

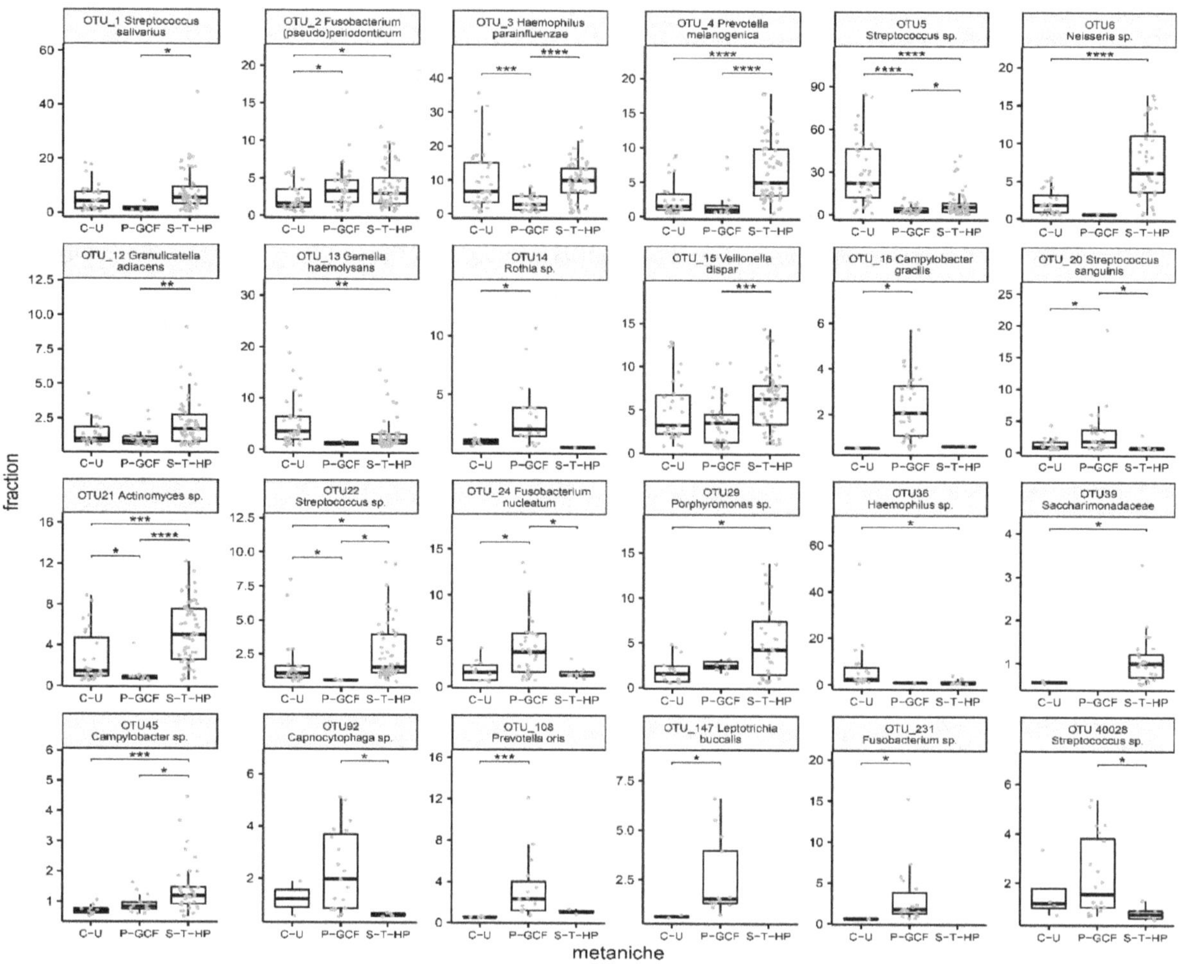

Figure 3. Characteristic operational taxonomic units (OTUs) for three different defined metaniches "plaque and gingival crevicular fluid" (P-GCF), "saliva, tongue and hard palate" (S-T-HP) and "cheek-sublingual" (C-U) are shown. The data is presented as median, 25 and 75 percentiles (box) and 1.5 × interquartile range of the 25 and 75 percentiles (whiskers). Raw data (n = 0-59) is displayed as overlaying grey points. Statistical analysis was performed using Mann-Whitney U-tests and was adjusted for sample size using the Benjamin–Hochberg algorithm. * $0.01 \leq p < 0.05$, ** $0.001 \leq p < 0.01$, *** $0.0001 \leq p < 0.001$, **** $p < 0.0001$.

Concerning **metaniche "C-U"**, a smaller number of OTUs allowed discrimination from "S-T-HP" and "P-GCF": **OTU_3** (*Haemophilus parainfluenzae*); **OTU_5** (*Streptococcus* sp.); **OTU_13** (*Gemella haemolysans*) and **OTU_36** (*Haemophilus* sp.).

Taken together, species like *Rothia* sp., *Campylobacter gracilis*, *Streptococcus sanguinis*, *Fusobacterium nucleatum*, *Capnocytophaga* sp., *Streptococcus* sp. and *Prevotella oris* were characteristic for metaniche **"P-GCF"**, *Streptococcus salivarius*, *Fusobacterium (pseudo)periodonticum*, *Prevotella melanogenica*, *Granulicatella adiacens*, *Veillonella dispar*, *Actinomyces* sp., *Streptococcus* sp., *Porphyromonas* sp., *Saccharimonadaceae* and *Campylobacter* sp. were peculiar for metaniche **"S-T-HP"** and *Haemophilus parainfluenzae*, *Streptococcus* sp., *Gemella haemolysans* and *Haemophilus* sp. distinctive for metaniche **"C-U"**.

2.2. Cytokine Profile

In our first approach, we compared the overall concentration of cytokines in 140 samples of the 7 described oral niches. Subsequently, we analyzed whether each oral niche shows a characteristic pattern of cytokine expression and whether it is related to certain microbial metaniches.

2.2.1. Cytokine Concentration in Different Oral Niches

The concentration (pg/mL) of granulocyte-macrophage colony-stimulating-factor (GM-CSF), IFN-γ, IL-2, IL-4, IL-6, IL-8 and IL-10 as well as TNF was measured in all oral niches (P, GCF, D, T, HP, C, U) and summed up (Figure S2). We observed significantly higher expression of cytokines in the gingival crevicular fluid with a mean value of 13,284.78 ± 2869.64 pg/mL compared to the hard palate (292.40 ± 73.38 pg/mL, $p < 0.0001$), plaque (768.20 ± 182.90 pg/mL, $p < 0.0001$), saliva (241.70 ± 60.53 pg/mL, $p < 0.0001$), sublingual area (27.31 ± 7.05 pg/mL, $p < 0.0001$), cheek (61.48 ± 13.83 pg/mL, $p < 0.0001$) and tongue (201.50 ± 69.20 pg/mL, $p < 0.0001$), respectively. Plaque (768.20 ± 182.90 pg/mL) showed significantly higher values compared to hard palate (292.4 ± 73.38 pg/mL), tongue (201.50 ± 69.20 pg/mL) and saliva (292.40 ± 73.38), while the lowest concentrations were found in cheek (61.48 ± 13.83 pg/mL) and sublingual area (27.31 ± 7.05 pg/mL).

To conclude, the highest cytokine concentrations were found in the gingival crevicular fluid, while plaque also showed higher values. Saliva, tongue and hard palate showed similar median values, whereas cheek and sublingual area contained the lowest cytokine concentration. Notably, the cytokine pattern somewhat correlated with the microbial metaniches "P-GCF", "S-T-HP" and "C-U", while GCF had a uniquely high cytokine concentration. Therefore, GCF was excluded from the further comparison of the anti- and pro-inflammatory cytokines in the different oral sites.

Considering the anti-inflammatory cytokines IL-10 and IL-4 [19], highest concentrations were found in supragingival plaque (IL-10: 14.38 ± 2.53; IL-4: 0.47 ± 0.08; both in pg/mL), while all other niches present significantly lower values (saliva 0.72 ± 0.12 IL-10 and 0.19 ± 0.02 IL-4; tongue 0.53 ± 0.67 IL-10 and 0.10 ± 0.04 IL-4; hard palate 0.28 ± 0.15 IL-10 and 0.14 ± 0.07 IL-4; cheek 0.30 ± 0.05 IL-10 and 0.07 ± 0.02 IL-4; sublingual area 0.39 ± 0.13 IL-10 and 0.22 ± 0.09 IL-4; all in pg/mL).

Regarding the measured pro-inflammatory cytokines [19], we found the highest concentrations of GM-CSF, IFN-γ, IL-6/-8 and TNF in supragingival plaque (3.62 ± 0.84 GM-CSF; 38.08 ± 8.14 IFN-γ; 17.87 ± 4.31 IL-6; 5,979 ± 1,072 IL-8; 11.03 ± 1.63 TNF; all in pg/mL). Notably, we detected the highest expression of IL-1β in the hard palate (1,533 ± 456.70 pg/mL) and the highest values of IL-2 in the sublingual area (2.28 ± 0.98 pg/mL).

In accordance with the microbial metaniche "S-T-HP" similar cytokine concentrations were found in saliva, tongue and hard palate for the following cytokines:

GM-CSF: saliva 1.27 ± 0.59, tongue 0.99 ± 0.29, hard palate 0.97 ± 0.46;

IFN-γ: saliva 6.45 ± 0.55, tongue 5.27 ± 2.04, hard palate 9.39 ± 4.05;

IL-6: saliva 5.54 ± 1.42, tongue 10.44 ± 6.05, hard palate 8.59 ± 2.50 (all in pg/mL).

Fitting with the microbial metaniche "C-U" similar and overall lowest cytokine concentrations were seen in cheek and sublingual area for the following cytokines:

GM-CSF: cheek 0.49 ± 0.12, sublingual area 0.71 ± 0.27;

IL-1β: cheek 38.49 ± 8.24, sublingual area 10.28 ± 2.27;

IL-6: cheek 4.17 ± 0.93, sublingual area 2.46 ± 0.69;

IL-8: cheek 501 ± 68.16, sublingual area 216.90 ± 45.16;

TNF: cheek 1.72 ± 0.26, sublingual area 2.28 ± 0.53 (all in pg/mL).

In summary, gingival crevicular fluid presented the highest values of all measured cytokines compared to other niches, while higher values were also found in plaque for most measured anti- and proinflammatory cytokines (GM-CSF, IFN-γ, IL-4/-6/-8/-10). Conforming to the microbial metaniche "S-T-HP" saliva, tongue and hard palate showed similar amounts of GM-CSF, IFN-γ and IL-6. In accordance with the microbial metaniche "C-U" cheek and sublingual area presented similar and the overall lowest cytokine concentrations of GM-CSF, IL-1β/-6/-8 and TNF.

2.2.2. Characteristic Cytokine Expression Pattern

In a second approach, we analyzed whether metaniches as seen in the microbial patterns also exist with respect to the concentrations and relative quantities of the measured cytokines at the different sites of sampling (Figures 4 and 5).

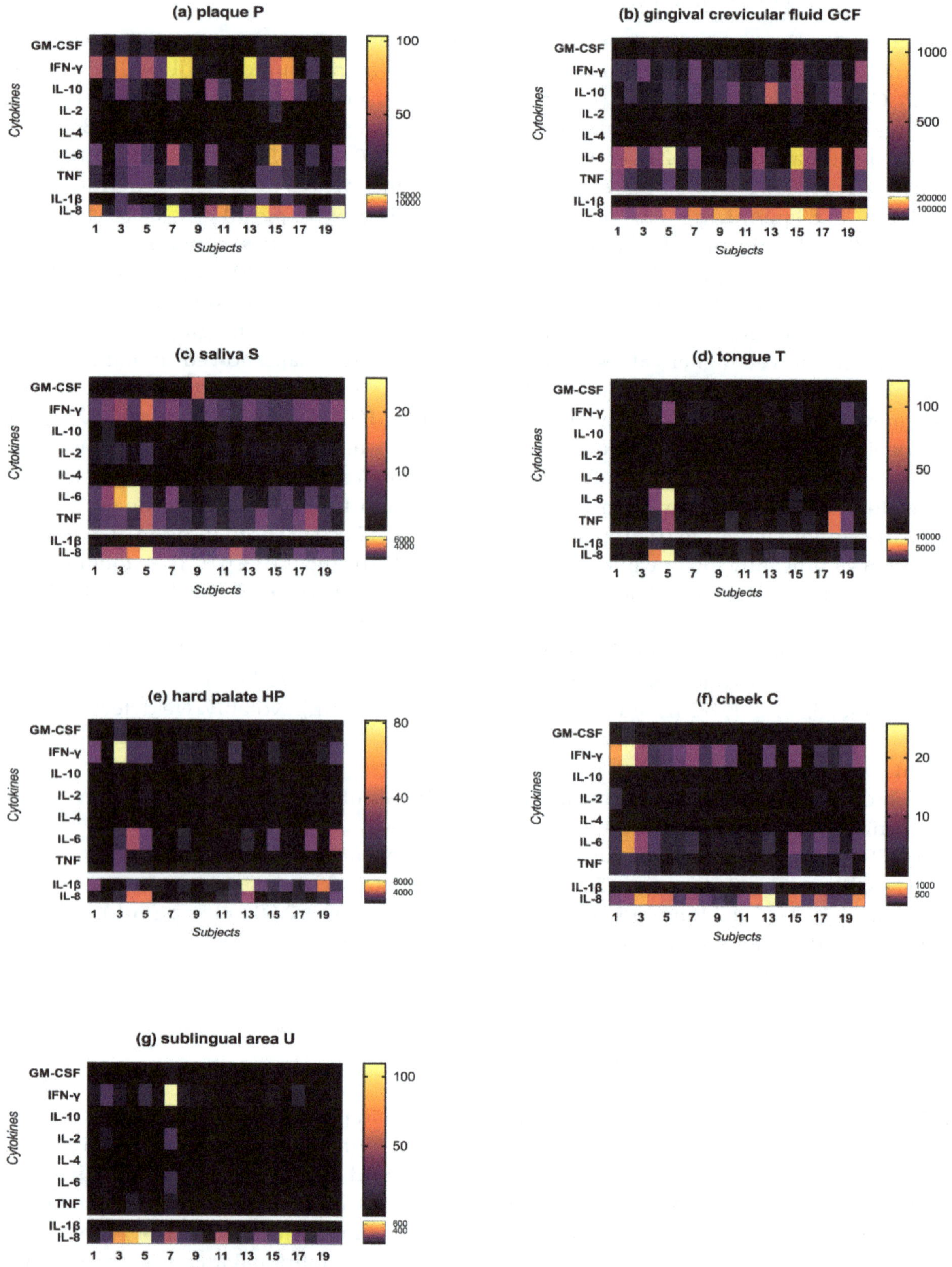

Figure 4. Heat map visualization of the cytokine concentration in different analyzed oral cavity sites including (**a**) supragingival plaque P, (**b**) gingival crevicular fluid GCF, (**c**) saliva S, (**d**) tongue T, (**e**) hard palate HP, (**f**) cheek C and (**g**) sublingual area U with the expression pattern of the pro- and anti-inflammatory cytokines. The cytokine concentration of GM-CSF, IFN-γ, IL-10, IL-2, IL-4, IL-6, TNF, IL-8 and IL-1β is shown. The inferno colour scale indicates the abundance of each cytokine in each subject, from black (zero, not observed) to very light yellow (highly abundant).

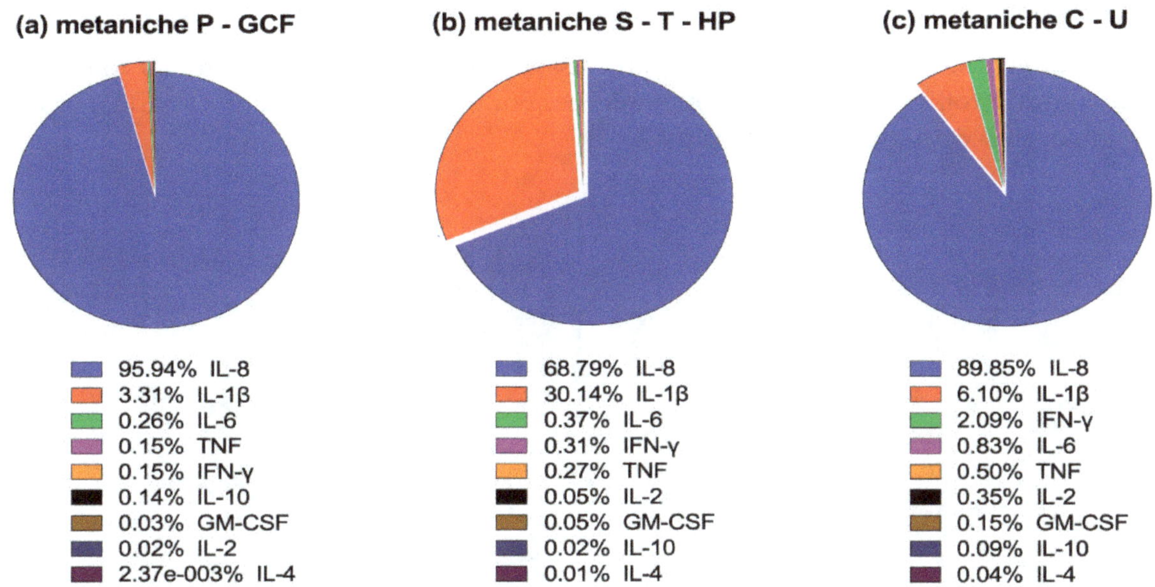

Figure 5. Relative quantities of cytokines in the defined microbial metaniches P-GCF, S-T-HP and C-U are given as a percentage of the total cytokine level measured. (**a**) metaniche P-GCF, (**b**) metaniche S-T-HP and (**c**) metaniche C-U.

Across all oral niches, the most dominant cytokine was IL-8, while IL-1β was also highly prevalent in most sites (Figure 4). Regarding IL-8 and IL-1β, similarities between hard palate and tongue were found with comparable concentrations of IL-1β and IL-8 showing similarities to the microbial metaniche "saliva-tongue-hard palate" (S-T-HP). Cheek and sublingual area also presented the lowest overall concentrations of IL-1β and IL-8 with similarities to the microbial metaniche "cheek-sublingual area" (C-U).

Regarding the other measured cytokines, similarities were also found for the immunological metaniche supragingival plaque and gingival crevicular fluid (P-GCF) with high concentrations of IL-10, IFN-γ, IL-6 and TNF and low concentrations of GM-CSF, IL-2 and IL-4 (Figure 4a,b). An "immunological metaniche" was also formed by tongue and hard palate (T-HP without S), which showed similar cytokine patterns with medium concentrations of IFN-γ, IL-6 and TNF and very low values of GM-CSF, IL-10, IL-2 and IL-4 (Figure 4d,e). Saliva took an intermediate position between the immunological metaniches "P-GCF", "T-HP" and "C-U", with high concentrations of IFN-γ, IL-6 and TNF similar to "P-GCF", but barely detectable IL-10 as observed in "T-HP" and "C-U", which are also characterized by relatively low IL-10 values (Figure 4a–f). Moreover, some samples of saliva showed high concentrations of GM-CSF and IL-2, which was not seen in other niches (Figure 4c). Cheek and sublingual area presented varying concentrations of IFN-γ, IL-6 and TNF with very low values of GM-CSF, IL-10, IL-2 and IL-4. However, a definitive correlation was not seen probably due to the low absolute cytokine concentrations in the sublingual area (Figure 4f,g).

In summary, by analyzing the relative quantities of cytokines measured in the defined microbial metaniches, we discovered characteristic cytokine profiles (Figure 5): Metaniche P-GCF is dominated by IL-8 with a low relative distribution of IL-1β, while all other measured cytokines ranged below 0.04%. Compared to P-GCF and C-U, metaniche S-T-HP showed a high proportion of IL-1β, being the second most abundant cytokine after IL-8. All other measured cytokines were also below 0.04%. While metaniche C-U was also dominated by IL-8, it was interesting to see that not only IL-1β but also IFN-γ, IL-6 and TNF showed relatively high values, whereas the values for IL-2, GM-CSF, IL-10 and IL-4 were again below 0.04%.

2.3. Correlation Between the Microbial Composition and Immunological Profile

In a final analysis, we investigated a possible association between the microbial composition and the immunological profiles of the defined metaniches. For that purpose, relative abundances of genera were correlated with cytokine levels (Figure 6).

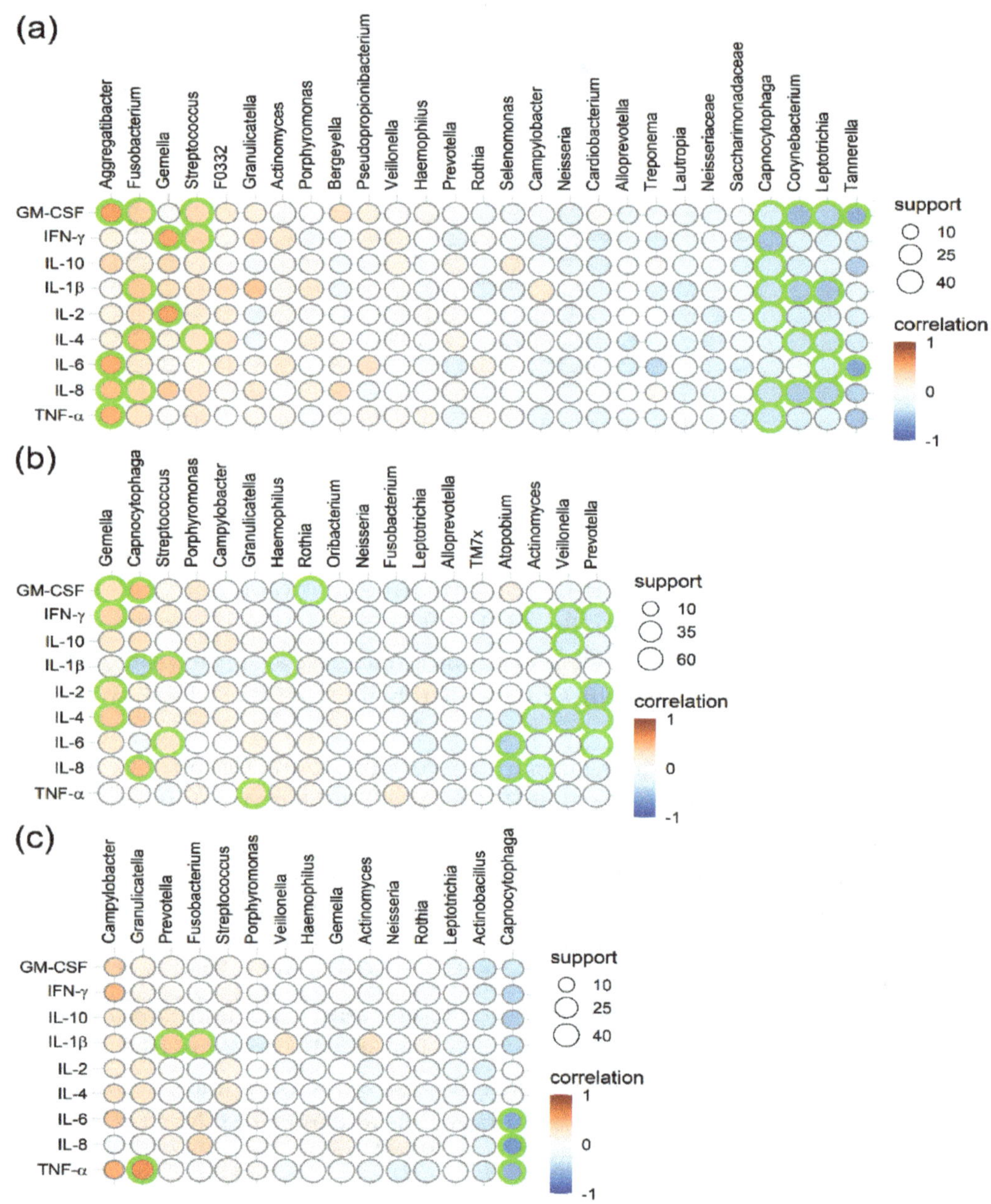

Figure 6. Pearson correlation plot between the cytokine concentrations and microbial composition (genus level) are given for the defined metaniches: (**a**) "plaque and gingival crevicular fluid" (P-GCF), (**b**) "saliva, tongue and hard palate" (S-T-HP) and (**c**) "cheek-sublingual" (C-U). The cytokines GM-CSF, IFN-ɣ, IL-10, IL-1ß, IL-2, -4, IL-6, IL-8, and TNF are given vertically on the left side, while genera are indicated horizontally on top of each figure. A colour key was used for the strength of correlation, ranging from highly positive (+1, red) to no correlation (0, white) to highly negative (−1, blue). The number of samples on which the results are based is depicted by the size of the circles, with a minimum of 10 and a maximum of 40 or 60 samples per metaniche. Shown are genera with a significant Pearson correlation ($p < 0.05$). Samples with significant correlation after Benjamin–Hochberg adjustment for sample size (adj. $p < 0.05$) were highlighted with bright green circles.

The following correlations between the cytokine profiles and the defined microbial metaniches were seen:

Regarding metaniche "P-GCF", positive correlations with high to highest support were found between cytokine levels and relative amounts of the genera *Aggregatibacter*, *Fusobacterium*, *Gemella* and *Streptococcus*, while negative correlations were seen with *Tannerella*, *Leptotrichia*, *Corynebacterium*, *Capnocytophaga*, *Saccharimononadae* and *Neisseriacae* (Figure 6a). In the metaniche "S-T-HP", positive correlations with the highest support were found for *Gemella* spp., while variable positive connections were identified for the genera *Capnocytophaga*, *Streptococcus*, *Porphyromonas* and *Campylobacter* (Figure 6b). Cytokine levels negatively correlated with relative amounts of *Prevotella*, *Veillonella* and *Actinomyces* species (Figure 6b). In the metaniche "C-U", we identified positive correlations with high to highest support for the genera *Campylobacter*, *Granulicatella* and *Prevotella*, while *Capnocytophaga*, *Actinobacillus* and *Leptotrichia* sp. negatively correlated with cytokine levels (Figure 6c).

3. Discussion

Regarding the pathogenesis of periodontal disease, previous theories relied on culture-based methods: Socransky et al. [29] divided bacterial species according to their pathogenicity into five microbial complexes and regarded the presence of the "red complex" consisting of *Porphyromonas gingivalis*, *Tannerella forsythia* and *Treponema denticola* as highly associated with periodontal inflammation. However, as mentioned above a new explanatory model defined periodontal health as a state of "symbiosis" and periodontal disease as a "dysbiotic inflammatory disease" [2]. To characterize the oral microbiota to its full complexity, the sequencing of the 16S rRNA genes has become an acknowledged, culture-independent method [1,3,4]. As the oral cavity contains several anatomically diverse oral niches, characterisation of the oral microbiota should not only focus on its whole complexity but also on their distinct niches.

3.1. Microbial Composition in Different Oral Niches

The first aim of this study was to investigate the microbial composition in different oral niches of young adults with excellent periodontal health and oral hygiene. To this aim, we analyzed the microbial composition in samples gained from 7 distinct oral niches (plaque (P), gingival crevicular fluid (GCF), saliva (S), tongue (T), hard palate (HP), cheek (C) and sublingual area (U)) using next generating sequencing.

We detected differences in the relative abundances of microbial genera between different oral niches. Moreover, with cluster analyses of the microbial composition of individual samples, we could define three specific microbial "metaniches": "P-GCF", "S-T-HP" and "C-U". A previous report also observed the formation of groups between seven diverse habitats of the digestive tract, which partly matched our results [30]. Here, four groups were defined: (1) buccal mucosa, keratinized gingiva and hard palate; (2) saliva, tongue, tonsils and throat; (3) sub- and supra-gingival plaques; (4) stool. In analogy to our results, clustering between saliva and tongue and differences in the microbial compositions between buccal mucosa, saliva/tongue and plaque were observed [30]. However, in contrast to our results, buccal mucosa and hard palate showed distinct clustering [30].

Regarding the microbial composition in different oral niches, another previous study analyzed the tongue dorsum, hard palate, buccal mucosa, keratinized gingiva, supragingival and subgingival plaque, and saliva with or without rinsing in 20 healthy subjects and demonstrated that no significant differences were seen between the study participants [4]. Consistent with this publication, no subject-related clustering was observed in our study. However, other previous studies detected not only site-specific but also subject-specific bacterial species in a study population of 5 subjects with a broad range of age (23 to 55 years) [17]. This dissimilarity might be explained by age-related alterations of the oral microbiota leading to "subject"-specific bacterial compositions. Also in line with our results, another investigation presented a "core microbiota" in health with strong similarities between unrelated individuals and pointed out that niche-specific microbiotas might exist [16]. However, only five niches (dental surfaces, cheek, hard palate, tongue and saliva) from three subjects were analyzed.

The similarities between plaque and gingival crevicular fluid and the clustering into metaniche "P-GCF" might be explained by their anatomical proximity to dental structures and direct contact to the gingival margin. Plaque can be found on the supra- or subgingival surface of teeth as a structurally and functionally organized complex microbial community with specific formation stages and has been referred to as "dental biofilm" [31]. This biofilm is considered the primary etiologic factor for polymicrobial inflammatory disease [32]. It was shown that the presence of a plaque/dental biofilm induces the production of the gingival crevicular fluid [33], which is a physiological fluid originating from blood vessels in the gingiva underlying the epithelium lining of the gingival sulcus [20,21]. Moreover, GCF serves as nutrition for biofilms in gingivitis and periodontitis and sulcus fluid flow rate (SFFR) increases dependent on the quantity and diversity of dental biofilm [34].

The origin and distribution of the saliva and the "salivary pellicles" found on tongue, hard palate, cheek and sublingual area are likely to account for the microbial similarities seen between "S-T-HP" and "C-U". Salivary glands can be differentiated into "major" and "minor" glands with varying quality and quantity of saliva [35]. Major glands are located in the buccal cheek (region of the first upper molar) and the sublingual area [35], which might explain the correlation seen between "C" and "U". Minor glands are found in the tongue, palate, lower lip [35], which might explain the microbial relationship between "T" and "HP". Considering anatomical variations, salivary flow is not constant, with the highest flow rate in the sublingual area and lowest in the anterior region of the maxillary front teeth [35]. The high clearance rate in the sublingual area and cheek with a constant salivary flow from major glands offers a plausible explanation for the least microbial diversity found in the metaniche "C-U".

Moreover, the close microbial relationship between saliva, tongue and hard palate and their clustering into metaniche "S-T-HP" might result from the functional tasks of hard palate and tongue, which are in close contact almost constantly.

In our study, most samples of the metaniche P-GCF comprised higher fractions of *Actinomyces, Aggregatibacter, Fusobacterium, Leptotrichia, Capnocytophaga, Corynebacterium, Lautropia, Campylobacter* and *Tannerella* and exhibited a high alpha diversity. Consistent with our results, a previous study demonstrated that plaque showed a high diversity including *Actinomyces, Fusobacterium, Corynebacterium, Capnocytophaga* and that saliva as well as tongue showed a high prevalence of Prevotella and *Neisseria* [30]. Partly similar results for plaque were found in a later consensus report, which indicated that the dental biofilm in periodontal health is dominated by the genera *Neisseria, Streptococcus, Actinomyces, Veillonella* and *Granulicatella*, but shifts to a more diverse and higher specialized form in gingivitis and periodontitis [34]. Samples from the metaniche S-T-HP showed a relatively high abundance of *Prevotella, Neisseria, Veillonella, Porphyromonas, Granulicatella* and *Alloprevotella*. Findings were partly similar to a previous report demonstrating the presence of *Veillonella, Prevotella, Neisseria* and *Granulicatella* in the hard palate and tongue dorsum. However, the highest values were found for *Streptococcus* [17]. The metaniche C-U presented a high relative abundance of *Streptococcus, Haemophilus, Gemella* and *Actinobacillus* with a very high abundance of *Streptococcus*, which was consistent with a previous study indicating that *Streptococcus* was dominant in the cheek [30].

On the species level, Campylobacter gracilis, Streptococcus sanguinis, Fusobacterium nucleatum, Capnocytophaga and Prevotella oris were characteristic for the metaniche "P-GCF", Streptococcus salivarius, Fusobacterium (pseudo)periodonticum, Prevotella melanogenica, Granulicatella adiacens, Veillonella dispar and Saccharimonadaceae were typical for "S-T-HP", and Haemophilus parainfluenzae and Gemella haemolysans signified "C-U". Similar findings were reported in a previous study [17], e.g., for (1) tooth surface/plaque (Streptococcus sanguinis); (2) tongue dorsum (Streptococcus salivarius); and (3) cheek (Gemella haemolysans). Our results are also in accordance with another recent publication demonstrating that the microbial diversity was significantly different between oral niches [4]; however, in this study, characteristic OTUs were only analyzed in each oral niche without grouping into metaniches.

3.2. Cytokine Expression in Different Oral Niches

Pathogenesis of periodontitis includes a complex interaction between microbial communities and the host immune response, resulting in the production of inflammatory mediators that alter connective tissue and bone metabolism [2,19,36]. Cytokines are soluble proteins that bind to specific receptors on target cells, activate intracellular signalling cascades and play important roles in acute-phase response, a primary defence reaction that protects the body against bacterial products in periodontal tissue breakdown [22,28,37]. In the diagnosis of periodontal disease, an increase in the amount of GCF and the presence of certain pro-inflammatory cytokines such as IL-1β, IL-6, IL-8, IFN-γ and TNF has been correlated with the progression of periodontitis, while pro-inflammatory cytokine levels decreased after periodontal therapy [19,23,24,38–40]. While cytokine expression in GCF has been investigated in periodontal disease [19], it has rarely been analyzed in other oral niches like the salivary pellicle on different soft tissue surfaces and has not yet been related to the oral microbiota.

In our study, we focused on the expression patterns of nine different cytokines, including the pro-inflammatory cytokines IL-1β, IL-2, IL-6, TNF and IFN-γ, the chemokine IL-8 and the anti-inflammatory mediators IL-4 and IL-10 [19]. Therefore, we performed a broad analysis in 20 age-matched young adults with excellent oral health (10 males and 10 females) providing characterisation of cytokine profiles of the aforementioned oral niches.

Regarding the microbial metaniche "P-GCF", similarities were also found for the "immunological metaniche" supragingival plaque and gingival crevicular fluid: First of all, cytokine concentrations were significantly higher in the gingival crevicular fluid compared to all other niches followed by supragingival plaque which was found to be significantly higher compared to saliva, tongue, hard palate, cheek and sublingual area. Very high concentrations of IL-8, high concentrations of IL-10, IFN-γ, IL-6, TNF and low concentrations of GM-CSF, IL-2 and IL-4 were detected in "P-GCF". The high cytokine concentration in GCF might originate from the enclosed area in the gingival sulcus, which is protected from salivary clearance and dilution effects. GCF is synthesized in the connective tissue, which is part of the dental attachment and secretes directly into the gingival sulcus where it can be collected [19]. In periodontal health, the sulcus fluid flow rate is low and GCF is described as a transudate following an osmotic gradient, while in periodontitis, GCF is comparable to an inflammatory exudate showing high sulcus fluid flow rates [20]. Moreover, GCF serves as a transport medium carrying nutrients for subgingival bacteria and several immune cells like neutrophils, which are the most common leukocytes recruited in periodontal disease [41]. Anatomically, plaque accumulation is often located on the gingival margin inducing the production of the gingival crevicular fluid [33], which might be the reason for the second-highest cytokine concentrations as part of the immune response. Bacterial components found in supragingival plaque, e.g., lipopolysaccharides, stimulate various inflammatory mediators and immune cells found in the connective tissue [19]. Initially, mast cells produce TNF triggering vasodilatation and the recruitment of polymorphonuclear leukocytes (PMNs), which can induce tissue destruction in periodontitis by the release of lysosomal enzymes [19]. Simultaneously, resident cells in the connective tissue, which are mainly gingival fibroblasts, release pro-inflammatory cytokines like IFN-γ, IL-1β, IL-6, IL-8 and PGE_2 activating a cascade of events in the host response [19]. Moreover, antigen-presenting cells stimulate differentiation of naïve T cells into various cell types, which release different cytokines like type 1 T helper (Th1) cells (production of IFN-γ, IL-2 and TNF), Th2 cells (e.g., IL-4, IL-10, IL-13), regulatory T cells (e.g., IL-10) and Th17 cells (e.g., IL-6, TNF- and IL-17) [19].

Considering the percentage of cytokine expression in all niches, IL-8 was found to be the most dominant cytokine. Similar to our results, high IL-8 levels were previously described in GCF of healthy individuals [42]. We observed similarities in the cytokine expression pattern between hard palate and tongue, with a relatively low percentage of IL-8 (<75%) and a high percentage of IL-1β (>20%), which might result from similar fluids produced by minor glands found in hard palate and tongue [35]. Cheek and sublingual area presented lowest cytokine concentrations, which matches the lowest microbial diversity found in metaniche "C-U" and can also be explained by the highest salivary flow due to the presence of salivary glands in those niches [35]. The highest relative quantities of IFN-γ, IL-6, GM-CSF, and IL-2 were found in the sublingual area and the cheek, indicating analogies between the cheek and sublingual area and the presence of an immunological metaniche "C-U".

Cytokine concentrations in saliva suggested similarities to "P-GCF" but also to "T-HP" and "C-U". On the one hand, similarities of tongue/hard palate and cheek/sublingual area with the salivary compartment probably originate from the formation of the "salivary pellicle", which builds a thin conditioning layer on all soft tissues in the oral cavity [43–45]. As mentioned before, saliva is mainly produced by salivary glands found not only in the cheek and in the sublingual area but also in the hard palate and tongue [35]. Saliva also contains gingival crevicular fluid [35], which is crucial in antimicrobial defence and maintenance of periodontal health by flushing microbial components and bacteria out of the gingival sulcus [46]. Taken together, it is plausible that cytokine concentrations in saliva show properties of all oral niches.

3.3. Correlation between Microbiota Composition and Cytokine Expression

Higher pro-inflammatory cytokine levels and a change in the microbial composition have not only been detected in periodontal disease, but have also been connected to other oral conditions. Regular smoking, which is a predisposing factor for oral and lung cancer, correlated with higher levels of the proinflammatory cytokine IL-2 and with a higher microbial prevalence of *Proteobacteria, Firmicutes, Bacteroidetes, Fusobacteria* and *Actinobacteria* [26]. Moreover, there is evidence that *Porphyromonas gingivalis* might play an important role in the development of oral squamous cell carcinoma [47]. Therefore, salivary biomarkers like the pro-inflammatory cytokines IL-1β, IL-2 and TNF might be used as a future diagnostic tool for oral squamous cell carcinoma [27].

Notably, the present investigation in healthy volunteers revealed positive correlations between increased relative quantities of cytokines (GM-CSF, IFN-γ, IL-10, IL-1β, IL-2, IL-4, IL-6, IL-8 and TNF) and specific microbial genera within the defined metaniches: Positive correlations with *Aggregatibacter* and *Fusobacterium* were characteristic for the metaniche "P-GCF", which are typical commensals of the dental biofilm. These associations might result from the properties of *Fusobacterium nucleatum*, which can stimulate the production of IL-6 and IL-8 in the gingiva [48], and the immunoregulatory potential of *Aggregatibacter actinomycetemcomitans* inducing expression of IFN-γ [49,50]. A moderate up-regulation of these cytokines might help in the defence of pathogens and the maintenance of "symbiosis" between microbial players and the immunity of the host, while high and uncontrolled up-regulation correlated with periodontitis [19]. In contrast, dysbiosis and inflammation mutually amplify each other in periodontitis: the innate immune system responds to colonization by pivotal pathogens (e.g., *P. gingivalis*) with dysregulated and increased production of GCF, which contains specific molecules from periodontal tissue destruction, and finally inhibits the growth of eubiotic species and fosters the growth of periodontitis associated taxa [41,51].

Positive correlations were also seen for *Gemella* and *Capnocytophaga* in the metaniche "S-T-HP" and for *Campylobacter* and *Granulicatella* in the metaniche "C-U". The genera *Campylobacter*, *Capnocytophaga* and *Gemella* were previously associated with periodontal health [52]. The genus *Granulicatella* is also a common and frequent component of healthy oral microbiotas [53]. However, little is known to date about the aforementioned microbes in the oral context and possible immune-stimulating properties.

Regarding associations between microbial composition and immunological features in different oral niches, only a small amount of data are available for periodontal health except comparisons with oral inflammatory disease: Higher levels of pro-inflammatory cytokines like IL-6 and TNF in GCF have been linked to the presence of "red complex" bacteria in supragingival plaque [54] or other periodontal pathogens in deep periodontal pockets [55]. However, to our best knowledge, no other studies are available that have investigated more than two oral niches with regard to their microbial composition and cytokine profile and/or correlations between immune response and bacterial composition. It was shown that tongue cleaning, which might lead to a reduction of microbial colonization, correlated with decreased levels of IL-1β and IL-8 in GCF in patients with gingivitis [56], suggesting that "health" of one oral niche can even lead to less inflammation in other oral niches. In line with these findings, we detected similarities in the oral microbiota and cytokine profile of anatomical adjunct niches or niches in direct contact facilitating the interaction between them.

4. Materials and Methods

The study was designed as a prospective, exploratory observational clinical trial. The study was performed in accordance with the Helsinki protocol and the local ethics committee of the Friedrich-Alexander-University Erlangen-Nürnberg (Krankenhausstraße 12, 91054 Erlangen, Vote number: 111_20 B). After written informed consent and fulfilment of the inclusion criteria, study participants were enrolled in the study. The inclusion and exclusion criteria are given in Table 1.

Table 1. List of inclusion and exclusion criteria for subject enrolment in the clinical study.

Inclusion	Exclusion	
• young adults • male and female • age: 20–35 years • excellent oral health • dentistry students, dentists, orthodontists or scientific assistants of the university hospital of Erlangen • signed declaration of consent by the patient	• systemic or metabolic disease that are related to gingivitis (e.g., diabetes) or could possibly influence the oral microbiota • gingivitis or periodontitis (PSI $\geq$ 3) • missing teeth due to extraction because of carious lesions • more than 6 missing teeth (including third molar extractions or hypodontia/congenitally missing teeth) • active carious lesions, peri-/apical lesions, fistulas, oral abscesses • pregnancy, regular smoking	• presence of orthodontic appliances, except fixed retainers to the incisors • obesity: body mass index (BMI) > 30 kg/m^2 • eating disorder or underweight: BMI < 18.5 kg/m^2 • intake of antibiotics or dietary supplementation in the last 6 months • disconfirmation of the declaration of consent by the patient

4.1. Study Population

Twenty healthy study participants (10 males, 10 females) with a mean age of 27.20 years (range 23 to 32) fulfilling the inclusion and not meeting the exclusion criteria given in Table 1 were enrolled in the study. To ensure excellent oral hygiene, all study participants were either dentistry students, dentists, orthodontists or scientific assistants at the university hospital of Erlangen-Nürnberg. The mean number of teeth was 29 (range 26–32) without apparent mobility (Grade 0) (Table S1). The periodontal probing depth (PPD) was measured with a periodontal probe (WHO probe) on six sites per tooth and ranged from 1.4 mm to 2.3 mm with a mean value of 1.8 mm without signs of pathological pockets. Periodontal and gingival health were evaluated with the bleeding on probing index (BOP), which was measured at six sites per tooth. The average BOP was 0.7%. In accordance with the definition of periodontal health [57], all subjects presented excellent periodontal health. For determination of the approximal plaque index (API) the Mira-2-Ton®disclosing agent was used, which is a two-tone erythrosine-free disclosing dye solution Mira-2-Ton®(Hager & Werken, Duisburg, Germany) that can help to distinguish blue-dyed older plaque from pink-dyed newer plaque. The mean API was 13% (range 7–18%) representing in only pink-dyed newer plaque as the old blue-dyed plaque was not detectable. In accordance with the definition of good oral hygiene with API < 25% [58,59], all subjects presented excellent oral hygiene. All subjects used a powered toothbrush and additionally interproximal hygiene devices. Eleven subjects used dental floss regularly, whereas nine subjects used dental floss only on an occasional basis. All participants are part of a dental recall system, which includes regular professional prophylaxis at a dental practice or dental clinic.

4.2. Sample Collection

After obtaining informed consent, 280 samples were collected from 7 different oral niches (2 samples per niche) of each study participant to analyse the composition of the oral microbiota and the cytokine expression in each oral niche. Individuals were instructed not to eat or drink anything except water up to three hours before saliva collection. Unstimulated saliva samples were gained by the spitting method and collected in microtubes. After collection of saliva, soft tissue samples were collected in sterile tubes from the hard palate (middle part), the tongue (middle and anterior part), the sublingual area (middle part) and the cheek (right side, molar region), using sterile swabs wiping over the area several times for about 30 s. Moreover, hard tissue samples of supragingival plaque were taken by sterile curettes and wiped off using sterile swabs. Samples of gingival sulcus fluid were collected from 6 periodontal pockets of the mesiobuccal side of defined teeth (Ramfjord teeth: 16, 21, 24, 36, 41, 44) using sterile paper strips. The samples were collected using a standardized protocol, which was modified to prior described protocols [60,61]: draining with cotton rolls, careful air-drying of the area, mild insertion of paper strip (ProFlow, Amityville, NY, USA) in the gingival sulcus for 30 s in the premolar and molar region and for 60 s in the incisor region (as study population consisted of healthy individuals, insertion for 30 s in the incisor region was not suitable for the collection of adequate amounts of sulcus fluid). After calibration of the Periotron 8000 before each usage, measurement of the amount of sulcus fluid flow rate (SFFR) were conducted subsequently for one sample each niche using Periotron 8000 according to the manufacturer's instructions to determine the cytokine concentration. To ensure that paper strips and oral sterile culture swabs were free from bacterial DNA, all materials were tested in advance.

After collection of samples and immediate storage on dry ice, clinical measurements were performed on all study participants using a standardized working process and diagnosis sheet: dental notation including the number of teeth (missing teeth due to extraction or agnesia), full mouth probing of periodontal pockets (periodontal probing depth, PPD), bleeding-on-probing (BOP)-positive sites and approximal plaque index (API) were measured and calculated.

Patient recruitment and sample collection were performed at the department of orthodontics and orofacial orthopedics of the university hospital of Erlangen. Storage of samples as well as isolation of bacterial DNA was performed in the research laboratory of the department of orthodontics and orofacial orthopedics.

4.3. Determination of Cytokine Concentrations

For determination of cytokine concentrations, collected samples were isolated from swabs by centrifugation (1 min at 23,000× g at 4 °C), volume was measured and samples were diluted with diluent 43 (Mesoscale Discovery, R50AG-2) to a volume of >100 µL. Saliva samples were directly diluted 1:3 with diluent 43. For recovery of cytokines from crevicular samples, sterile paper stripes of each test person were sequentially shaken in 150 µL diluent 43 at 4 °C for 5 min each. Residual volume was measured. The dilution factor was calculated by dividing the residual volume by the total volume of crevicular fluid as determined by Periotron measurements. Plaque samples were suspended in 125 µL diluent 43. As weighing of plaque samples was not feasible due to variation of test tube weight, we assigned these samples into three groups according to their pellet size after centrifugation of diluted suspensions: large, medium size and small plaque samples, corresponding 8 µL, 4 µL or 2 µL, respectively. Dilution factors for plaque samples were calculated from these assignments.

Cytokine concentrations were determined by multiplex immunoassay in 96 well plates with a U-PLEX Biomarker Group 1 (hu) assay (Mesoscale discovery; K15067L-2) on a MESO QuickPlex SQ 120 instrument (Mesoscale discovery). The assay was performed according to the manufacturer's instructions, standard dilution series (one per each plate) and samples were measured in duplicates.

4.4. Microbiota Analysis

DNA of samples was extracted with a ZymoBIOMICS DNA Microprep Kit (Zymo Research, Freiburg, Germany) in combination with a BeadRupter 24 (Omni International, Kennesaw, GA, USA). The bacterial 16S rRNA gene was amplified with primers 27Fmod 5′-AGRGTTTGATCMTGGCTCAG-3′ and 519R 5′-GWATTACCGCGGCKGCTG-3′ [62]. A total of 12 primer pairs, each modified with different 0-11 bp heterogeneity spacers and adapters for the Illumina Nextera XT system were synthesized (IDT, Munich, Germany) and used to amplify the 16S V1-V3 region. For PCR the KAPA HiFi HotStart ReadyMix (Roche, Mannheim, Germany) was used in a Mastercycler nexus Gradient (Eppendorf, Hamburg, Germany) with the following program: 3′ 95 °C, 25 cycles of 30″ 95 °C, 30″ 55 °C, 35″ 72 °C and finally 5′ 95 °C. Fragments were purified with AMPure XP beads (Beckman-Coulter, Krefeld, Germany). A second indexing PCR was performed (8 cycles) using the Nextera Index Kit v2 Sets A and B (Illumina, Munich, Germany). After final purification (AMPure XP), equal molarities of the samples were pooled and subjected to 2 × 300 bp paired-end sequencing on a MiSeq system (Illumina).

Sequence data were demultiplexed according to the index sequences with the "Generate Fastq" workflow in MiSeq Reporter (Illumina). Sequencing files in the fastq format are available through the National Center for Biotechnology Information (NCBI) Sequence Read Archive (SRA) under BioProject PRJNA668021. Sequences were filtered based on quality using Trimmomatic v0.39 [63] and primer sequences were removed with Cutadapt v2.9 [64]. For OTU-based classification with the USEARCH v8 algorithm [65] sequences were re-multiplexed using a Perl script (I. Lagkouvardos, available from www.imngs.org) and submitted to the IMNGS server [66]. We obtained in median 45,338 OTU counts per sample (range 2334–112,749). Taxonomic classification of the identified OTUs was done using the SILVA alignment, classification and tree service [67] with SILVA database release 138.1 and NCBI nucleotide BLAST [68]. All further analyses were performed using the R-based pipeline "Rhea" [69] and ggplot2 [70] (for visualization) within R v4.0.2 [71].

4.5. Statistics

The statistical analysis of cytokine concentrations was done with Microsoft Excel 365 (Microsoft, Redmond, WAUSA), R v4.0.2 [71] and GraphPad Prism 8 statistical software (GraphPad Software, San Diego, CA, USA). If not stated otherwise, data are presented as mean ± Standard Error of Mean (SEM) and fraction of total. The data sets were analyzed by using the Kruskal–Wallis test and Dunn's multiple comparisons test. Differences were considered significant with p-values < 0.05.

5. Conclusions

The presented investigations allowed the definition of three distinct metaniches: (1) plaque and gingival crevicular fluid; (2) saliva, tongue and hard palate; and (3) cheek and sublingual area according to their microbial composition. These metaniches were associated with defined cytokine profiles, except saliva, which showed relationships to the cytokine profile of all oral niches. These defined metaniches provide new insights into microenvironmental similarities between anatomically diverse oral niches and indicate possible interactions between niches and their defined metaniches. The metaniches in the oral cavity are formed and influenced by (1) the anatomical proximity and interactions in host defence (dental biofilm can be found on the gingival margin and stimulates the production of gingival crevicular fluid leading to flushing out of bacterial products); (2) the function (permanent contact between tongue and saliva—also during swallowing and speech); (3) the salivary glands and flow rate of saliva (major glands found in the cheek and sublingual area with highest salivary flow, while minor glands are present in hard palate and tongue); and (4) the mixed composition of saliva (fluids from salivary glands found in diverse oral niches and GCF), building a "salivary pellicle" on hard and soft tissues. The understanding of these metaniches is crucial when analysing changes in the composition of the oral microbiota or immune responses associated with treatment or oral diseases. Hence, future studies are necessary to improve our knowledge of site-specific alterations, e.g., in periodontitis. This knowledge might help to define the state of "dysbiosis" more precisely and detect future biomarkers in periodontal disease. It might also help to improve potential site-specific preventive or therapeutic strategies, which not only have an impact on the directly treated oral niche but also associated or distant niche(s).

Author Contributions: Conceptualization, C.L.S., M.W., R.G.G., C.B. and L.G.; methodology, C.L.S., M.W., R.G.G. and G.R.; formal analysis, C.L.S., M.W., P.W. and R.G.G; investigation C.L.S, P.W. and G.R.; resources M.H., B.F. and U.S.G.; visualization, C.L.S., P.W. and R.G.G.; writing—original draft preparation; C.L.S., R.G.G., M.W. and P.W.; writing—review F.C., C.K., A.B., U.S.G., C.B. and L.G.; supervision C.B. and L.G.; project administration; C.L.S., M.W., R.G.G. and P.W. All authors have read and agreed to the published version of the manuscript.

Acknowledgments: We want to thank Isabel Enderle for the laboratory support.

Abbreviations

API	Approximal Plaque Index
BMI	Body Mass Index
BOP	Bleeding on Probing
C	Cheek
GCF	Gingival crevicular fluid
GM-CSF	Granulocyte-macrophage colony-stimulating factor
HOMD	Human Oral Microbiota Database
HP	Hard palate
IL-1β	Interleukin 1 beta
IL-2	Interleukin 2
IL-4	Interleukin 4
IL-6	Interleukin 6
IL-8	Interleukin 8
IL-10	Interleukin 10
IL-32	Interleukin 32
IL-33	Interleukin 33
IFN-γ	Interferon gamma
MDS	Multidimensional scaling
OTU	Operational taxonomic unit
P	Plaque
PPD	Periodontal probing depth
PSI	Periodontal Screening Index
S	Saliva
SEM	Standard error of mean
SFFR	Sulcus fluid flow rate
spp.	Species
T	Tongue
TNF	Tumor-necrosis-factor
U	Sublingual area

References

1. Dewhirst, F.E.; Chen, T.; Izard, J.; Paster, B.J.; Tanner, A.C.; Yu, W.H.; Lakshmanan, A.; Wade, W.G. The human oral microbiome. *J. Bacteriol.* **2010**, *192*, 5002–5017. [CrossRef] [PubMed]
2. Hajishengallis, G. Periodontitis: From microbial immune subversion to systemic inflammation. *Nat. Rev. Immunol.* **2015**, *15*, 30–44. [CrossRef] [PubMed]
3. Du Teil Espina, M.; Gabarrini, G.; Harmsen, H.J.M.; Westra, J.; van Winkelhoff, A.J.; van Dijl, J.M. Talk to your gut: The oral-gut microbiome axis and its immunomodulatory role in the etiology of rheumatoid arthritis. *FEMS Microbiol. Rev.* **2019**, *43*, 1–18. [CrossRef] [PubMed]
4. Caselli, E.; Fabbri, C.; D'Accolti, M.; Soffritti, I.; Bassi, C.; Mazzacane, S.; Franchi, M. Defining the oral microbiome by whole-genome sequencing and resistome analysis: The complexity of the healthy picture. *BMC Microbiol.* **2020**, *20*, 120. [CrossRef]
5. Glöckner, F.O.; Yilmaz, P.; Quast, C.; Gerken, J.; Beccati, A.; Ciuprina, A.; Bruns, G.; Yarza, P.; Peplies, J.; Westram, R.; et al. 25 years of serving the community with ribosomal RNA gene reference databases and tools. *J. Biotechnol.* **2017**, *261*, 169–176. [CrossRef] [PubMed]
6. Quast, C.; Pruesse, E.; Yilmaz, P.; Gerken, J.; Schweer, T.; Yarza, P.; Peplies, J.; Glöckner, F.O. The SILVA ribosomal RNA gene database project: Improved data processing and web-based tools. *Nucleic Acids Res.* **2013**, *41*, D590–D596. [CrossRef]
7. Costello, E. The application of ecological theory toward an understanding of the human microbiome. *Science* **2012**, *336*, 1255–1262. [CrossRef]
8. Kononen, E. Development of oral bacterial flora in young children. *Ann. Med.* **2000**, *32*, 107–112. [CrossRef]
9. Kononen, E.; Asikainen, S.; Saarela, M.; Karjalainen, J.; Jousimies-Somer, H. The oral gram-negative anaerobic microflora in young children: Longitudinal changes from edentulous to dentate mouth. *Oral. Microbiol. Immunol.* **1994**, *9*, 136–141. [CrossRef]
10. Kononen, E.; Kanervo, A.; Takala, A.; Asikainen, S.; Jousimies-Somer, H. Establishment of oral anaerobes during the first year of life. *J. Dent. Res.* **1999**, *78*, 1634–1639. [CrossRef]
11. Sundstrom, K.; Mishra, P.P.; Pyysalo, M.J.; Lehtimaki, T.; Karhunen, P.J.; Pessi, T. Similarity of salivary microbiome in parents and adult children. *PeerJ* **2020**, *8*, e8799. [CrossRef]
12. Tamburini, S.; Shen, N.; Wu, H.C.; Clemente, J.C. The microbiome in early life: Implications for health outcomes. *Nat. Med.* **2016**, *22*, 713–722. [CrossRef]
13. Paster, B.J.; Boches, S.K.; Galvin, J.L.; Ericson, R.E.; Lau, C.N.; Levanos, V.A.; Sahasrabudhe, A.; Dewhirst, F.E. Bacterial diversity in human subgingival plaque. *J. Bacteriol.* **2001**, *183*, 3770–3783. [CrossRef]
14. Wei, Y.; Shi, M.; Zhen, M.; Wang, C.; Hu, W.; Nie, Y.; Wu, X. Comparison of subgingival and buccal mucosa microbiome in chronic and aggressive periodontitis: A pilot study. *Front. Cell Infect. Microbiol.* **2019**, *9*, 53. [CrossRef]
15. Cieplik, F.; Zaura, E.; Brandt, B.W.; Buijs, M.J.; Buchalla, W.; Crielaard, W.; Laine, M.L.; Deng, D.M.; Exterkate, R.A.M. Microcosm biofilms cultured from different oral niches in periodontitis patients. *J. Oral Microbiol.* **2019**, *11*, 1551596. [CrossRef] [PubMed]
16. Zaura, E.; Keijser, B.J.; Huse, S.M.; Crielaard, W. Defining the healthy "core microbiome" of oral microbial communities. *BMC Microbiol.* **2009**, *9*, 259. [CrossRef]
17. Aas, J.A.; Paster, B.J.; Stokes, L.N.; Olsen, I.; Dewhirst, F.E. Defining the normal bacterial flora of the oral cavity. *J. Clin. Microbiol.* **2005**, *43*, 5721–5732. [CrossRef]
18. Lundmark, A.; Hu, Y.O.O.; Huss, M.; Johannsen, G.; Andersson, A.F.; Yucel-Lindberg, T. Identification of salivary microbiota and its association with host inflammatory mediators in periodontitis. *Front Cell Infect. Microbiol.* **2019**, *9*, 216. [CrossRef]
19. Yucel-Lindberg, T.; Bage, T. Inflammatory mediators in the pathogenesis of periodontitis. *Expert. Rev. Mol. Med.* **2013**, *15*, e7. [CrossRef]
20. Barros, S.P.; Williams, R.; Offenbacher, S.; Morelli, T. Gingival crevicular fluid as a source of biomarkers for periodontitis. *Periodontology 2000* **2016**, *70*, 53–64. [CrossRef]
21. Tsuchida, S.; Satoh, M.; Takiwaki, M.; Nomura, F. Current Status of Proteomic Technologies for Discovering and Identifying Gingival Crevicular Fluid Biomarkers for Periodontal Disease. *Int. J. Mol. Sci.* **2018**, *20*, 86. [CrossRef]

22. Delima, A.J.; Karatzas, S.; Amar, S.; Graves, D.T. Inflammation and tissue loss caused by periodontal pathogens is reduced by interleukin-1 antagonists. *J. Infect. Dis.* **2002**, *186*, 511–516. [CrossRef]
23. Thunell, D.H.; Tymkiw, K.D.; Johnson, G.K.; Joly, S.; Burnell, K.K.; Cavanaugh, J.E.; Brogden, K.A.; Guthmiller, J.M. A multiplex immunoassay demonstrates reductions in gingival crevicular fluid cytokines following initial periodontal therapy. *J. Periodontal Res.* **2010**, *45*, 148–152. [CrossRef]
24. Holmlund, A.; Hänström, L.; Lerner, U.H. Bone resorbing activity and cytokine levels in gingival crevicular fluid before and after treatment of periodontal disease. *J. Clin. Periodontol.* **2004**, *31*, 475–482. [CrossRef]
25. Syrjäläinen, S.; Gursoy, U.K.; Gursoy, M.; Pussinen, P.; Pietiäinen, M.; Jula, A.; Salomaa, V.; Jousilahti, P.; Könönen, E. Salivary Cytokine Biomarker Concentrations in Relation to Obesity and Periodontitis. *J. Clin. Med.* **2019**, *8*, 2152. [CrossRef]
26. Rodríguez-Rabassa, M.; López, P.; Rodríguez-Santiago, R.E.; Cases, A.; Felici, M.; Sánchez, R.; Yamamura, Y.; Rivera-Amill, V. Cigarette Smoking Modulation of Saliva Microbial Composition and Cytokine Levels. *Int. J. Environ. Res. Public Health* **2018**, *15*, 2479. [CrossRef]
27. Khurshid, Z.; Zafar, M.S.; Khan, R.S.; Najeeb, S.; Slowey, P.D.; Rehman, I.U. Role of Salivary Biomarkers in Oral Cancer Detection. *Adv. Clin. Chem.* **2018**, *86*, 23–70. [CrossRef]
28. Preshaw, P.M.; Taylor, J.J. How has research into cytokine interactions and their role in driving immune responses impacted our understanding of periodontitis? *J. Clin. Periodontol.* **2011**, *38* (Suppl. 11), 60–84. [CrossRef]
29. Socransky, S.S.; Haffajee, A.D.; Cugini, M.A.; Smith, C.; Kent, R.L., Jr. Microbial complexes in subgingival plaque. *J. Clin. Periodontol.* **1998**, *25*, 134–144. [CrossRef] [PubMed]
30. Segata, N.; Haake, S.K.; Mannon, P.; Lemon, K.P.; Waldron, L.; Gevers, D.; Huttenhower, C.; Izard, J. Composition of the adult digestive tract bacterial microbiome based on seven mouth surfaces, tonsils, throat and stool samples. *Genome Biol.* **2012**, *13*, R42. [CrossRef]
31. Marsh, P.D. Dental plaque as a microbial biofilm. *Caries Res.* **2004**, *38*, 204–211. [CrossRef] [PubMed]
32. Kinane, D.F.; Attström, R. Advances in the pathogenesis of periodontitis. Group B consensus report of the fifth European Workshop in Periodontology. *J. Clin. Periodontol.* **2005**, *32* (Suppl. 6), 130–131. [CrossRef]
33. Stathopoulou, P.G.; Benakanakere, M.R.; Galicia, J.C.; Kinane, D.F. Epithelial cell pro-inflammatory cytokine response differs across dental plaque bacterial species. *J. Clin. Periodontol.* **2010**, *37*, 24–29. [CrossRef]
34. Sanz, M.; Beighton, D.; Curtis, M.A.; Cury, J.A.; Dige, I.; Dommisch, H.; Ellwood, R.; Giacaman, R.A.; Herrera, D.; Herzberg, M.C.; et al. Role of microbial biofilms in the maintenance of oral health and in the development of dental caries and periodontal diseases. Consensus report of group 1 of the Joint EFP/ORCA workshop on the boundaries between caries and periodontal disease. *J. Clin. Periodontol.* **2017**, *44* (Suppl. 18), S5–S11. [CrossRef]
35. Humphrey, S.P.; Williamson, R.T. A review of saliva: Normal composition, flow, and function. *J. Prosthet. Dent.* **2001**, *85*, 162–169. [CrossRef]
36. Page, R.C.; Kornman, K.S. The pathogenesis of human periodontitis: An introduction. *Periodontology 2000* **1997**, *14*, 9–11. [CrossRef]
37. Silva, T.A.; Garlet, G.P.; Fukada, S.Y.; Silva, J.S.; Cunha, F.Q. Chemokines in oral inflammatory diseases: Apical periodontitis and periodontal disease. *J. Dent. Res.* **2007**, *86*, 306–319. [CrossRef]
38. Gamonal, J.; Acevedo, A.; Bascones, A.; Jorge, O.; Silva, A. Levels of interleukin-1 beta, -8, and -10 and RANTES in gingival crevicular fluid and cell populations in adult periodontitis patients and the effect of periodontal treatment. *J. Periodontol.* **2000**, *71*, 1535–1545. [CrossRef]
39. Ertugrul, A.S.; Sahin, H.; Dikilitas, A.; Alpaslan, N.; Bozoglan, A. Comparison of CCL28, interleukin-8, interleukin-1β and tumor necrosis factor-alpha in subjects with gingivitis, chronic periodontitis and generalized aggressive periodontitis. *J. Periodontal Res.* **2013**, *48*, 44–51. [CrossRef]
40. Fujita, Y.; Ito, H.; Sekino, S.; Numabe, Y. Correlations between pentraxin 3 or cytokine levels in gingival crevicular fluid and clinical parameters of chronic periodontitis. *Odontology* **2012**, *100*, 215–221. [CrossRef] [PubMed]
41. Lamont, R.J.; Koo, H.; Hajishengallis, G. The oral microbiota: Dynamic communities and host interactions. *Nat. Rev. Microbiol.* **2018**, *16*, 745–759. [CrossRef] [PubMed]
42. Gamonal, J.; Acevedo, A.; Bascones, A.; Jorge, O.; Silva, A. Characterization of cellular infiltrate, detection of chemokine receptor CCR5 and interleukin-8 and RANTES chemokines in adult periodontitis. *J. Periodontal Res.* **2001**, *36*, 194–203. [CrossRef]

43. Marsh, P.D.; Do, T.; Beighton, D.; Devine, D.A. Influence of saliva on the oral microbiota. *Periodontology 2000* **2016**, *70*, 80–92. [CrossRef] [PubMed]
44. Rudney, J.D. Saliva and dental plaque. *Adv. Dent. Res.* **2000**, *14*, 29–39. [CrossRef]
45. Lynge Pedersen, A.M.; Belstrøm, D. The role of natural salivary defences in maintaining a healthy oral microbiota. *J. Dent.* **2019**, *80* (Suppl. 1), S3–S12. [CrossRef]
46. Subbarao, K.C.; Nattuthurai, G.S.; Sundararajan, S.K.; Sujith, I.; Joseph, J.; Syedshah, Y.P. Gingival Crevicular Fluid: An Overview. *J. Pharm. Bioallied Sci.* **2019**, *11*, S135–S139. [CrossRef]
47. Lafuente Ibáñez de Mendoza, I.; Maritxalar Mendia, X.; García de la Fuente, A.M.; Quindós Andrés, G.; Aguirre Urizar, J.M. Role of *Porphyromonas gingivalis* in oral squamous cell carcinoma development: A systematic review. *J. Periodontal Res.* **2020**, *55*, 13–22. [CrossRef]
48. Brennan, C.A.; Garrett, W.S. *Fusobacterium nucleatum*—Symbiont, opportunist and oncobacterium. *Nat. Rev. Microbiol.* **2019**, *17*, 156–166. [CrossRef] [PubMed]
49. Herbert, B.A.; Novince, C.M.; Kirkwood, K.L. *Aggregatibacter actinomycetemcomitans*, a potent immunoregulator of the periodontal host defense system and alveolar bone homeostasis. *Mol. Oral Microbiol.* **2016**, *31*, 207–227. [CrossRef]
50. Garlet, G.P.; Avila-Campos, M.J.; Milanezi, C.M.; Ferreira, B.R.; Silva, J.S. *Actinobacillus actinomycetemcomitans*-induced periodontal disease in mice: Patterns of cytokine, chemokine, and chemokine receptor expression and leukocyte migration. *Microbes Infect.* **2005**, *7*, 738–747. [CrossRef]
51. Marsh, P.D.; Zaura, E. Dental biofilm: Ecological interactions in health and disease. *J. Clin. Periodontol.* **2017**, *44* (Suppl. 18), S12–S22. [CrossRef]
52. Kumar, P.S.; Griffen, A.L.; Moeschberger, M.L.; Leys, E.J. Identification of candidate periodontal pathogens and beneficial species by quantitative 16S clonal analysis. *J. Clin. Microbiol.* **2005**, *43*, 3944–3955. [CrossRef] [PubMed]
53. Bik, E.M.; Long, C.D.; Armitage, G.C.; Loomer, P.; Emerson, J.; Mongodin, E.F.; Nelson, K.E.; Gill, S.R.; Fraser-Liggett, C.M.; Relman, D.A. Bacterial diversity in the oral cavity of 10 healthy individuals. *ISME J.* **2010**, *4*, 962–974. [CrossRef]
54. Rescala, B.; Rosalem, W., Jr.; Teles, R.P.; Fischer, R.G.; Haffajee, A.D.; Socransky, S.S.; Gustafsson, A.; Figueredo, C.M. Immunologic and microbiologic profiles of chronic and aggressive periodontitis subjects. *J. Periodontol.* **2010**, *81*, 1308–1316. [CrossRef]
55. Dosseva-Panova, V.T.; Popova, C.L.; Panov, V.E. Subgingival microbial profile and production of proinflammatory cytokines in chronic periodontitis. *Folia Med.* **2014**, *56*, 152–160. [CrossRef]
56. Acar, B.; Berker, E.; Tan, Ç.; İlarslan, Y.D.; Tekçiçek, M.; Tezcan, İ. Effects of oral prophylaxis including tongue cleaning on halitosis and gingival inflammation in gingivitis patients-a randomized controlled clinical trial. *Clin. Oral Investig.* **2019**, *23*, 1829–1836. [CrossRef]
57. Caton, J.G.; Armitage, G.; Berglundh, T.; Chapple, I.L.C.; Jepsen, S.; Kornman, K.S.; Mealey, B.L.; Papapanou, P.N.; Sanz, M.; Tonetti, M.S. A new classification scheme for periodontal and peri-implant diseases and conditions—Introduction and key changes from the 1999 classification. *J. Periodontol.* **2018**, *89* (Suppl. 1), S1–S8. [CrossRef]
58. Lange, D.E.; Plagmann, H.C.; Eenboom, A.; Promesberger, A. Clinical methods for the objective evaluation of oral hygiene. *Dtsch. Zahnarztl. Z.* **1977**, *32*, 44–47. [PubMed]
59. Lange, D.E. New aspects of diagnosis and therapy of periodontal diseases for dental practitioners. *Quintessenz* **1986**, *37*, 521–532.
60. Twetman, S.; Derawi, B.; Keller, M.; Ekstrand, K.; Yucel-Lindberg, T.; Stecksen-Blicks, C. Short-term effect of chewing gums containing probiotic *Lactobacillus reuteri* on the levels of inflammatory mediators in gingival crevicular fluid. *Acta Odontol. Scand.* **2009**, *67*, 19–24. [CrossRef]
61. Yucel-Lindberg, T.; Twetman, S.; Skold-Larsson, K.; Modeer, T. Effect of an antibacterial dental varnish on the levels of prostanoids, leukotriene B4, and interleukin-1 beta in gingival crevicular fluid. *Acta Odontol. Scand.* **1999**, *57*, 23–27. [CrossRef]
62. Lane, D.J.; Pace, B.; Olsen, G.J.; Stahl, D.A.; Sogin, M.L.; Pace, N.R. Rapid determination of 16S ribosomal RNA sequences for phylogenetic analyses. *Proc. Natl. Acad. Sci. USA* **1985**, *82*, 6955–6959. [CrossRef]
63. Bolger, A.M.; Lohse, M.; Usadel, B. Trimmomatic: A flexible trimmer for Illumina sequence data. *Bioinformatics* **2014**, *30*, 2114–2120. [CrossRef]

64. Martin, M. Cutadapt removes adapter sequences from high-throughput sequencing reads. *EMBnet. J.* **2011**, *17*, 10–12. [CrossRef]
65. Edgar, R.C. Search and clustering orders of magnitude faster than BLAST. *Bioinformatics* **2010**, *26*, 2460–2461. [CrossRef]
66. Lagkouvardos, I.; Joseph, D.; Kapfhammer, M.; Giritli, S.; Horn, M.; Haller, D.; Clavel, T. IMNGS: A comprehensive open resource of processed 16S rRNA microbial profiles for ecology and diversity studies. *Sci. Rep.* **2016**, *6*, 33721. [CrossRef]
67. Pruesse, E.; Peplies, J.; Glöckner, F.O. SINA: Accurate high-throughput multiple sequence alignment of ribosomal RNA genes. *Bioinformatics* **2012**, *28*, 1823–1829. [CrossRef]
68. Altschul, S.F.; Gish, W.; Miller, W.; Myers, E.W.; Lipman, D.J. Basic local alignment search tool. *J. Mol. Biol.* **1990**, *215*, 403–410. [CrossRef]
69. Lagkouvardos, I.; Fischer, S.; Kumar, N.; Clavel, T. Rhea: A transparent and modular R pipeline for microbial profiling based on 16S rRNA gene amplicons. *PeerJ* **2017**, *5*, e2836. [CrossRef]
70. Wickham, H. *ggplot2: Elegant Graphics for Data Analysis*; Springer: New York, NY, USA, 2016. [CrossRef]
71. R Core Team. *R: A Language and Environment for Statistical Computing*; R Foundation for Statistical Computing: Vienna, Austria, 2020.

2

Effects of Oral Commensal Streptococci on *Porphyromonas gingivalis* Invasion into Oral Epithelial Cells

Alyssa N. Hanel [1,2], Hannah M. Herzog [1], Michelle G. James [1] and Giancarlo A. Cuadra [1,*]

1 Department of Biology, Muhlenberg College, 2400 W. Chew Street, Allentown, PA 18104, USA; ah3573@cumc.columbia.edu (A.N.H.); hmherzog@muhlenberg.edu (H.M.H.); mgjames@muhlenberg.edu (M.G.J.)

2 College of Dental Medicine, Columbia University, 622 W 168th St, New York, NY 10032, USA

* Correspondence: giancarlocuadra@muhlenberg.edu;

Abstract: The objective of this study was to determine if the interaction between common oral commensal bacteria and oral epithelial cells would provide protective effects against the invasion of periodontopathogen *Porphyromonas gingivalis*. Oral epithelial OKF6/Tert cells were used in co-cultures with *Streptococcus gordonii*, *Streptococcus oralis*, *Streptococcus mitis*, and *Streptococcus intermedius*. The viability of OKF6/Tert cells following a bacterial challenge was evaluated by trypan blue exclusion. The adherence of commensal species was determined by CFU counts. *P. gingivalis* invasion in OKF6/Tert cells was assessed before and after exposure to commensal species according to CFU counts. Viability assays show that only *S. gordonii* and *S. intermedius* display low toxicity toward OKF6/Tert cells. Both commensals adhere to OKF6/Tert cells at an average ratio of 1 CFU to 10 cells. *P. gingivalis* invasion into host cells is significantly reduced by 25% or 60% after exposure to *S. gordonii* or *S. intermedius*, respectively. The results suggest that these commensal species bind to host cells and diminish *P. gingivalis* invasion. This is important in the context of periodontal disease since *P. gingivalis* primarily acts on the host by invading it. Therefore, efforts to decrease invasion will eventually lead to future therapies harnessing the mechanisms employed by oral commensal bacteria.

Keywords: oral; commensal; streptococci; *P. gingivalis*; invasion; protection

---

1. Introduction

Periodontal disease (PD) is an oral inflammatory condition induced by the diffusion of bacteria into the epithelium surrounding the tooth. PD affects 47.2% of adults over the age of 30 in some capacity, and approximately 70.1% of adults 65 years of age and older have a form of PD [1]. This is exceedingly important, as the number of adults aged 65 and older is increasing markedly and periodontal health is a key contributor to systemic health [2]. PD can cause tooth loss, pain, discomfort and difficulty speaking, chewing and swallowing, which could ultimately lead to poor nutrition [2]. The first stage of PD is caused by a disruption of bacterial homeostasis in the areas that surround and support the tooth, leading to the inflammation and infection of the gums, or gingivitis [3]. The inflammation associated with gingivitis and periodontitis can lead to a proliferation and dilation of the vasculature, which provide a greater opportunity for oral bacteria to enter the bloodstream. While this bacteremia is often transient, it has the potential to reach a variety of target organs [4]. Bacteria that originate in the oral cavity are also associated with several severe systemic conditions including cardiovascular disease [5,6], respiratory infections [7], arthritis [8], diabetes [9,10], and Alzheimer's disease [11,12].

The oral cavity contains a rich microbiota which, in healthy individuals, remains in homeostasis. The health of periodontal tissues is determined by the composition of this microbiota and the antagonistic and synergistic relationships therein [13]. Pathogenic bacteria within this microbial environment lead to tissue destruction by subverting the host immune response and disrupting the microbial–host homeostasis [14]. Gram-negative anaerobes, most notably *Porphyromonas gingivalis*, are found in large quantities in the subgingival sulcus of patients suffering from periodontitis [15]. Growing evidence suggests that these pathogens have an exceedingly complex relationship with both the host [16] and the nearby commensal microbiota [17,18]. In healthy individuals, several species of streptococci take part in the early colonization of the oral cavity by inhibiting the growth of pathogenic bacteria [19,20]. For instance, *Streptococcus gordonii*, which is regarded as a species of commensal bacteria, is found more frequently in healthy tissue than in areas affected by PD. This commensal species does not alter transcription in oral epithelial cells as significantly as pathogenic strains [21,22]. *S. gordonii* is one of the first species to re-colonize after brushing or antibacterial rinses, which makes it a candidate for the exclusion of pathogenic microbes from tooth surfaces. In fact, oral streptococci constitute over 80% of early oral biofilm and plaque [23]. Commensal streptococci include several groups with multiple species. Examples of these groups and species are the Anginosus group (*Streptococcus intermedius*), Sanguinis group (*Streptococcus gordonii*), and Mitis group (*Streptococcus mitis* and *Streptococcus oralis*) [24]. The four species mentioned have been found to be ubiquitous in healthy and PD-affected individuals [25].

P. gingivalis has been studied extensively in the context of its role in the progression of PD. This pathogen is known to adhere to and invade both monolayers and multilayers of primary gingival epithelial cells (GEC) [26–29] The adherence of *P. gingivalis* is mediated by the major fimbriae, a key virulence factor [30]. Fimbrillin (FimA), a subunit of these filamentous components, interacts with both the host tissue and other bacteria to allow for association [30]. β1 integrins have been identified as epithelial cell cognate receptors for these *P. gingivalis* fimbriae [29]. After *P. gingivalis* initially adheres, with the predominant adhesins being the major fimbriae, an integrin-associated signaling cascade is initiated. Actin microfilaments and microtubule structures in the cell accommodate the entry of the bacteria. This, along with the recruitment of lipid raft components and host-cell signaling events, is required for the internalization of *P. gingivalis* [15]. Once *P. gingivalis* invades, several virulence factors including FimA, RgpA/B and Kgp show decreased expression, and stress-associated proteins such as peroxidases and heat shock proteins are upregulated [15]. These changes result from a need for *P. gingivalis* to adapt to the intracellular environment.

ArcA is a conserved gene found in several oral commensal species and encodes for arginine deaminase [31]. Some studies have investigated ArcA as a factor that potentially inhibits the interactions of *P. gingivalis* with the host tissue, disrupting the progression of periodontal disease. For instance, *Streptococcus cristatus* ArcA interferes with the colonization of *P. gingivalis* in mice [32]. Similarly, arginine deaminase of oral streptococci like *S. cristatus* and *S. intermedius* downregulates the expression of FimA in *P. gingivalis*, which allows for biofilm formation [13,31,33,34]. In addition, commensal bacteria including *S. gordonii*, *S. mitis* and *S. intermedius* were capable of antagonizing the growth of pathogenic species including *P. gingivalis* [20,35]. H_2O_2 released by these streptococci appeared to be the most prevalent antimicrobial substance that inhibited the growth of the pathogens [20,36].

The invasive capabilities of commensal streptococci have not been investigated to a great extent. *S. intermedius* interacts with and, to a certain extent, seems to invade hepatic cell models [37]. While *S. gordonii* is known to invade endothelial cells [38], it does not exhibit detectable invasion of gingival epithelial cell (GEC) multilayers [26]. Previous research suggests that *S. gordonii* has the ability to invade human aortic endothelial cells [38], but to date, there is scant research regarding the invasion of *S. gordonii* or any other commensal strain into oral epithelial cells. Conversely, *S. gordonii* tends to induce an immune response in GECs, leading to the secretion of IL-1ß, IL-6, IL-8 and TNF-α and ultimately contributing to gingival health via immunosurveillance [26]. Additionally, this commensal improved paracellular barrier function by increasing the expression of genes encoding the tight junction components ZO-1, ZO-2, JAM-A, and occludin [39].

To date, it remains unclear if commensal bacteria can interfere with the ability of *P. gingivalis* to invade host cells. If so, this means that the commensal bacteria promote a protective effect in the context of pathogenic invasion. The aim of this study is to determine whether commensal bacteria can slow *P. gingivalis* invasion into host cells in sequential co-cultures. We are investigating the effect of a pre-exposure to commensal bacteria on oral epithelial cells to determine if that interaction protects epithelial cells from a subsequent *P. gingivalis* invasion. We hypothesize that the interaction between commensal bacteria and oral epithelial cells will directly hinder *P. gingivalis* invasion.

2. Materials and Methods

2.1. Cell Line and Bacterial Cultures

The immortal human oral keratinocyte OKF6/Tert cell line was kindly provided by Dr. Gill Diamond from the University of Florida, College of Dentistry (Gainesville, FL, USA) [40]. Cells were cultured in tissue culture plates at 37 °C in 5% CO_2 (standard conditions) with complete Keratinocyte Serum-Free Growth Medium (KSFM) prepared following the methods described by Brice et al. [40]. Briefly, KSFM base medium plus 30 µg/mL of bovine pituitary extract, 0.3 mM calcium chloride, 1 mM glutamine, and 100 U/mL of penicillin and streptomycin was used. Cells were sub-cultured every 4 to 6 days. All experiments were conducted between passages 21 and 37.

Streptococcus gordonii DL1, *Streptococcus intermedius* 0809, *Streptococcus mitis* UF2, and *Streptococcus oralis* SK139 were grown in Brain Heart Infusion Broth (BHI) with 5 µg/mL hemin or in BHI agar at 37 °C in 5% CO_2 (standard conditions). All four commensal species were kindly provided by Dr. Robert Burne from the University of Florida, College of Dentistry (Gainesville, FL, USA). *Porphyromonas gingivalis* 33277 was kindly provided by Dr. Richard Lamont at the University of Louisville, School of Dentistry (Louisville, KY, USA). *P. gingivalis* 33277 was grown in Trypticase soy broth with yeast extract (1 mg/mL), hemin (5 µg/mL), and menadione (1 µg/mL) (TSBY) or in blood agar with menadione (1 µg/mL) anaerobically at 37 °C in a Bactron 300 anaerobic incubator from Sheldon Manufacturing, Inc. (Cornelius, OR, USA).

2.2. Bacterial Growth Curves

Starter cultures of *S. gordonii* DL1, *S. mitis* UF2, *S. intermedius* 0809, and *S. oralis* SK139 were grown in BHI media overnight at 37 °C in 5% CO_2. The following day, starter cultures were adjusted to $OD_{595nm} = 1.0$, and 1% inoculum was used to grow new cultures in BHI and KSFM without antibiotics. The cultures were incubated at 37 °C in 5% CO_2, and absorbance was read every 2 h for 12 h and at 24 h post-inoculation.

2.3. Streptococcal Cytotoxicity Assay

OKF6/Tert cells were grown in 12-well plates with 1 mL of complete KSFM/well to at least 90% confluency. Streptococci were grown to late exponential phase, and cultures of each species were adjusted to $OD_{595nm} = 1.0$. Bacteria were diluted separately in antibiotic-free KSFM. OKF6/Tert cells were washed three times with 1 mL of sterile PBS per well to remove excess antibiotics. Bacteria in their spent media were diluted in antibiotic-free KSFM to ensure that the microbes and their products were involved in all assays, mimicking in vivo interactions as close as possible. After diluting, all streptococcal strains and their extracellular products were added to OKF6/Tert cells at a multiplicity of infection (MOI) of 100 in a final volume of 1 mL in separate wells. In addition, matching volumes of filtered-sterile spent BHI media were diluted in KSFM, or KSFM alone was added to OKF6/Tert cells as controls for cytotoxicity. All co-cultures and corresponding controls were then incubated for 1 or 2 h post-infection under standard conditions. Then, OKF6/Tert cells were washed three times with 1 mL of sterile PBS per well to remove unbound streptococci, and an antibiotic protection assay was performed. Briefly, OKF6/Tert cells were incubated for an hour with 1 mL of KSFM containing 300 µg/mL of gentamicin and 200 µg/mL of metronidazole to kill extracellular bacteria [27–29,41,42]. Then, cultures were incubated for 48 h post-infection in complete KSFM (containing penicillin and streptomycin) under standard conditions. To assess cellular morphology during and after host–bacteria interactions, images of the keratinocyte monolayers were acquired at 200X magnification using a Nikon Eclipse TE2000-U inverted microscope equipped with a Nikon Digital Sight DS-Fi1 camera and NIS Elements Imagine Software (Nikon Instruments Inc, Melvin, NY, USA) at indicated time-points. After 48 h post-infection, cells were trypsinized and mixed with an equal volume of trypan blue, which diffuses inside dead cells, thus staining them blue under the light microscope. Live (unstained) cells were counted using the hemocytometer and light microscopy.

2.4. *Streptococcal Adherence and Invasion Assays*

Co-cultures of OKF6/Tert cells with either *S. gordonii* DL1 or *S. intermedius* 0809 at MOI = 100 were incubated for 1 h as above. Excess bacteria were then washed three times with 1 mL of PBS per well, and OKF6/Tert cells were either lysed with 1 mL of sterile diH_2O per well or subjected to an antibiotic protection assay as described above. After the hour of killing, OKF6/Tert cells were washed and lysed as above. Lysates before and after the antibiotic protection assay were plated on BHI agar for CFU counts to quantify commensal bacteria adherence and invasion, respectively.

2.5. *P. gingivalis Invasion Assays*

OKF6/Tert cells were incubated for 1 h with either *S. gordonii* DL1 or *S. intermedius* 0809 as above. Then, cells were washed three times with 1 mL of PBS per well to remove excess commensal bacteria. To ensure the streptococci that adhered to the OKF6/Tert cells remained alive, no antibiotic protection assay was performed at this point. The *P. gingivalis* 33277 overnight culture was adjusted to OD = 1.0, diluted in antibiotic-free KSFM, and added to cells pre-exposed to streptococci at MOI = 100. Equal quantities of *P. gingivalis* 33277 were also added to OKF6/Tert cells that were not exposed to streptococci (control). Co-cultures were incubated for 30 min under standard conditions [28,43]. Then, cells were washed three times with 1 mL of PBS per well, and an antibiotic protection assay was performed to kill all extracellular bacteria, as described above. Cells were washed and lysed as indicated above. Lysates were serially diluted in sterile PBS, plated on blood agar plates with menadione, and incubated for about 5 days anaerobically before counting *P. gingivalis* colonies.

2.6. *Streptococcal Inhibition of P. gingivalis Growth*

Growth inhibition experiments were conducted following the methodology of Herrero et al. [20]. *Escherichia coli* does not have any effect on *P. gingivalis* growth [20] and therefore was used as a negative control for inhibition experiments. Late exponential phase cultures of *S. gordonii* DL1, *S. intermedius* 0809, and *E. coli* OP50 grown in BHI (OD = 1.0) were diluted to 1:100 in TSBY. Ten microliters of each strain were plated on separate blood agar plates with 1 μg/mL of menadione and allowed to dry. Bacteria were cultured for 24 h. *P. gingivalis* was grown overnight in TSBY anaerobically, the OD was adjusted to 1.0, the cultures were diluted 1:10 in TSBY, and 10 μL were plated on the same blood agar approximately 1 mm away from the spots of the already existing strains. Bacteria were cultured for about three days anaerobically, and the plates were photographed to observe *P. gingivalis* growth patterns.

2.7. *Statistical Analyses*

Every experiment was repeated at least three times. Figures represent the mean and standard deviation of the data. T-tests and ANOVAs were performed, and p values < 0.05 were noted as significant.

3. Results

3.1. KSFM Supports Growth of Commensal Bacteria

In order to compare growth patterns, all commensals were grown in BHI and KSFM without antibiotics. As shown in Figure 1, *S. gordonii* had the most rapid growth in BHI, followed by *S. mitis*, *S. oralis* and *S. intermedius*. *S. gordonii* and *S. mitis* entered the exponential phase of growth by 2 h and continued growing, reaching the late-exponential phase at 4 h. For these species, the stationary phase lasted from Hour 4 to the end of the experiment (Figure 1). *S. oralis* grew exponentially from Hours 2 to 6 and then continued into the stationary phase for the remainder of the experiment (Figure 1). *S. intermedius* reached the end of exponential phase at 12 h. Similar growth patterns were observed in KSFM. However, for all species, absorbance values throughout the experiment remained below 0.5 in this medium. Once again, *S. gordonii* and *S. mitis* grew the fastest in KSFM compared to the other two species (Figure 1). *S. intermedius* also experienced the slowest growth in KSFM. Our data indicate that these four streptococci are not harmed in KSFM. This cell culture medium supports their growth but to a limited absorbance value when compared to growth in BHI broth (Figure 1).

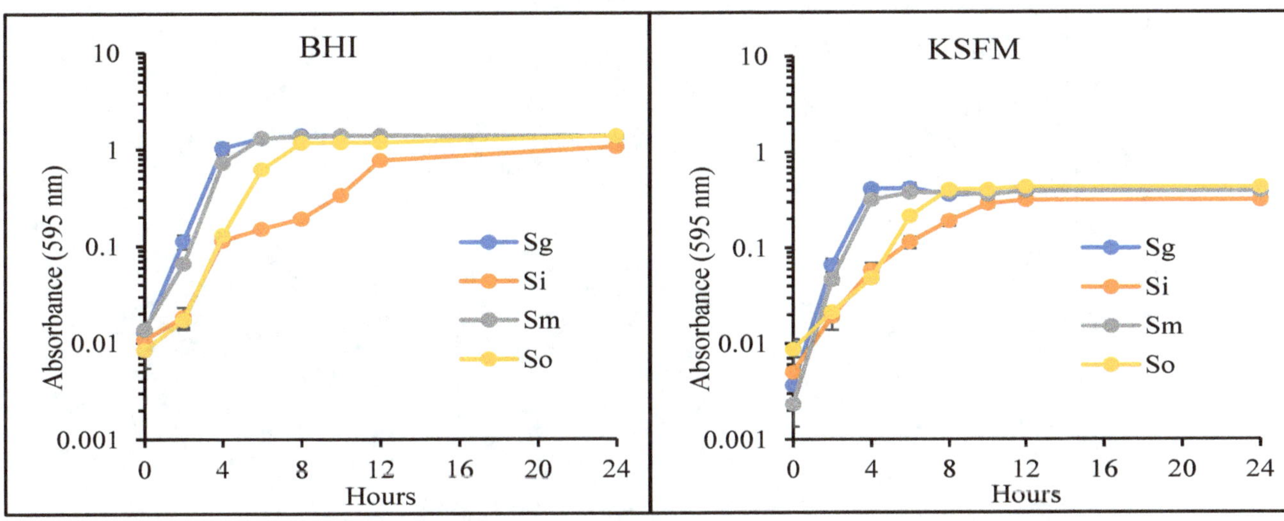

Figure 1. Growth of commensal bacteria in Brain Heart Infusion Broth (BHI) and Keratinocyte Serum-Free Growth Medium (KSFM). *S. gordonii* (Sg), *S. intermedius* (Si), *S. mitis* (Sm) and *S. oralis* (So) were grown in KSFM and BHI. Absorbance was measured at indicated time-points ($n = 3$).

3.2. OKF6 Cell Viability after Commensal Challenge

Prior to any further studies, we determined the periods of time for which OKF6/Tert cells can withstand each of the oral streptococci at MOI = 100. Figure 2 shows the cellular morphology at 0, 24 and 48 h after exposure with all four commensals for 1 h of host–bacteria interactions in 24-well plates. The results show that the cells were nearly 100% confluent at the time of exposure to bacteria and remained at high confluency until 48 h post-exposure. The cellular morphology seems to be intact, but some cellular changes begin to appear after exposure to *S. mitis*, *S. intermedius* and *S. oralis* at 24 h of incubation (Figure 2). However, by 48 h of incubation, cellular morphologies in all conditions seem comparable to each other and to control. To assess the viability of cells, trypan blue exclusion assays were performed. *S. gordonii* did not cause significant OKF6/Tert cell death after 1 h of bacterial exposure. However, this commensal did cause significant cell death after 2 h of exposure (Figure 3). Cells remained viable following challenge by *S. intermedius* at a MOI of 100 for up to 2 h (Figure 3). Exposure to *S. oralis* and *S. mitis* resulted in significant cell death after 1 and 2 h compared to untreated controls ($p < 0.05$). The effect of these two commensals is time-dependent as more cell death is observed over prolonged periods of challenge. In every case, OKF6 cells remained viable when exposed, for up to 2 h, to the spent BHI media of any of the four strains. These results indicate that, under the conditions tested, cytotoxicity only occurs when three of the four streptococci are present and physically interacting for at least 2 h with the OKF6/Tert cells. Based on these results, the remainder of the study was performed using only *S. gordonii* and *S. intermedius* for up to 1 h of interaction.

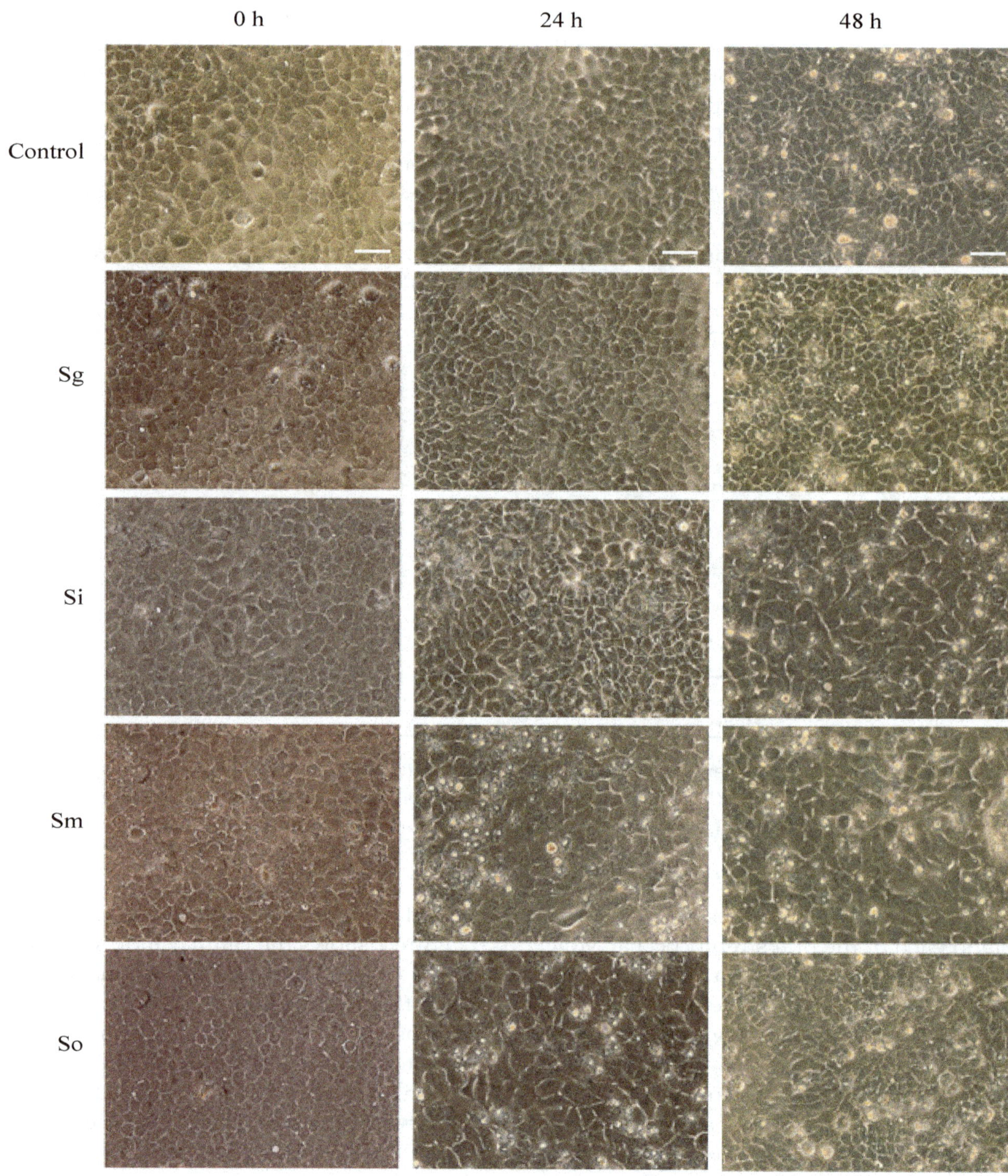

Figure 2. OKF6/Tert cellular morphology after exposure to *S. gordonii* (Sg), *S. intermedius* (Si), *S. mitis* (Sm), and *S. oralis* (So) at MOI = 100 for 1 h of interaction. Light microscopy images were obtained at a magnification of 200×. Bars = 100 μm. Representative images from three independent experiments.

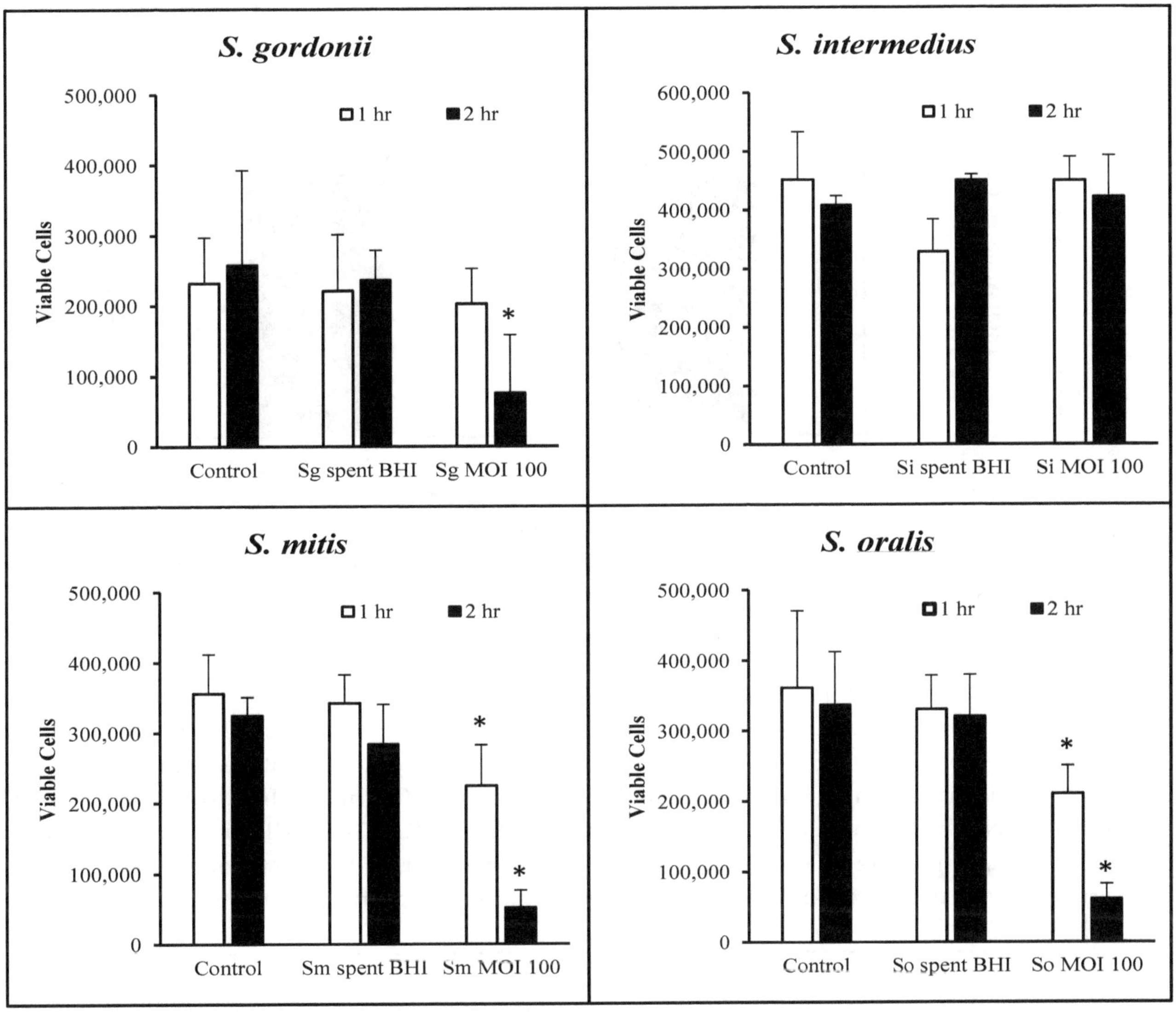

Figure 3. Viability of OKF6/Tert cells following exposure to commensal streptococci. Cell viability reflects the number of live OKF6 cells two days after exposure to *S. gordonii* (Sg), *S. intermedius* (Si), *S. mitis* (Sm), or *S. oralis* (So) or their spent media. Live cells were quantified using the trypan blue exclusion assay. Graphs represent the average and SD of four independent experiments. * = $p < 0.05$ compared to control.

3.3. Commensal Bacteria Adherence Assay

OKF6/Tert cells were exposed to *S. gordonii* and *S. intermedius*. Figure 4 displays the total number of CFUs per well for both streptococci after incubation for 1 h. Following thorough washing, 27,574 +/− 1539 CFUs of *S. gordonii* per well were recovered. Similarly, 30,203 +/− 4883 CFUs of *S. intermedius* were quantified after adherence to OKF6/Tert cells (Figure 4). This suggests that, when contrasting the number of OKF6/Tert cells per well in Figure 3 to the number of adhered CFUs per well, roughly one streptococcal CFU of either of these species adheres to every 10 to 15 cells on average (Figure 4). In addition, following antibiotic protection assays, an average of 96 or 99 CFUs of *S. gordonii* and *S. intermedius*, respectively, were found for every 100,000 host cells (data not shown). These results suggest that these two oral commensal streptococci invade at extremely low rates or not at all.

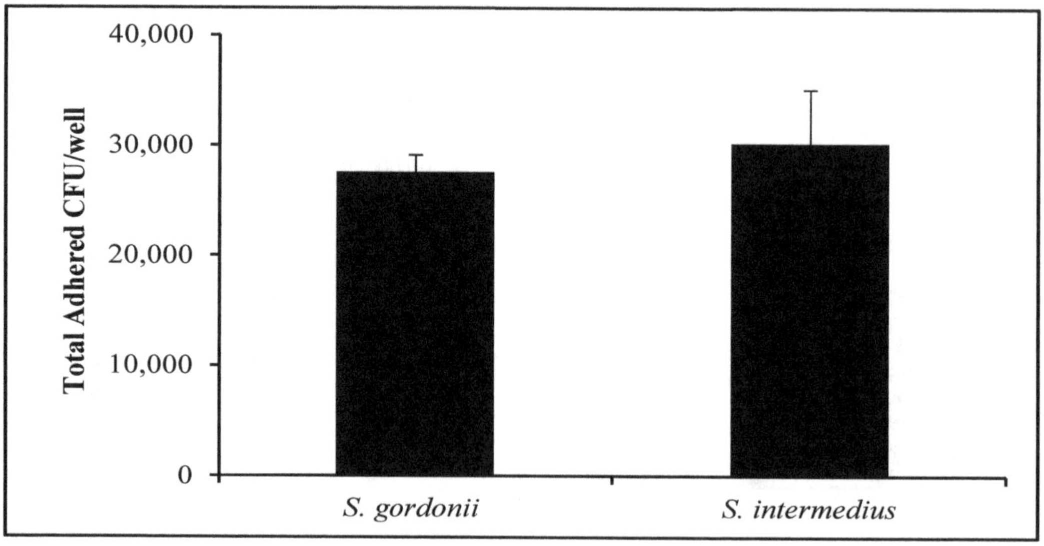

Figure 4. Adherence of commensal bacteria. Quantification of oral commensal streptococci CFUs after adherence to OKF6/Tert cells (MOI = 100) in 24-well plates. Graph represents the average and SD of six independent experiments.

3.4. P. gingivalis Invasion Post-Commensal Co-Cultures

P. gingivalis 33277 invasion into OKF6/Tert cells is around 370,000 bacteria into about 300,000 to 400,000 cells/well, which makes the bacterium/cell ratio around 1:1 (Figure 5). This result agrees with the results obtained by others [28,41–43]. *S. gordonii* and *S. intermedius* pre-treatments of OKF6/Tert cells reduced *P. gingivalis* invasion to about 75% and 40%, respectively (Figure 5). In addition, *S. intermedius* treatment reduced the amount of *P. gingivalis* invasion into OKF6/Tert cells significantly less than *S. gordonii* treatment (p value < 0.05). Our results indicate that during the host–bacteria interactions of OKF6/Tert cells with either commensal, *P. gingivalis* invasion is significantly reduced.

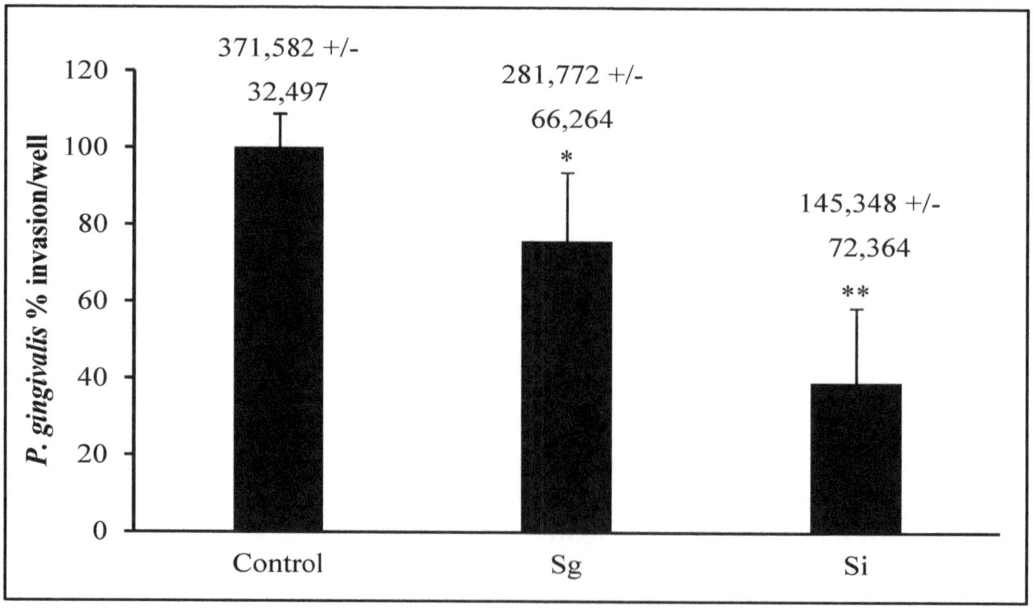

Figure 5. Invasion of *P. gingivalis* following exposure to commensal bacteria. Percentage of *P. gingivalis* CFUs (absolute values +/− SD above each bar) that invaded OKF6/Tert cells after exposure to *S. gordonii* (Sg) or *S. intermedius* (Si). All bacteria were added to OKF6/Tert cells at MOI = 100. Graph represents the average and SD of four independent experiments. * = $p < 0.05$ compared to control. ** = $p < 0.05$ compared to control and Sg.

3.5. Commensal Antagonistic Properties against P. gingivalis

Figure 6 shows *S. gordonii* and *S. intermedius*'s inhibiting effects on *P. gingivalis*. *E. coli*, which has already been shown to have no effect on the growth of *P. gingivalis* [20], and TSBY (outlined in the black circle) were used as negative controls for inhibitory effects. Both oral commensal streptococci show antagonistic relationships with *P. gingivalis*, as indicated by the white arrows pointing at the areas of growth inhibition. Note that these areas are directly in front of the oral commensal streptococci spots. These results suggest that *S. gordonii* and *S. intermedius* produce inhibitory substances that diffuse through the medium and inhibit *P. gingivalis* growth. This antagonism may be related to the commensal streptococci's ability to decrease *P. gingivalis* invasion into the OKF6/Tert cells (Figure 5).

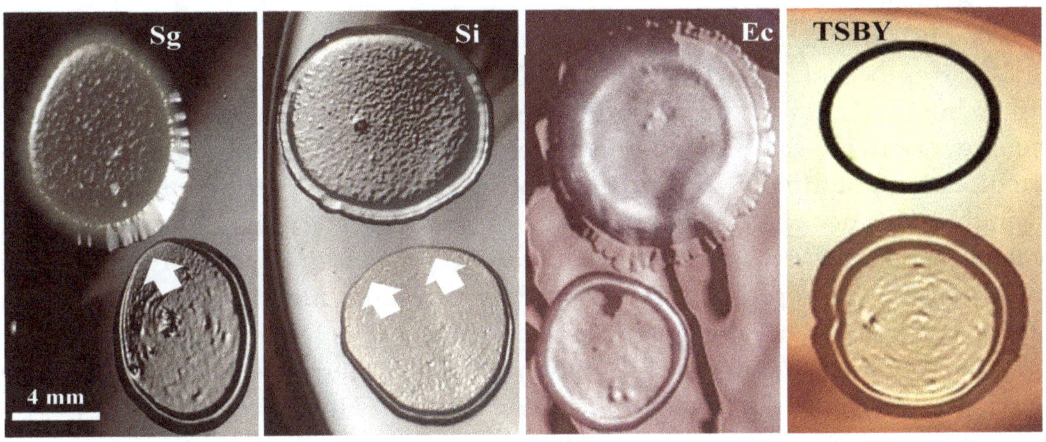

Figure 6. *S. gordonii* and *S. intermedius* antagonism against *P. gingvalis*. All bacteria were diluted in TSBY before plating. Spots for *S. gordonii* (Sg), *S. intermedius* (Si), *E. coli* (Ec), diluted 1:100, or TSBY are shown on the top of each image. Spots for *P. gingivalis*, diluted 1:10, are shown at the bottom of every image. White arrows point at areas of *P. gingivalis* spots with growth inhibition. Representative images from three independent experiments.

4. Discussion

Overall, our study demonstrates that commensal bacteria can provide a protective effect for the host in the context of pathogenic invasion. The specific mechanisms of commensal bacterial protection remain unknown. However, these mechanisms may serve as additional therapeutic methods to treat PD.

KSFM was used as the vehicle for bacteria to establish the MOI throughout the study. KSFM does support the growth of all commensals tested, albeit at a much slower pace than BHI. Therefore, some bacterial growth is expected to occur during the interaction with the host, and this may cause the MOI values to deviate slightly throughout the experiments. Interestingly, *S. gordonii* and *S. intermedius* are the commensal strains that grow the fastest and slowest, respectively (Figure 1). However, neither of these species appears to be harmful to the host within the first hour of host–bacteria interactions (Figure 3). Furthermore, even though *S. intermedius* can be expected to exist in lower quantities than *S. gordonii*, by the end of the hour of host–bacteria interactions, both species were bound to the host at similar levels (Figure 4). Nonetheless, *S. intermedius* is the strain that confers the best protection to the host cells (Figure 5).

Figure 2 shows that the cellular morphology of OKF6/Tert cells does not seem to change significantly after one hour of interactions. However, *S. oralis* and *S. mitis* lead to the substantial death of OKF6/Tert cells after the same treatment (Figure 3). The spent media of all commensals tested, on the other hand, did not harm the host cells, which may suggest that the death of OKF6/Tert cells requires direct contact or the activity of the species near the host. We tested the possibility of streptococcal invasion into OKF6/Tert cells (data not shown) and found extremely low levels to no invasion at all. We propose that the commensal strains *S. gordonii* and *S. intermedius* do not invade OKF6/Tert cells, which is in agreement with the little to no invasion observed with *S. gordonii* by others [26]. Interestingly, since *S. mitis* and *S. oralis* are cytotoxic, it is unclear if cells exposed to these bacteria may be more susceptible to *P. gingivalis* invasion or how this dynamic may affect the development of PD.

The methodology of CFU counts was used primarily because of its reliability in counting the live bacteria harvested at the end of every experiment. Quantitative PCR can also take account of the total bacteria per well but with the limitation of including live and dead bacteria. For example, commensal bacteria that are bound to OKF6/Tert cells and undergo antibiotic protection assays will still contain DNA, which will still be amplified during the qPCR assay. Similarly, in fluorescence-based microscopy techniques, fluorescent labels would not distinguish between live and dead bacteria, and therefore, the microscopic images would present all bacteria associated with OKF6/Tert cells. Because of the limitations of all those other techniques, we chose CFU counts as a dependable method for measuring live bacteria only.

Streptococci CFUs do not necessarily reflect one bacterium, but often a chain of bacteria that may include 10 to 20 streptococci. This explains the CFU/cell ratio of roughly 1 CFU corresponding to roughly 10 to 15 host cells, which means that a given chain of commensal bacteria could have been bound to one of every twelve cells on average. It becomes plausible that several commensal bacteria in a chain are blocking potential *P. gingivalis* receptors, decreasing pathogenic invasion into the host cells. However, this does not explain the decrease in invasion in the neighboring host cells. In order to decrease invasion, other mechanisms must be in place to prevent *P. gingivalis* from entering these host cells. Such mechanisms of streptococcal host protection from *P. gingivalis* invasion remain unknown.

Figure 6 demonstrates that both *S. gordonii* and *S. intermedius* have antagonistic relationships with *P. gingivalis*. These results are in concordance with the results of Herrero et al., where *S. gordonii* inhibited *P. gingivalis* growth via the production of hydrogen peroxide. Herrero et al. report the production of peroxide by several species of oral commensal bacteria, inhibiting the growth of pathogens including *P. gingivalis*, *Aggregatibacter actinomycetemcomitans*, and *Prevotella intermedia* [20]. In accordance, we also report *S. gordonii* and *S. intermedius*'s inhibition of *P. gingivalis* growth (Figure 6), which could suggest a putative mechanism by which peroxide production may deter *P. gingivalis* from approaching the host. An additional mechanism could be the streptococcal binding to and concealing of common host receptors. In order to address this point, studies aiming to (i) identify the surface molecules on *S. intermedius* that serve as anchoring agents for host epithelial tissues and (ii) add these surface molecules to the host in competition assays with *P. gingivalis* may be considered. Molecules from a commensal species that prevent the colonization and invasion of *P. gingivalis* may be used to enhance therapies for PD. Lastly, in healthy individuals who maintain good oral health, commensal streptococci create a beneficial oral biofilm that contributes to the host immune response [19,44]. Therefore, it is possible that these commensal species are protective against the invasion of pathogens in vivo.

Our study agrees with other studies where commensal bacteria work in cooperation with the host to inhibit the pathogenesis of disease-causing bacteria [45,46]. For example, several species of commensal gut bacteria show protective effects against airway infections by *Klebsiella pneumoniae* and *Streptococcus pneumoniae* [47]. An interesting study demonstrates that *Akkermansia muciniphila* from the gut decreases *P. gingivalis*-based periodontitis in vivo [48]. Furthermore, *S. gordonii* itself promotes the improvement of the epithelial barrier (tight junctions) [39], as well as the expression of cytokines, human defensins, and other immunological mediators [26,44,49,50]. Our results align well with other studies demonstrating that commensal bacteria can slow pathogenic activity.

Cytokine production could be an important parameter to measure. However, we feel that it falls outside of the aim of this study because cytokines are relevant to the cellular immune response. Our study is most concerned with the interactions between commensal bacteria and the host leading to protection from invasive *P. gingivalis*. Several other studies address this inquiry [26,38,44,51–54]

In conclusion, we have observed that *S. gordonii* and *S. intermedius* do not cause cell death when compared to the other two commensal species tested. Both species adhere to our oral epithelial cell model and significantly decrease the invasion of periodontopathogen *P. gingivalis*, offering protection to the host. *S. intermedius* reduced *P. gingivalis* invasion by more than 60%. The mechanisms of this protective effect are still unknown.

The invasion of *P. gingivalis* plays a large role in the initiation and progression of PD and therefore the oral health of individuals [55]. Oral health is important in maintaining overall health [15,56–58]. At a higher risk for PD, Americans 65 years of age and older may experience tooth loss, pain, discomfort, the inability to properly chew and swallow food, and ultimately poor nutrition [2]. The role of *P. gingivalis* in systemic diseases further heightens the gravity of this pathogen. Our work is innovative in the context of using the oral commensal microbiota against pathogens such as *P. gingivalis* in an effort to decrease the chances of periodontal disease.

Author Contributions: Conceptualization, G.A.C.; Methodology, G.A.C. and A.N.H.; Formal analysis, G.A.C.; Investigation, A.N.H., H.M.H., M.G.J.; Writing—Original Draft Preparation, A.N.H. and G.A.C.; Writing—Review and Editing, G.A.C., A.N.H., H.M.H., M.G.J.; Funding Acquisition, G.A.C. All authors have read and agreed to the published version of the manuscript.

Acknowledgments: The authors would like to thank faculty members from the biology department at Muhlenberg College and Dominic Palazzolo from Lincoln Memorial University for their assistance in the preparation of this manuscript.

References

1. Periodontal Disease Division of Oral Health CDC. Available online: https://www.cdc.gov/oralhealth/periodontal_disease/index.htm (accessed on 23 May 2018).
2. Eke, P.I.; Wei, L.; Borgnakke, W.; Zhang, X.; McGuire, L.C.; Genco, R.J.; Thornton-Evans, G.; Lu, H. Periodontitis prevalence in adults? 65 years of age, in the USA. *Periodontology 2000* **2016**, *72*, 76–95. [CrossRef] [PubMed]
3. Periodontitis: MedlinePlus Medical Encyclopedia. Available online: https://medlineplus.gov/ency/article/001059.htm (accessed on 23 May 2018).
4. Parahitiyawa, N.B.; Jin, L.J.; Leung, W.; Yam, W.C.; Samaranayake, L.P. Microbiology of Odontogenic Bacteremia: Beyond Endocarditis. *Clin. Microbiol. Rev.* **2009**, *22*, 46–64. [CrossRef] [PubMed]
5. Kumar, P. Oral microbiota and systemic disease. *Anaerobe* **2013**, *24*, 90–93. [CrossRef] [PubMed]
6. Seymour, G.; Ford, P.J.; Cullinan, M.; Leishman, S.; Yamazaki, K. Relationship between periodontal infections and systemic disease. *Clin. Microbiol. Infect.* **2007**, *13*, 3–10. [CrossRef] [PubMed]
7. Zhou, X.; Han, J.; Liu, Z.; Song, Y.; Wang, Z.; Sun, Z. Effects of periodontal treatment on lung function and exacerbation frequency in patients with chronic obstructive pulmonary disease and chronic periodontitis: A 2-year pilot randomized controlled trial. *J. Clin. Periodontol.* **2014**, *41*, 564–572. [CrossRef]
8. Wu, Z.; Nakanishi, H. Lessons from Microglia Aging for the Link between Inflammatory Bone Disorders and Alzheimer's Disease. Available online: https://www.hindawi.com/journals/jir/2015/471342/ (accessed on 12 June 2018).
9. Scannapieco, F. The oral microbiome: Its role in health and in oral and systemic infections. *Clin. Microbiol. Newsl.* **2013**, *35*, 163–169. [CrossRef]
10. Borgnakke, W.; Ylöstalo, P.V.; Taylor, G.W., Genco, R.J. Effect of periodontal disease on diabetes: Systematic review of epidemiologic observational evidence. *J. Clin. Periodontol.* **2013**, *40*, 135–152. [CrossRef]
11. Gaur, S.; Agnihotri, R. Alzheimer's disease and chronic periodontitis: Is there an association? *Geriatr. Gerontol. Int.* **2014**, *15*, 391–404. [CrossRef]
12. Singhrao, S.K.; Harding, A.; Poole, S.; Kesavalu, L.; Crean, S. Porphyromonas Gingivalis Periodontal Infection and Its Putative Links with Alzheimer's Disease. Available online: https://www.hindawi.com/journals/mi/2015/137357/ (accessed on 12 June 2018).

13. Ho, M.-H.; Lamont, R.J.; Xie, H. Identification of Streptococcus cristatus peptides that repress expression of virulence genes in Porphyromonas gingivalis. *Sci. Rep.* **2017**, *7*, 1413. [CrossRef]
14. Hajishengallis, G.; Liang, S.; Payne, M.A.; Hashim, A.; Jotwani, R.; Eskan, M.A.; McIntosh, M.L.; Alsam, A.; Kirkwood, K.L.; Lambris, J.D.; et al. Low-Abundance Biofilm Species Orchestrates Inflammatory Periodontal Disease through the Commensal Microbiota and Complement. *Cell Host Microbe* **2011**, *10*, 497–506. [CrossRef]
15. Tribble, G.; Lamont, R.J. Bacterial invasion of epithelial cells and spreading in periodontal tissue. *Periodontology 2000* **2010**, *52*, 68–83. [CrossRef] [PubMed]
16. Hoppe, T.; Kraus, D.; Probstmeier, R.; Jepsen, S.; Winter, J. Stimulation with Porphyromonas gingivalis enhances malignancy and initiates anoikis resistance in immortalized oral keratinocytes. *J. Cell. Physiol.* **2019**, *234*, 21903–21914. [CrossRef]
17. Lamont, R.J.; El-Sabaeny, A.; Park, Y.; Cook, G.S.; Costerton, J.W.; DeMuth, D.R. Role of the Streptococcus gordonii SspB protein in the development of Porphyromonas gingivalis biofilms on streptococcal substrates. *Microbiology* **2002**, *148*, 1627–1636. [CrossRef] [PubMed]
18. Park, Y.; Simionato, M.R.; Sekiya, K.; Murakami, Y.; James, D.; Chen, W.; Hackett, M.; Yoshimura, F.; DeMuth, D.R.; Lamont, R. Short Fimbriae of Porphyromonas gingivalis and Their Role in Coadhesion with Streptococcus gordonii. *Infect. Immun.* **2005**, *73*, 3983–3989. [CrossRef] [PubMed]
19. Gutt, B.; Ren, Q.; Hauser-Gerspach, I.; Kardas, P.; Stübinger, S.; Astasov-Frauenhoffer, M.; Waltimo, T. Beneficial Oral Biofilms as Smart Bioactive Interfaces. *Front. Microbiol.* **2018**, *9*, 9. [CrossRef] [PubMed]
20. Herrero, E.R.; Slomka, V.; Bernaerts, K.; Boon, N.; Hernandez-Sanabria, E.; Passoni, B.B.; Quirynen, M.; Teughels, W. Antimicrobial effects of commensal oral species are regulated by environmental factors. *J. Dent.* **2016**, *47*, 23–33. [CrossRef]
21. Handfield, M.; Mans, J.J.; Zheng, G.; Lopez, M.C.; Mao, S.; Progulske-Fox, A.; Narasimhan, G.; Baker, H.V.; Lamont, R.J. Distinct transcriptional profiles characterize oral epithelium-microbiota interactions. *Cell. Microbiol.* **2005**, *7*, 811–823. [CrossRef]
22. Hasegawa, Y.; Mans, J.J.; Mao, S.; Lopez, M.C.; Baker, H.V.; Handfield, M.; Lamont, R.J. Gingival Epithelial Cell Transcriptional Responses to Commensal and Opportunistic Oral Microbial Species. *Infect. Immun.* **2007**, *75*, 2540–2547. [CrossRef]
23. Rosan, B.; Lamont, R.J. Dental plaque formation. *Microbes Infect.* **2000**, *2*, 1599–1607. [CrossRef]
24. Facklam, R. What Happened to the Streptococci: Overview of Taxonomic and Nomenclature Changes. *Clin. Microbiol. Rev.* **2002**, *15*, 613–630. [CrossRef]
25. Colombo, A.V.; Da Silva, C.M.; Haffajee, A.; Colombo, A.P.V. Identification of intracellular oral species within human crevicular epithelial cells from subjects with chronic periodontitis by fluorescence in situ hybridization. *J. Periodontal Res.* **2007**, *42*, 236–243. [CrossRef] [PubMed]
26. Dickinson, B.C.; Moffatt, C.E.; Hagerty, D.; Whitmore, S.E.; A Brown, T.; Graves, D.T.; Lamont, R.J. Interaction of oral bacteria with gingival epithelial cell multilayers. *Mol. Oral Microbiol.* **2011**, *26*, 210–220. [CrossRef] [PubMed]
27. Lee, K.; Roberts, J.S.; Choi, C.H.; Atanasova, K.; Yilmaz, Ö. Porphyromonas gingivalis traffics into endoplasmic reticulum-rich-autophagosomes for successful survival in human gingival epithelial cells. *Virulence* **2018**, *9*, 845–859. [CrossRef] [PubMed]
28. Lamont, R.J.; Chan, A.; Belton, C.M.; Izutsu, K.T.; Vasel, D.; Weinberg, A. Porphyromonas gingivalis invasion of gingival epithelial cells. *Infect. Immun.* **1995**, *63*, 3878–3885. [CrossRef] [PubMed]
29. Yilmaz, Ö.; Watanabe, K.; Lamont, R.J. Involvement of integrins in fimbriae-mediated binding and invasion by Porphyromonas gingivalis. *Cell. Microbiol.* **2002**, *4*, 305–314. [CrossRef] [PubMed]
30. Nakagawa, I.; Amano, A.; Kuboniwa, M.; Nakamura, T.; Kawabata, S.; Hamada, S. Functional Differences among FimA Variants of Porphyromonas gingivalis and Their Effects on Adhesion to and Invasion of Human Epithelial Cells. *Infect. Immun.* **2002**, *70*, 277–285. [CrossRef]
31. Cugini, C.; Stephens, D.N.; Nguyen, D.; Kantarci, A.; Davey, M.E. Arginine deiminase inhibits Porphyromonas gingivalis surface attachment. *Microbiology* **2013**, *159*, 275–285. [CrossRef]
32. Xie, H.; Hong, J.; Sharma, A.; Wang, B. Streptococcus cristatus ArcA interferes with Porphyromonas gingivalis pathogenicity in mice. *J. Periodontal Res.* **2012**, *47*, 578–583. [CrossRef]
33. Christopher, A.B.; Arndt, A.; Cugini, C.; Davey, M.E. A streptococcal effector protein that inhibits Porphyromonas gingivalis biofilm development. *Microbiology* **2010**, *156*, 3469–3477. [CrossRef]

34. Wang, B.-Y.; Wu, J.; Lamont, R.J.; Lin, X.; Xie, H. Negative Correlation of Distributions of Streptococcus cristatus and Porphyromonas gingivalis in Subgingival Plaque. *J. Clin. Microbiol.* **2009**, *47*, 3902–3906. [CrossRef]
35. Kreth, J.; Zhang, Y.; Herzberg, M.C. Streptococcal Antagonism in Oral Biofilms: Streptococcus sanguinis and Streptococcus gordonii Interference with Streptococcus mutans. *J. Bacteriol.* **2008**, *190*, 4632–4640. [CrossRef] [PubMed]
36. Wang, B.-Y.; Kuramitsu, H.K. Interactions between Oral Bacteria: Inhibition of Streptococcus mutans Bacteriocin Production by Streptococcus gordonii. *Appl. Environ. Microbiol.* **2005**, *71*, 354–362. [CrossRef]
37. Sukeno, A.; Nagamune, H.; Whiley, R.A.; Jafar, S.I.; Opoku, A.; Ohkura, K.; Maeda, T.; Hirota, K.; Miyake, Y.; Kourai, H. Intermedilysin Is Essential for the Invasion of Hepatoma HepG2 Cells byStreptococcus intermedius. *Microbiol. Immunol.* **2005**, *49*, 681–694. [CrossRef]
38. Nagata, E.; De Toledo, A.; Oho, T. Invasion of human aortic endothelial cells by oral viridans group streptococci and induction of inflammatory cytokine production. *Mol. Oral Microbiol.* **2010**, *26*, 78–88. [CrossRef] [PubMed]
39. Ye, P.; Harty, D.; Commandeur, Z.; Hunter, N. Binding of Streptococcus gordonii to oral epithelial monolayers increases paracellular barrier function. *Microb. Pathog.* **2013**, *56*, 53–59. [CrossRef] [PubMed]
40. Brice, D.C.; Figgins, E.; Yu, F.; Diamond, G. Type I interferon and interferon-stimulated gene expression in oral epithelial cells. *Mol. Oral Microbiol.* **2019**, *34*, 245–253. [CrossRef]
41. Ho, M.-H.; Lamont, R.J.; Xie, H. A novel peptidic inhibitor derived from Streptococcus cristatus ArcA attenuates virulence potential of Porphyromonas gingivalis. *Sci. Rep.* **2017**, *7*, 16217. [CrossRef]
42. Saito, A.; Inagaki, S.; Ishihara, K. Differential ability of periodontopathic bacteria to modulate invasion of human gingival epithelial cells by Porphyromonas gingivalis. *Microb. Pathog.* **2009**, *47*, 329–333. [CrossRef]
43. Jauregui, C.; Robinson, B.; De Moya, A.V.; Brockman, R.D.; Roman, A.V.; Cash, M.N.; Culp, D.J.; Lamont, R.J. Establishment and characterization of a telomerase immortalized human gingival epithelial cell line. *J. Periodontal Res.* **2013**, *48*, 713–721. [CrossRef]
44. Dommisch, H.; Reinartz, M.; Backhaus, T.; Deschner, J.; Chung, W.; Jepsen, S. Antimicrobial responses of primary gingival cells to Porphyromonas gingivalis. *J. Clin. Periodontol.* **2012**, *39*, 913–922. [CrossRef]
45. O'Callaghan, A.; Corr, S. Establishing Boundaries: The Relationship That Exists between Intestinal Epithelial Cells and Gut-Dwelling Bacteria. *Microorganisms* **2019**, *7*, 663. [CrossRef] [PubMed]
46. Dumas, A.; Bernard, L.; Poquet, Y.; Lugo-Villarino, G.; Neyrolles, O. The role of the lung microbiota and the gut-lung axis in respiratory infectious diseases. *Cell. Microbiol.* **2018**, *20*, e12966. [CrossRef] [PubMed]
47. Brown, R.L.; Sequeira, R.P.; Clarke, T.B. The microbiota protects against respiratory infection via GM-CSF signaling. *Nat. Commun.* **2017**, *8*, 1512. [CrossRef] [PubMed]
48. Huck, O.; Mulhall, H.; Rubin, G.; Kizelnik, Z.; Iyer, R.; Perpich, J.D.; Haque, N.; Cani, P.D.; De Vos, W.M.; Amar, S. Akkermansia muciniphila reduces Porphyromonas gingivalis -induced inflammation and periodontal bone destruction. *J. Clin. Periodontol.* **2019**, *47*, 202–212. [CrossRef] [PubMed]
49. Ji, S.; Kim, Y.; Min, B.-M.; Han, S.H.; Choi, Y. Innate immune responses of gingival epithelial cells to nonperiodontopathic and periodontopathic bacteria. *J. Periodontal Res.* **2007**, *42*, 503–510. [CrossRef]
50. Chung, W.O.; Dale, B.A. Innate Immune Response of Oral and Foreskin Keratinocytes: Utilization of Different Signaling Pathways by Various Bacterial Species. *Infect. Immun.* **2004**, *72*, 352–358. [CrossRef]
51. Sliepen, I.; Van Damme, J.; Van Essche, M.; Loozen, G.; Quirynen, M.; Teughels, W. Microbial Interactions Influence Inflammatory Host Cell Responses. *J. Dent. Res.* **2009**, *88*, 1026–1030. [CrossRef]
52. Peyyala, R.; Kirakodu, S.S.; Novak, K.F.; Ebersole, J.L. Oral epithelial cell responses to multispecies microbial biofilms. *J. Dent. Res.* **2013**, *92*, 235–240. [CrossRef]
53. Stathopoulou, P.G.; Benakanakere, M.R.; Galicia, J.C.; Kinane, D.F. Epithelial cell pro-inflammatory cytokine response differs across dental plaque bacterial species. *J. Clin. Periodontol.* **2010**, *37*, 24–29. [CrossRef]
54. Zhang, G.; Chen, R.; Rudney, J. Streptococcus cristatus attenuates Fusobacterium nucleatum-induced interleukin-8 expression in oral epithelial cells. *J. Periodontal Res.* **2008**, *43*, 408–416. [CrossRef]
55. Lamont, R.J.; Jenkinson, H.F. Life Below the Gum Line: Pathogenic Mechanisms ofPorphyromonas gingivalis. *Microbiol. Mol. Boil. Rev.* **1998**, *62*, 1244–1263. [CrossRef]
56. Daalderop, L.; Wieland, B.; Tomsin, K.; Reyes, L.; Kramer, B.; Vanterpool, S.; Been, J.V. Periodontal Disease and Pregnancy Outcomes: Overview of Systematic Reviews. *JDR Clin. Transl. Res.* **2017**, 3, 10–27. [CrossRef] [PubMed]

57. Hajishengallis, G.; Lamont, R.J. Beyond the red complex and into more complexity: The polymicrobial synergy and dysbiosis (PSD) model of periodontal disease etiology. *Mol. Oral Microbiol.* **2012**, *27*, 409–419. [CrossRef] [PubMed]
58. Holmlund, A.; Lampa, E.; Lind, L. Oral health and cardiovascular disease risk in a cohort of periodontitis patients. *Atherosclerosis* **2017**, *262*, 101–106. [CrossRef] [PubMed]

3

Influence of Probiotics on the Salivary Microflora Oral Streptococci and their Integration into Oral Biofilm

Nicole B. Arweiler [1,*], Thorsten M. Auschill [1], Christian Heumann [2], Elmar Hellwig [3] and Ali Al-Ahmad [3]

1 Department of Periodontology and Peri-Implant Diseases, Philipps-University, 35039 Marburg, Germany; auschill@med.uni-marburg.de
2 Department of Statistics, Ludwig-Maximilians University, 80539 Munich, Germany; chris@stat.uni-muenchen.de
3 Department of Operative Dentistry & Periodontology, Center for Dental Medicine, Faculty of Medicine, University of Freiburg, 79106 Freiburg, Germany; elmar.hellwig@uniklinik-freiburg.de (E.H.); ali.al-ahmad@uniklinik-freiburg.de (A.A.-A.)
* Correspondence: arweiler@med.uni-marburg.de;

Abstract: Probiotics' ability to integrate into dental biofilms is not yet clarified. The aim of this trial was to detect probiotic bacteria from probiotic products in dental biofilm and saliva during and after intake. In this parallel, randomized clinical trial, 39 subjects wore customized appliances to build up intra-oral biofilms (72-h periods). The trial was divided into screening (S) to determine baseline biofilm flora, intervention (I), and wash out (WO). During I (28 days), subjects consumed a product containing (a) *Enterococcus faecalis* (b) *Lactobacillus casei*, or (c) *Lactobacillus rhamnosus* GG. Probiotic bacteria and Streptococci spp. were detected in the biofilms and saliva of the 35 subjects that were included in the analysis. During I and WO, the ratio of probiotics in the biofilm was very low compared to total bacterial load, while saliva had slightly but not significantly higher values. No significant changes of probiotic bacteria ($p > 0.05$) were found at any visit during I or WO. The proportion of streptococci was significantly reduced ($p < 0.05$) during I and even lower in WO, compared to S. Probiotic bacteria could neither integrate nor persist in dental biofilm and saliva but did influence the growth of streptococci in biofilm and saliva.

Keywords: biofilms; probiotics; *Streptococcus mutans*; saliva; bacteria; oral microbiology

---

1. Introduction

The global probiotics market size was valued at 48.88 billion USD in 2019 and is projected to reach USD 94.48 billion USD by 2027, exhibiting a compound annual growth rate (CAGR) of 7.9% during the forecast period [1].

While probiotics have been praised for having a positive influence on the immune system and regarding some gut-related diseases [2,3], most health claims are still unsupported and systematic reviews reached no definite conclusions about their significant effects [4–7]. This is mostly due to the heterogeneity of yeasts, products, doses, and vehicles. The underlying mechanisms are seen in the competition with other yeasts, the interaction with virulence factors of other pathogens, the provision of nutrients and cofactors, and the stimulation of the host's immune response.

Meanwhile, probiotics have also been scientifically evaluated according to their effect on oral health [8–12] because the oral cavity presents conditions similar to the gastrointestinal system regarding the high diversity of the microbiota and exposure to food components.

As to microbiome research in general, most research so far has focused on the gut microbiome [13], but recently the oral microbiome and its implication in oral [14] and systemic diseases [15] have been the subject of investigation. The oral microbiome is a highly dynamic community undergoing multiple changes in composition during childhood, with a more stable microbiota in adults. Dysbiosis characterized by overgrowth, e.g., by periopathogenic species, is seen as the cause of periodontal diseases like gingivitis and periodontitis, a chronic inflammation of the tooth-supporting structures with progressive alveolar bone loss [16]. Many studies have found clinical and inflammatory relationships between chronic periodontitis and other chronic metabolic, inflammatory, and vascular disease such as diabetes, cardiovascular diseases, chronic obstruction pulmonary disease (COPD), and metabolic syndrome and obesity [17–20]. Regarding caries, a further frequent oral disease, the total oral biofilm and especially oral streptococci play an important role as etiological agents [21].

Since dental diseases, especially periodontal diseases, are a major challenge to the immune system and general health [22], antipathogenic strategies are important pillars of prevention. Several agents, including antiseptics and antibiotics, have proven their preventive and therapeutic efficacy [23,24]. While studies have examined the effects of probiotic bacteria on salivary microbiota, gingivitis, and periodontitis [8,9,12,25], the underlying (explanatory) mechanisms of probiotic bacteria, such as their ability to integrate into dental biofilms resulting in displacement of other oral cavity bacteria, remain postulations and have only been shown in vitro [26–28]. So far, the few clinical studies on microbiological implication have only examined 10 subjects or less, were only of 14 days duration or applied probiotic bacteria only outside the mouth and only on glass slabs [29,30]. Thus, the aim of this randomized, three-armed clinical trial was to detect probiotic bacteria from probiotic products in in situ dental biofilms and saliva during and after 28 days of intake. The fate of the probiotics, as well as the proportion of oral streptococci, the major causative agents of caries, were examined in the supragingival biofilm and saliva using fluorescent in situ hybridization (FISH) and the culture technique.

2. Materials and Methods

2.1. Sample Size Calculation

Assuming $\alpha = 0.05$, $\beta = 0.2$ and an effect size of 0.9, the paired Wilcoxon signed rank test (two-tailed) required a sample size of 13 (GPower 3.1.9.7).

2.2. Study Design and Population

The observer-blind, parallel, randomized clinical trial took place at the Department of Periodontology and Peri-Implant Diseases of the Philipps-University, Marburg, Germany. It was approved by the Medical Ethics Committee of Philipps University (no. 44/11) and conducted in accordance with the ICH, Good Clinical Practice guidelines, and the Declaration of Helsinki (1964). The clinical trial was registered as 'DRKS 00017822'. Sixty potential participants took part in an initial screening visit to assess their eligibility; the main inclusion criterion was a DMFT (number of decayed, missing, and/or filled teeth) of 0–5, corresponding to low caries experience. Patients had to be over 18 years of age, in good health, without any allergies to the products used in the study and had to be non-smokers (less than five cigarettes per day). They received participant information and signed an informed consent form. Exclusion criteria were any systemic diseases, smoking, untreated periodontal disease with signs of destructive periodontitis or inflammatory symptoms, caries, systemic antibiotic therapy within the last 6 months, a history of probiotic intake, or pregnancy. Furthermore, the use of any of the following drugs within the last 6 months: oral, intravenous, intramuscular, nasal or inhaled corticosteroids, and/or a history of viral infection (i.e., HBV, HCV, HIV) was excluded. In the end, 39 participants (aged 18–32 years) were included. A flow chart of the study is presented in Figure 1.

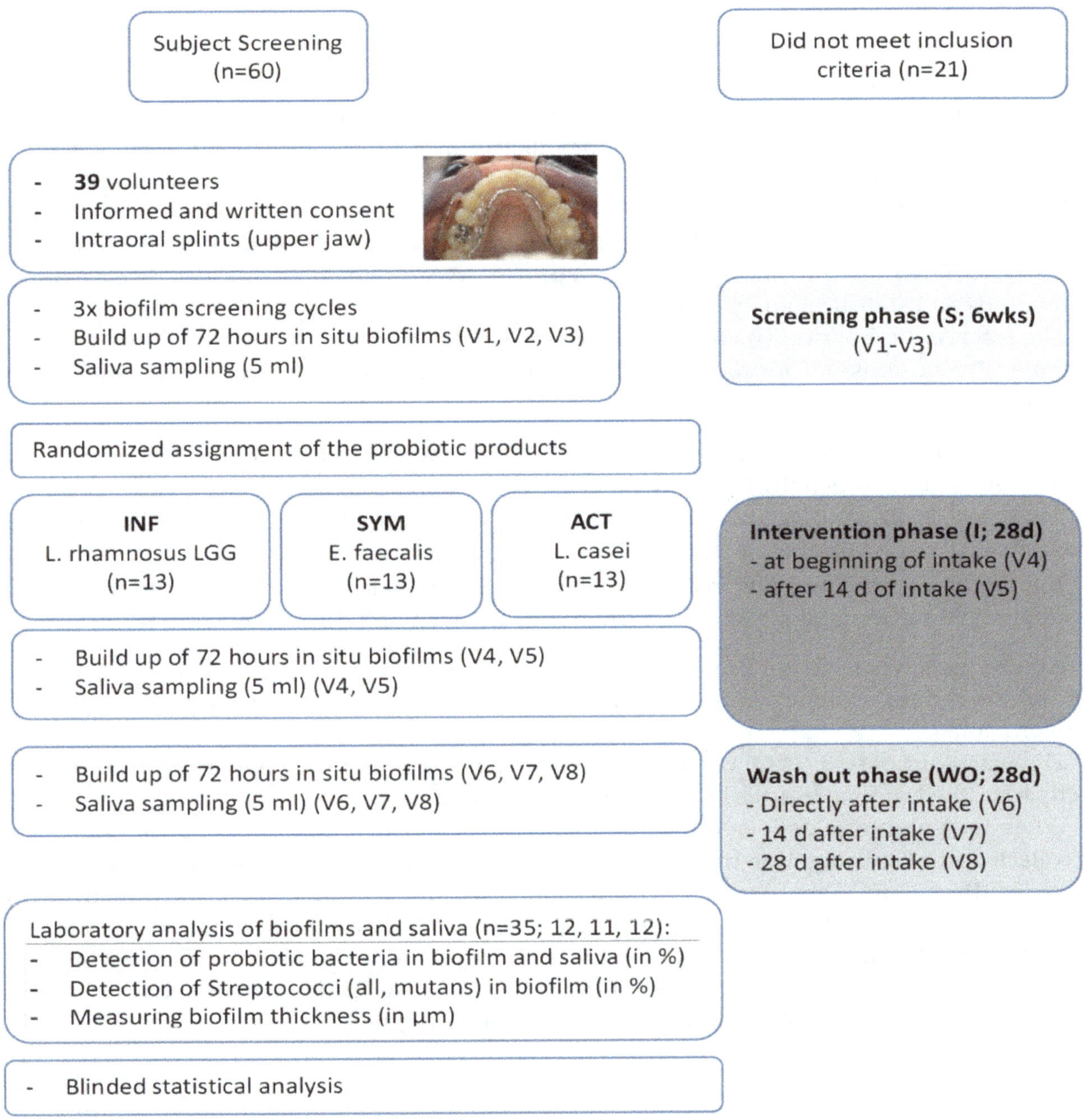

Figure 1. Flow chart of the study.

2.3. *Grow-up of In Situ Biofilms*

All volunteers received individually customized acrylic appliances for the upper jaw into which six plasma sterilized bovine enamel discs (diameter 3 mm, height 2 mm) were inserted. The three discs on each side were positioned towards the interdental area of two teeth in order to generate and mimic approximal biofilms (for details see [31] and Figure 1). A total of 1872 enamel discs were prepared for the eight wearing cycles. The appliances had to be worn continuously for 72 h (3 days) except during eating and oral hygiene measures (twice daily for 2 min each, using only an allocated toothpaste and toothbrush), during which the appliances were put into a dish filled with tap water.

2.4. Study Course and Products

The study was organized into a screening period (S), intervention period (I), and wash out period (WO). The screening period (S) consisted of three weekly visits (V1–V3), to determine the baseline biofilm and salivary flora. After S, the subjects were randomly allocated to the three different treatments ($n = 13$ each), according to a random allocation table and numbers assigned by the order of their attendance for the initial treatment phase. While the investigator and statistician were blinded, the participants were aware of the product since blinding of the products was not possible. The participants received the allocated product from a laboratory assistant not otherwise involved in the study. The randomization code was kept in a sealed envelope and was disclosed after all examinations and statistical analyses had been finished.

The intervention period (I) comprised two visits (V4: 72 h after beginning of intake, V5: after 14 days + 72 h of intake). During the 28 days of intervention, subjects had to consume one of the following products:

- Treatment 1: *Enterococcus faecalis* (SYM), Symbioflor 1 (SymbioPharm GmbH, Herborn, Germany); 30 drops, three times daily (=5 × 50 mL bottles);
- Treatment 2: *Lactobacillus casei* DN-114 001 (ACT), Actimel Classic (Danone GmbH, Munich, Germany); once daily, before lunch (=28 bottles during intervention);
- Treatment 3: *Lactobacillus rhamnosus* GG (INF); InfectoDiarrstop (InfectoPharm GmbH, Heppenheim, Germany), twice daily (morning and evening), diluted in water (=56 sachets).

All products were used or prepared according to the manufacturer's instructions but had to be rinsed in the mouth for 2 min before swallowing, to allow a prolonged period of contact with the oral microbiota.

The wash out period (WO) consisted of three visits (V6–V8); the appliances were again worn directly after the last intake, after 14 and after 28 days, for 72 h each.

When the volunteers delivered their appliance at each visit, a 5 mL unstimulated saliva sample was collected in a centrifugation tube (Nunc IVF; ORIGIO GmbH, Berlin, Germany) and centrifuged with g = 1431 for 5 min (Labofuge 300, Kendro Laboratory Products GmbH, Langenselbold, Germany). Sampling of unstimulated saliva was chosen since oral microbiome analysis from unstimulated saliva performs equally to stimulated saliva or mouthwash rinse [32,33]. Supernatant was frozen immediately and stored at −80 °C in reduced transport fluid (RTF) [21]. The biofilm-covered enamel specimens were removed from the splints and processed for further analysis.

2.5. Fluorescence In Situ Hybridization (FISH)

The different probiotic bacteria, total oral streptococci, *Streptococcus mutans* and *Streptococcus sobrinus* were detected and their percentage compared to eubacteria, in biofilm and saliva, were calculated using the following specific gene probes, each on one enamel disc per subject.

- EUB 338 (5′-GCTGCCTCCGTAGGAGT-3′) for eubacteria (total count of all bacteria, [34]);
- LGC358a (5′-CCA TTG TGG AAG ATT CCC T-3′) for *Lactobacillus* spp. [35];
- Efs 129 (5′-CCCTCTGATGGGTAGGTT-3′) for *Enterococcus faecalis* [36];
- STR 405 (5′-TAG CCG TCC CTT TCT GGT-3′) for *Streptococcus* spp. [37];
- MUT590 (5′ ACT CCA GAC TTT CCT GAC-3′) for *S. mutans* [37,38];
- L-Ssob440-2 (5′ CAC ACG TTC TTC CCC TAC-3′) for *S. sobrinus* [35].

Briefly, the biofilms and saliva samples were fixed in 4% paraformaldehyde in phosphate-buffered saline (PBS, 1.7 mM KH_2PO_4—5mM Na_2HPO_4 with 0.15 M sodium chloride, pH 7.2) for 12 h at 4 °C. In order to minimize cell loss during the following hybridization and washing steps, the saliva samples were coated with agarose and spotted onto microscope slides (Erie Scientific Company, Portsmouth, NH, USA). Samples were further processed using FISH, as has been described in detail elsewhere [39].

2.6. CLSM Analysis

The labelled biofilms were visualized in a chambered cover glass (μ Slide 8 well; ibidi GmbH, Munich, Germany) with confocal laser scanning microscopy (Leica TCS SP2 AOBS, Mannheim, Germany) using a 63× water immersion objective (HCX PL APO lbd.BL 63.0 × 1.2W, Leica, Mannheim, Germany). The areas measured were from three representative locations on the biofilm and averaged for statistical analysis. The quantification of the different microbial targets within the biofilm (in %) and the measurement of biofilm thickness (BT in μm) were carried out as has previously been described [40].

2.7. Confirmation of Probiotic Bacteria by Culture Technique, MALDI-TOF and DNA Fingerprinting

In order to cultivate and identify the different probiotic bacteria *E. faecalis*, *L. casei* DN-114 001, and *L. rhamnosus* GG in the products, serial dilutions were incubated, and isolates analyzed and identified using MALDI-TOF-MS or the VITEK®2 microbial identification system and 16S rDNA gene sequencing. For details see [41]. To confirm the origin of the probiotic bacteria in the subjects' biofilms and saliva from probiotic products supplied, pulsed-field gel electrophoresis (PFGE) was performed as described by Matushek et al. [42] and Klare et al. [43] with modifications as described by Al-Ahmad et al. [44]. The control strain *Staphylococcus aureus* NCTC 8325 was used as a molecular size standard for normalization.

2.8. Statistical Analysis

All parameters were analyzed for groups SYM, INF, ACT. The statistical analysis was conducted by C.H. using SAS. The intra group differences compared to screening were tested using the two-sided Wilcoxon signed rank test for paired samples (significance level $\alpha = 0.05$). No multiple comparison adjustments were made.

3. Results

Of the 39 subjects, 35 (mean age 23.66 ± 3.44) completed all visits; in Group INF $n = 12$ (8 female, 4 male; age 23.17 ± 2.21), in group ACT $n = 12$ (4 female, 8 male; age 24.17 ± 4.61), group SYM $n = 11$ (6 female, 5 male: age 23.64 ± 3.29). One subject in the SYM group did not want to continue intake, three participants (one in each group) stated that they had underestimated the effort.

3.1. Detection and Percentage of Probiotic Bacteria by Multiplex FISH in Biofilm

Figure 2a shows the percentage of probiotic bacteria (*Lactobacillus* spp. for treatments 1 and 2, treatment 3: *E. faecalis*) during screening (V1–V3; blue bars), during intake (V4, V5; green bars), and during wash out (V6–V8; red bars). The proportion of *Lactobacillus* spp. throughout the biofilm (see also CLSM images in Figure 3) was low for INF and ACT, with percentages not exceeding 2%. To compare the treatment products with the baseline, the screening visits (V1–V3) were averaged since they did not differ significantly ($p > 0.05$; Table 1). The I and WO percentages did not differ significantly within any of the treatment products compared to the baseline ($p > 0.05$). There were no significant differences between the three treatment groups ($p > 0.05$).

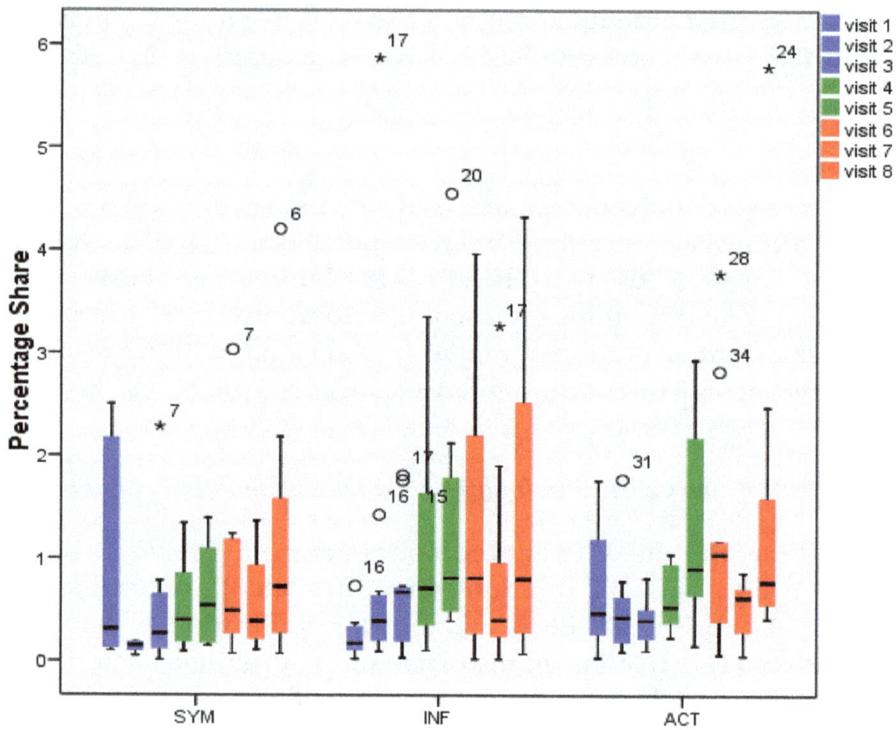

(a)

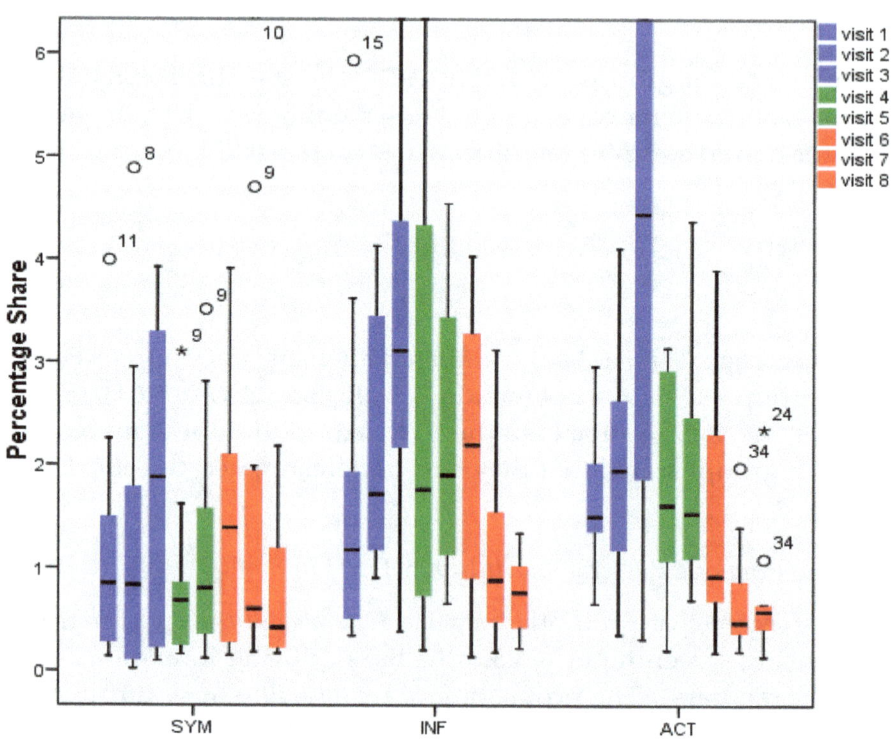

Figure 2. Percentage of lactobacilli/*Enterococcus faecalis* in 72-h dental biofilm (**a**) and saliva (**b**). °: Outliers with values between 1.5 and 3 times the interquartile range (IQR) above the 75%-quantile (Q3) ($Q3 + 1.5 \times IQR \leq value \leq Q3 + 3 \times IQR$); *: Extremes with values more than 3 times the IQR higher than Q3 ($value > Q3 + 3 \times IQR$).

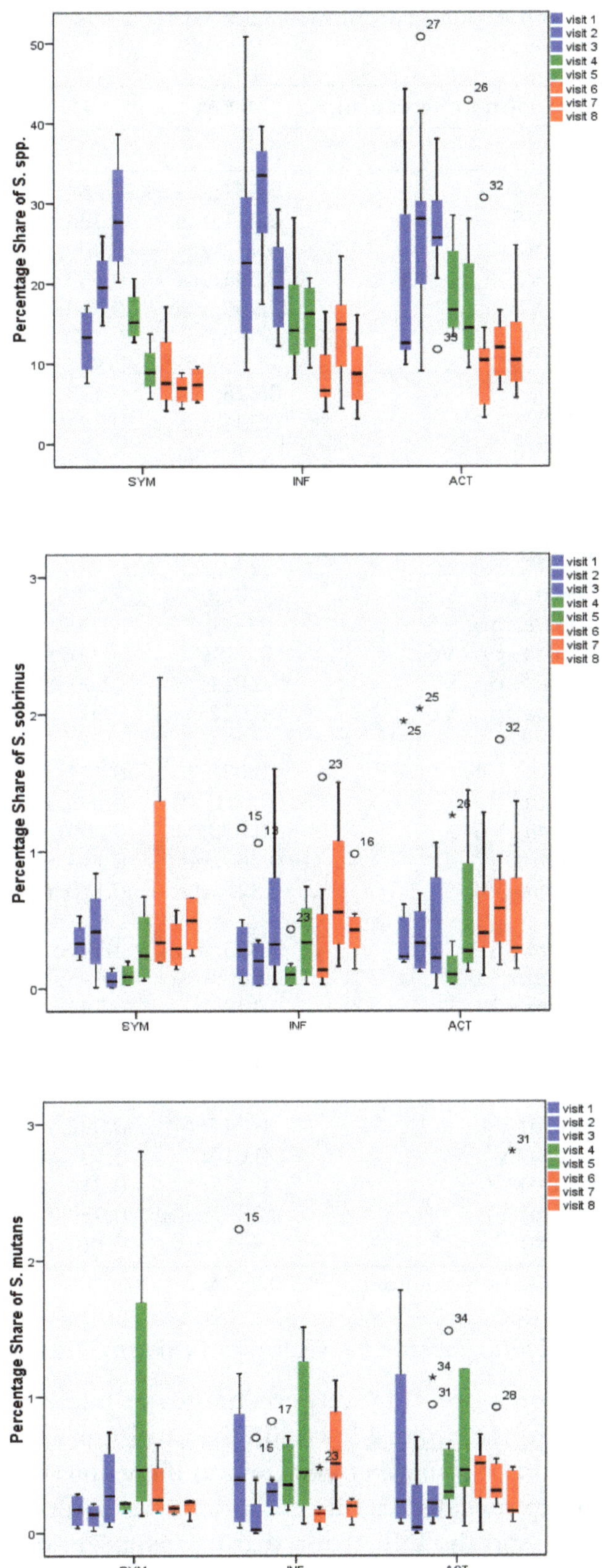

(a)

(b)

(c)

Figure 3. Percentage of all *Streptococcus* spp. (**a**), *Streptococcus sobrinus* (**b**), and *Streptococcus mutans* (**c**) in 72-h dental biofilm. °: Outliers with values between 1.5 and 3 times the interquartile range (IQR) above the 75%-quantile (Q3) (Q3 + 1.5 × IQR ≤ value ≤ Q3 + 3 × IQR); *: Extremes with values more than 3 times the IQR higher than Q3 (value > Q3 + 3 × IQR).

Table 1. Statistical analysis (p-value) of all parameters, comparing visits with screening period in the different groups.

Parameter (in Comparison to Screening)	SYM	INF	ACT
Biofilm			
% PB V4	0.477; n.s.	0.754; n.s.	0.347; n.s.
% PB V5	0.241; n.s.	0.286; n.s.	0.155; n.s.
% PB V6	0.477; n.s.	0.209; n.s.	0.286; n.s.
% PB V7	0.594; n.s.	0.530; n.s.	0.110; n.s.
% PB V8	0.959; n.s.	0.308; n.s.	0.239; n.s.
Saliva			
% PB V4	0.328; n.s.	0.433; n.s.	0.182; n.s.
% PB V5	0.534; n.s.	0.388; n.s.	0.091; n.s.
% PB V6	0.790; n.s.	0.272; n.s.	0.034; *
% PB V7	0.790; n.s.	0.010; **	0.003; **
% PB V8	0.142; n.s.	0.002; **	0.003; **
Biofilm			
% *Streptococcus* spp. V4	0.028; *	0.003; **	0.091; n.s.
% *Streptococcus* spp. V5	0.008; **	0.002; **	0.328; n.s.
% *Streptococcus* spp. V6	0.008; **	0.002; **	0.010; **
% *Streptococcus* spp. V7	0.011; *	0.005; **	0.003; **
% *Streptococcus* spp. V8	0.012; *	0.003; **	0.007; **
% *S. mutans* V4	0.028; *	0.754; n.s.	0.657; n.s.
% *S. mutans* V5	0.021; **	0.099; n.s.	0.286; n.s.
% *S. mutans* V6	0.038; *	0.099; n.s.	0.424; n.s.
% *S. mutans* V7	0.260; n.s.	0.114; n.s.	1.000; n.s.
% *S. mutans* V8	0.327; n.s.	0.110; n.s.	0.838; n.s.
% *S. sobrinus* V4	0.333; n.s.	0.008; **.	0.182; n.s.
% *S. sobrinus* V5	0.260; n.s.	0.695; n.s.	0.824; n.s.
% *S. sobrinus* V6	0.123; n.s.	0.583; n.s.	0.959; n.s.
% *S. sobrinus* V7	0.260; n.s.	0.114; n.s.	0.213; n.s.
% *S. sobrinus* V8	0.036; *	0.477; n.s.	0.314; n.s.
BT (in µm) V4	0.047; *	0.092; n.s.	0.575; n.s.
BT (in µm) V5	0.015; *	0.505; n.s.	0.131; n.s.
BT (in µm) V6	0.021; *	0.814; n.s.	1.000; n.s.
BT (in µm) V7	0.086; n.s.	0.959; n.s.	0.062; n.s.
BT (in µm) V8	0.401; n.s.	0.110; n.s.	0.374; n.s.

n.s.: non significant; *: $p \leq 0.05$; **: $p \leq 0.01$.

3.2. Detection and Percentage of Probiotic Bacteria by Multiplex FISH in Saliva

Saliva (Figure 2b) showed somewhat higher percentages of bacteria than biofilm (Figure 2a). *Lactobacillus* spp. were found at values of up to 4.5% (with the exception of V3 in ACT: 6.5%). While for the SYM group, no differences could be found between any of the visits (V4–V8) compared to baseline screening ($p > 0.05$), the ACT group revealed significant reductions in lactobacilli counts during visits 6, 7, and 8 ($p = 0.034, 0.003, 0.003$) and the INF group during visits 7 and 8 ($p = 0.10, 0.002$). Proof of the bacteria's conformity during screening showed no match to the bacteria supplied. No significant differences could be found when the different groups were compared ($p > 0.05$).

3.3. Detection and Percentage of Streptococci by Multiplex FISH in Biofilm

The percentage share of *Streptococcus* spp., *S. mutans* and *S. sobrinus* in biofilm for all visits and all treatment groups is presented in Figure 3. Representative CLSM images for *Streptococcus* spp. are depicted in Figure 4. While SYM and INF groups showed significantly lower shares of *Streptococcus* spp. in all visits (V4–V8) compared to screening (p-values SYM V4:0.028, V5:0.008, V6:0.008, V7:0.011, V8:0.012; INF V4:0.003, V5:0.002, V6:0.002, V7:0.005, V8:0.003), reductions in ACT group were only significant for V6 ($p = 0.01$), V7 ($p = 0.003$), and V8 ($p = 0.007$) (Table 1). No significant reductions in *S. mutans* were found with the exception of the SYM group in V4 ($p = 0.028$), V5 (0.021), and V6 (0.038). *S. sobrinus* was not significantly reduced during these periods, with the only exception being V4 of the INF group ($p = 0.008$).

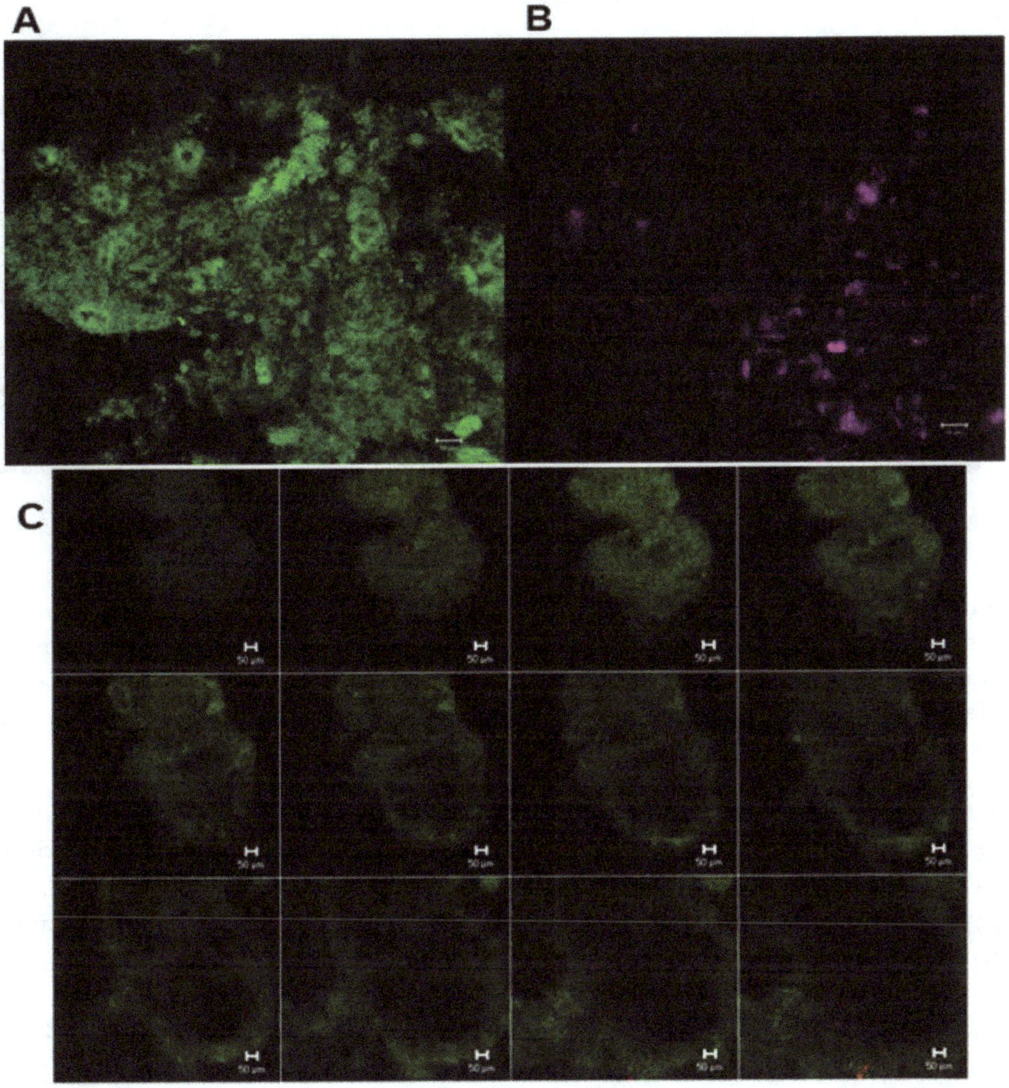

Figure 4. Confocal laser scanning microscopic (CLSM) images from different sections of in situ oral biofilm after the application of fluorescent in situ hybridization with different specific probes. (**A**) Green, eubacteria-specific; (**B**) *Streptococcus* spp.-specific probe; (**C**) Z-section galleries of representative CLSM images depicting a 3-day old biofilm hybridized with eubacteria-specific (green) and *Lactobacillus* spp.-specific probe (red).

3.4. Culture Technique and DNA Fingerprinting

The culture technique used with MALDI-TOF and DNA fingerprinting with PFGE showed that most subjects' biofilm and saliva did not include the original strain supplied during the different phases (S, I, WO) (Table 2, Figure 5).

Table 2. Detected putative probiotic bacteria in biofilm and saliva samples in the different phase.

	Lactobacillus casei		*Lactobacillus rhamnosus*		*Enterococcus faecalis*	
	Participant #	**Range/BES ***	**Participant #**	**Range/BES ***	**Participant #**	**Range/BES ***
Screening (S) /Biofilm	1	10–500	2	10–40		
Ingestion (I)/Biofilm	6	20–700	3	10–100		
Wash out (WO)/Biofilm	2	500	2	20–100	1	2×10^3
Screening (S)/Saliva	2	$200–10^4$	3	40–1000	1	10
Ingestion (I)/Saliva	4	$200–10^5$	7	$100–10^4$		
Wash out (WO)/Saliva	5	$30–2.2 \times 10^3$	4	20–2000		

(#: number; * BES: bovine enamel slab).

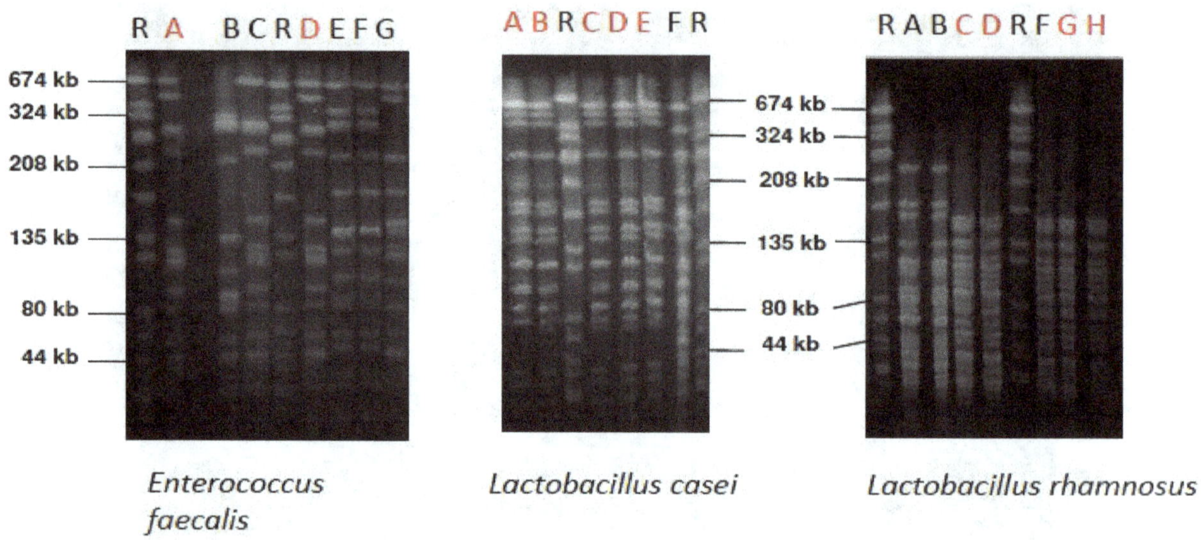

Figure 5. Pulsed-field gel electrophoresis (PFGE) patterns of *E. faecalis*, *L. casei*, and *L. rhamnosus* strains isolated from the supragingival biofilm of the different subjects. Red letters show the strains that were isolated from volunteers and genetically identical to the probiotic product strain. SYM strain: Lane A, ACT strain: Lane B, IINF strain: Lane H. Lane R above the PFGE indicates the reference strain *Staphylococcus aureus* NCTC 8325.

An oral *E. faecalis* isolate was only detected in one subject, in low proportion in WO; this was revealed to be identical with the strain isolated from SYM. *L. rhamnosus* was detected in low concentrations in two subjects during S, in three subjects during I, and in two subjects during WO. However, only two *L. rhamnosus* isolates found during I and two during WO were confirmed to be similar to those supplied in INF. A few colonies of *L. casei* were found in one subject's biofilm during S, for six subjects in I, and two subjects in WO. *L. casei* isolates from four subjects during I and two subjects during WO were revealed to be similar to those of ACT. All species were detected in most of the volunteers, at a low proportion of $10–10^3$ CFU/BES (bovine enamel slab).

L. casei, *L. rhamnosus*, and *E. faecalis* were also isolated in the saliva samples (Table 2). The concentration of *L. casei* in saliva was in the range of $30–10^5$ CFU/mL, whereas *L. rhamnosus* was detected at a concentration of $20–10^4$ CFU/mL. Only a few colonies of *E. faecalis* were revealed in saliva of one volunteer in S. *L. casei* was detected in two subjects' saliva samples during S, four volunteers during I, and five subjects during WO. Only the *L. casei* isolates from three volunteers' samples and only those collected during I, were similar to those isolated from ACT. *L. rhamnosus* was isolated from three volunteers' saliva samples during S, seven subjects during I, and four during WO. The PFGE revealed similarity between the isolated *L. rhamnosus* from two subjects during I and the original strain isolated from INF, whereas such confirmation was only shown in two volunteers' saliva samples during WO. *E. faecalis* was only detected in one subject during S but was not confirmed by PFGE.

Thus, when any lactobacilli or *E. faecalis* strains were found at all in FISH from I or WO, in biofilm or saliva, they were not derived from the products being tested, or were in negligible amounts, which supported the FISH conclusion (no significant increase due to intake).

3.5. Biofilm Thickness (in μm)

Mean thickness of the 3 day-old biofilms ranged between 11.00 (±3.04) and 20.85 (±7.71) μm in all treatments groups (Table 3) and did not change significantly between phases or treatment groups ($p > 0.05$).

Table 3. Biofilm thickness (BT in μm; mean ± SD).

	SYM	INF	ACT
Screening (V1–V3)	15.59 ± 5.41	15.54 ± 5.50	14.10 ± 4.54
Intake (V4)	11.00 ± 3.04	12.45 ± 3.34	13.03 ± 4.04
Intake (V5)	11.85 ± 5.44	14.89 ± 5.71	12.09 ± 5.42
Wash-out (V6)	11.18 ± 2.40	15.22 ± 6.57	13.82 ± 5.56
Wash-out (V7)	12.93 ± 5.05	15.93 ± 5.16	19.27 ± 6.77
Wash-out (V8)	16.75 ± 4.40	20.85 ± 7.71	18.76 ± 11.85

4. Discussion

The hypothesis that probiotic bacteria are significantly raised during and after intake in biofilm and saliva was rejected, while the hypothesis that the number of *Streptococcus* spp. are significantly reduced during and after intake could be confirmed for SYM and INF. For ACT, *Streptococcus* spp. numbers were only significantly reduced after intake (WO).

A combination of two microbiological methods was applied to detect probiotic bacteria in biofilm and saliva. Due to the possibility of a diverse source of similar bacterial species, e.g., from food, the culture technique was still required in order to characterize and compare the strains isolated with the original strains cultivated from the probiotic products themselves by using PFGE [44]. The use of FISH in combination with confocal laser scanning microscopy allows for the integration of different probiotics within the biofilm to be explored in situ without its destruction [39,40]. Microbiome analysis using next-generation sequencing would have been beneficial for examining total variations in the oral microbiota; however, a specific examination of the probiotic bacteria—as in the present study—cannot be achieved.

In contrast to some in vitro or laboratory based studies, the present clinical study could not detect an increase of probiotic bacteria in dental biofilm even when supplied daily.

The clinical demonstration of the inability of probiotic bacteria to integrate into dental biofilm and saliva, either during or after 1 month of intake, confirms former statements (e.g., [12]) that probiotic bacteria cannot change adults' residual oral microflora beyond the supply period. Teughels et al. [12] even recommend antibiotic therapy before probiotic supply, to improve their establishment in the microflora. This was not the case in the present study, which mimicked the normal situation when using commercially available probiotic preparations.

Lodi et al. [29] examined in a combined in vitro/in situ study the influence of two probiotic, fermented milk products, Batavito (B) and Yakult (Y), on biofilms, saliva microflora, and enamel. Ten subjects wore intraoral splints with enamel slabs for 14 days (on the palatal site) and either a 20% sugar solution or one of the probiotic products was applied eight times daily for 5 min outside the mouth and then the splints were worn again. After 7 days of wash out time, the other product was used (cross-over design). The biofilms were analyzed using classical cultivation on agar plates. Saliva was collected in a further experiment in which volunteers had to drink 80 g of one of the milk products. The authors could not detect any significant reduction in the total bacterial load (TBL) when comparing the probiotic to sugar application. The *S. mutans*, lactobacilli, and EPS (extracellular polysaccharides) concentration was similar in all the groups. Only in saliva was a significant reduction of TBL compared to the baseline seen, for B but not for Y.

An additional study using (similar to the present) a combination of CLSM and FISH analyzed a time series of samples from 6 to 72 h in two individuals and six participants that wore similar appliances (with glass slabs) for 48 and 72 h [30]. The individuals had to apply 5 mL of a probiotic milk product eight times a day (Cultura Dofilus® naturell) on each side of the top of the integrated glass slabs. This short-term study used varying time points in their individuals, an extraoral application of the probiotics, no enamel slabs, and thus no strict study protocol as in the present study; therefore, no statistically supported statement was possible. However, they also could not detect any of three probiotic bacteria contained in the product in their in situ biofilms. In their saliva samples (although not strictly in all volunteers) probiotic bacteria were sporadically recorded.

The present study was also unable to detect significant differences between the I and WO periods, suggesting that these probiotic bacteria have no adherence or coaggregation properties in the oral cavity. Taking a mean salivary flow rate of 1 mL min^{-1} of the volunteers into consideration, a retention of probiotic bacteria would only be possible if they could adhere to hard tissues or could coaggregate with other supragingival biofilm microorganisms. So far, a coaggregation of *Lactobacillus salivarius* with oral streptococci could only be proven in few in vitro studies [28,45]. However, adherence properties of lactobacilli are currently highly discussed. Stamatova et al. [46] revealed high variations in the ability of different yoghurt starter lactobacilli to adhere to saliva-coated surfaces. In this context, the tongue, with its distinct surface characteristics (fissures, crypts, papillae, saliva), could also be prone to the colonization, growth, and proliferation of microbiota [47]. It is a highly populated niche which has a significant impact on the colonization of other regions in the oral cavity [48] and could be a noninvasive biomarker for oral and systemic health [49]. Since it could be expected that colonization of the tongue by probiotics may have an impact on the microbiota and the health of the oral cavity, the fate of probiotics within tongue coatings should be considered in future clinical studies.

In dentistry, such properties of probiotic bacteria could be both a blessing and a curse: many studies have shown changes in different cariological aspects after the supply of probiotic products, for example, in rats [50], in children [51,52], and in vitro (partly with human isolates; [10,11,27,29]). In their review, Gruner et al. [8] concluded that there was insufficient evidence for recommending probiotics for managing dental caries and refer to only short-term studies or parameters with limited value for the caries process (such as TBL, instead of caries incidence). Schwendicke et al. [10] highlight the principal cariogenicity of lactobacilli, as in their biofilm model they found significant mineral loss in dentin cavities caused by *L. rhamnosus* GG during sucrose supply concurrent with a lack of *S. mutans* inhibition. Such potential caries risk was taken into account by the study inclusion criteria of DMFT < 5 (decayed, missed, or filled teeth) in the study volunteers.

In contrast to the feared caries risks, a concomitant significant reduction in *Streptococcus* spp. share in 72-h biofilm was found during intake, which was even more pronounced during wash out. Thus, the data are in accordance with earlier studies that probiotic bacteria can replace or, better, suppress *Streptococcus* spp. [27,53,54]. Laleman et al. [9] could only include two studies in their meta-analysis, but confirmed that groups with probiotic intake showed significantly more subjects with lower streptococci counts and fewer subjects with higher streptococci counts compared to control groups. A very interesting and unique result from the present study is that the species *S. mutans* and *S. sobrinus* were in general not reduced by probiotic bacteria, while *Streptococcus* group and therewith obviously other species were significantly reduced by the probiotic supply. This seems to be in contrast to Laleman et al. [9], who found reductions in *S. mutans*. However, Laleman confirmed (in personal communication) that the commercial *S. mutans* tests which were used in the reviewed studies examined nonspecific counts of the *S. mutans* group and were not as specific as the present FISH technique which aims to detect *S. mutans* itself.

A recent study using high throughput sequencing analysis and the same splint system as the present study showed that the role and abundance of *S. mutans* in the in vivo supragingival oral biofilm is overestimated [21].

Such reductions can be explained by bacteriocins which are generally held responsible for effects in the gut and which could also have an influence on dental biofilm, without the direct integration of probiotic bacteria. Furthermore, Laleman et al. [9] did not find any differences between the intake and control group in terms of higher or lower lactobacilli counts, which is also in accordance with the present data.

So far, changes in biofilm thickness under the influence of probiotics have not been examined and are therefore not comparable. Significant reductions in biofilm thickness were only found in the SYM group (*E. faecalis*) at visits 4–6 (I and first WO visit). The lactobacilli supplied in INF and ACT were obviously not capable of reducing the biofilm thickness. It is interesting to note that, especially in these visits, SYM was also able to reduce *S. mutans* significantly.

5. Conclusions

Probiotic bacteria from all products were not able to integrate or persist in dental biofilm and saliva, but they did influence the growth of streptococci in biofilm. Biofilm thickness was not influenced (with the exception of *E. faecalis* during intake and early wash out). The interaction obviously does not happen through replacement but by interaction with other virulence factors, competition with nutrients or cofactors, or possibly, by stimulation of the host's immune response. The present findings are initial steps to an explanation of the clinical effects of probiotic bacteria and products in oral cavity and further dental research.

The weak points of this clinical in situ study are intrinsically related to the small sample size and a targeted search for probiotic bacteria and oral streptococci, which could only provide an association and not determine a cause–effect relationship. Longitudinal studies with higher sample sizes and next-generation sequencing are required to examine the microbial fingerprint after (long-term) use of probiotics. Since oral bacteria are swallowed and translocated to the gut, affecting the intestinal health and disease [55], it is furthermore important to examine the influence of probiotic bacteria on both the oral and gut microbiota, which so far have not been studied in parallel.

Author Contributions: N.B.A.: principal investigator and contributed to the conception, design, data analysis and interpretation, drafted and critically revised the manuscript. T.M.A.: data analysis and interpretation, drafted and critically revised the manuscript. C.H.: performed all statistical analyses and provided data figures. E.H.: contribution to the conception and design of the study A.A.-A.: contribution to the conception and design of the study, CLSM and PFGE data analysis, drafted and critically revised the manuscript. All authors have read and agreed to the published version of the manuscript.

Acknowledgments: We thank Marie Follo (Lighthouse Core Facility) for her help during the CLSM image analysis, Lutz Netuschil for his contribution to data acquisition, and Petra Grimmelbein and Bettina Spitzmüller for their laboratory work.

References

1. Available online: https://www.fortunebusinessinsights.com/industry-reports/probiotics-market-100083 (accessed on 12 November 2020).
2. Sanders, M.E.; Merenstein, D.J.; Reid, G. Probiotics and prebiotics in intestinal health and disease: From biology to the clinic. *Nat. Rev. Gastroenterol. Hepatol.* **2019**, *16*, 605–616. [CrossRef] [PubMed]
3. Vitetta, L.; Vitetta, G.; Hall, S. Immunological tolerance and function: Associations between intestinal bacteria, probiotics, prebiotics, and phages. *Front. Immunol.* **2018**, *9*, 2240. [CrossRef] [PubMed]

4. Forsberg, A.; West, C.E.; Prescott, S.L.; Jenmalm, M.C. Pre- and probiotics for allergy prevention: Time to revisit recommendations? *Clin. Exp. Allergy J. Br. Soc. Allergy Clin. Immunol.* **2016**, *46*, 1506–1521. [CrossRef] [PubMed]
5. Haß, U.; Herpich, C.; Norman, K. Anti-inflammatory diets and fatigue. *Nutrients* **2019**, *11*, 2315. [CrossRef]
6. Kanauchi, O.; Andoh, A.; AbuBakar, S.; Yamamoto, N. Probiotics and paraprobiotics in viral infection: Clinical application and effects on the innate and acquired immune systems. *Curr. Pharm. Des.* **2018**, *24*, 710–717. [CrossRef]
7. Vuotto, C.; Longo, F.; Donelli, G. Probiotics to counteract biofilm-associated infections: Promising and conflicting data. *Int. J. Oral Sci.* **2014**, *6*, 189–194. [CrossRef]
8. Gruner, D.; Paris, S.; Schwendicke, F. Probiotics for managing caries and periodontitis: Systematic review and meta-analysis. *J. Dent.* **2016**, *48*, 16–25. [CrossRef]
9. Laleman, I.; Detailleur, V.; Slot, D.E.; Slomka, V.; Quirynen, M.; Teughels, W. Probiotics reduce mutans streptococci counts in humans: A systematic review and meta-analysis. *Clin. Oral Investig.* **2014**, *18*, 1539–1552. [CrossRef]
10. Schwendicke, F.; Dörfer, C.; Kneist, S.; Meyer-Lueckel, H.; Paris, S. Cariogenic effects of probiotic lactobacillus rhamnosus gg in a dental biofilm model. *Caries Res.* **2014**, *48*, 186–192. [CrossRef]
11. Schwendicke, F.; Korte, F.; Dörfer, C.E.; Kneist, S.; Fawzy El-Sayed, K.; Paris, S. Inhibition of streptococcus mutans growth and biofilm formation by probiotics in vitro. *Caries Res.* **2017**, *51*, 87–95. [CrossRef]
12. Teughels, W.; Loozen, G.; Quirynen, M. Do probiotics offer opportunities to manipulate the periodontal oral microbiota? *J. Clin. Periodontol.* **2011**, *38* (Suppl. 11), 159–177. [CrossRef] [PubMed]
13. Xu, F.; Fu, Y.; Sun, T.-Y.; Jiang, Z.; Miao, Z.; Shuai, M.; Gou, W.; Ling, C.W.; Yang, J.; Wang, J.; et al. The interplay between host genetics and the gut microbiome reveals common and distinct microbiome features for complex human diseases. *Microbiome* **2020**, *8*, 145. [CrossRef] [PubMed]
14. Costalonga, M.; Herzberg, M.C. The oral microbiome and the immunobiology of periodontal disease and caries. *Immunol. Lett.* **2014**, *162*, 22–38. [CrossRef] [PubMed]
15. Sampaio-Maia, B.; Caldas, I.M.; Pereira, M.L.; Pérez-Mongiovi, D.; Araujo, R. The Oral Microbiome in Health and Its Implication in Oral and Systemic Diseases. *Adv. Appl. Microbiol.* **2016**, *97*, 171–210. [PubMed]
16. Willis, J.R.; Gabaldón, T. The Human Oral Microbiome in Health and Disease: From Sequences to Ecosystems. *Microorganisms* **2020**, *8*, 308. [CrossRef]
17. Khumaedi, A.I.; Purnamasari, D.; Wijaya, I.P.; Soeroso, Y. The relationship of diabetes, periodontitis and cardiovascular disease. *Diabetes Metab. Syndr.* **2019**, *13*, 1675–1678. [CrossRef]
18. Sanz, M.; Marco Del Castillo, A.; Jepsen, S.; Gonzalez-Juanatey, J.R.; D'Aiuto, F.; Bouchard, P.; Chapple, I.; Dietrich, T.; Gotsman, I.; Graziani, F.; et al. Periodontitis and cardiovascular diseases: Consensus report. *J. Clin. Periodontol.* **2020**, *47*, 268–288. [CrossRef]
19. Sapey, E.; Yonel, Z.; Edgar, R.; Parmar, S.; Hobbins, S.; Newby, P.; Crossley, D.; Usher, A.; Johnson, S.; Walton, G.M.; et al. The clinical and inflammatory relationships between periodontitis and chronic obstructive pulmonary disease. *J. Clin. Periodontol.* **2020**, *47*, 1040–1052. [CrossRef]
20. Jepsen, S.; Suvan, J.; Deschner, J. The association of periodontal diseases with metabolic syndrome and obesity. *Periodontology* **2020**, *83*, 125–153. [CrossRef]
21. Anderson, A.C.; Rothballer, M.; Altenburger, M.J.; Woelber, J.P.; Karygianni, L.; Lagkouvardos, I.; Hellwig, E.; Al-Ahmad, A. In-vivo shift of the microbiota in oral biofilm in response to frequent sucrose consumption. *Sci. Rep.* **2018**, *8*, 14202. [CrossRef]
22. Pihlstrom, B.L.; Michalowicz, B.S.; Johnson, N.W. Periodontal diseases. *Lancet Lond. Engl.* **2005**, *366*, 1809–1820. [CrossRef]
23. Arweiler, N.B.; Auschill, T.M.; Sculean, A. Patient self-care of periodontal pocket infections. *Periodontology 2000* **2018**, *76*, 164–179. [CrossRef] [PubMed]
24. Zandbergen, D.; Slot, D.E.; Cobb, C.M.; Van der Weijden, F.A. The clinical effect of scaling and root planing and the concomitant administration of systemic amoxicillin and metronidazole: A systematic review. *J. Periodontol.* **2013**, *84*, 332–351. [CrossRef]
25. Teughels, W.; Van Essche, M.; Sliepen, I.; Quirynen, M. Probiotics and oral healthcare. *Periodontology 2000* **2008**, *48*, 111–147. [CrossRef] [PubMed]
26. Matsumoto, M.; Tsuji, M.; Sasaki, H.; Fujita, K.; Nomura, R.; Nakano, K.; Shintani, S.; Ooshima, T. Cariogenicity of the probiotic bacterium lactobacillus salivarius in rats. *Caries Res.* **2005**, *39*, 479–483. [CrossRef]

27. Twetman, L.; Larsen, U.; Fiehn, N.E.; Stecksén-Blicks, C.; Twetman, S. Coaggregation between probiotic bacteria and caries-associated strains: An in vitro study. *Acta Odontol. Scand.* **2009**, *67*, 284–288. [CrossRef]
28. Willcox, M.D.; Patrikakis, M.; Harty, D.W.; Loo, C.Y.; Knox, K.W. Coaggregation of oral lactobacilli with streptococci from the oral cavity. *Oral Microbiol. Immunol.* **1993**, *8*, 319–321. [CrossRef]
29. Lodi, C.S.; Oliveira, L.V.; Brighenti, F.L.; Delbem, A.C.; Martinhon, C.C. Effects of probiotic fermented milk on biofilms, oral microbiota, and enamel. *Braz. Oral Res.* **2015**, *29*. [CrossRef]
30. Ravn, I.; Dige, I.; Meyer, R.L.; Nyvad, B. Colonization of the oral cavity by probiotic bacteria. *Caries Res.* **2012**, *46*, 107–112. [CrossRef]
31. Arweiler, N.B.; Netuschil, L.; Beier, D.; Grunert, S.; Heumann, C.; Altenburger, M.J.; Sculean, A.; Nagy, K.; Al-Ahmad, A.; Auschill, T.M. Action of food preservatives on 14-days dental biofilm formation, biofilm vitality and biofilm-derived enamel demineralisation in situ. *Clin. Oral Investig.* **2014**, *18*, 829–838. [CrossRef]
32. Fan, X.; Peters, B.A.; Min, D.; Ahn, J.; Hayes, R.B. Comparison of the oral microbiome in mouthwash and whole saliva samples. *PLoS ONE* **2018**, *13*, e0194729. [CrossRef] [PubMed]
33. Jo, R.; Nishimoto, Y.; Umezawa, K.; Yama, K.; Aita, Y.; Ichiba, Y.; Murakami, S.; Kakizawa, Y.; Kumagai, T.; Yamada, T.; et al. Comparison of oral microbiome profiles in stimulated and unstimulated saliva, tongue, and mouth-rinsed water. *Sci. Rep.* **2019**, *9*, 16124. [CrossRef] [PubMed]
34. Amann, R.I.; Binder, B.J.; Olson, R.J.; Chisholm, S.W.; Devereux, R.; Stahl, D.A. Combination of 16s rrna-targeted oligonucleotide probes with flow cytometry for analyzing mixed microbial populations. *Appl. Environ. Microbiol.* **1990**, *56*, 1919–1925. [CrossRef]
35. Quevedo, B.; Giertsen, E.; Zijnge, V.; Lüthi-Schaller, H.; Guggenheim, B.; Thurnheer, T.; Gmür, R. Phylogenetic group- and species-specific oligonucleotide probes for single-cell detection of lactic acid bacteria in oral biofilms. *BMC Microbiol.* **2011**, *11*, 14. [CrossRef] [PubMed]
36. Behr, T.; Koob, C.; Schedl, M.; Mehlen, A.; Meier, H.; Knopp, D.; Frahm, E.; Obst, U.; Schleifer, K.; Niessner, R.; et al. A nested array of rrna targeted probes for the detection and identification of enterococci by reverse hybridization. *Syst. Appl. Microbiol.* **2000**, *23*, 563–572. [CrossRef]
37. Paster, B.J.; Bartoszyk, I.M.; Dewhirst, F.E. Identification of oral streptococci using pcr-based, reverse-capture, checkerboard hybridization. *Methods Cell Sci.* **1998**, *20*, 223–231. [CrossRef]
38. Thurnheer, T.; Gmür, R.; Giertsen, E.; Guggenheim, B. Automated fluorescent in situ hybridization for the specific detection and quantification of oral streptococci in dental plaque. *J. Microbiol. Methods* **2001**, *44*, 39–47. [CrossRef]
39. Al-Ahmad, A.; Roth, D.; Wolkewitz, M.; Wiedmann-Al-Ahmad, M.; Follo, M.; Ratka-Krüger, P.; Deimling, D.; Hellwig, E.; Hannig, C. Change in diet and oral hygiene over an 8-week period: Effects on oral health and oral biofilm. *Clin. Oral Investig.* **2010**, *14*, 391–396. [CrossRef]
40. Al-Ahmad, A.; Wunder, A.; Auschill, T.M.; Follo, M.; Braun, G.; Hellwig, E.; Arweiler, N.B. The in vivo dynamics of streptococcus spp., actinomyces naeslundii, fusobacterium nucleatum and veillonella spp. In dental plaque biofilm as analysed by five-colour multiplex fluorescence in situ hybridization. *J. Med. Microbiol.* **2007**, *56*, 681–687. [CrossRef]
41. Anderson, A.C.; Sanunu, M.; Schneider, C.; Clad, A.; Karygianni, L.; Hellwig, E.; Al-Ahmad, A. Rapid species-level identification of vaginal and oral lactobacilli using maldi-tof ms analysis and 16s rdna sequencing. *BMC Microbiol.* **2014**, *14*, 312. [CrossRef]
42. Matushek, M.G.; Bonten, M.J.; Hayden, M.K. Rapid preparation of bacterial DNA for pulsed-field gel electrophoresis. *J. Clin. Microbiol.* **1996**, *34*, 2598–2600. [CrossRef] [PubMed]
43. Klare, I.; Konstabel, C.; Mueller-Bertling, S.; Werner, G.; Strommenger, B.; Kettlitz, C.; Borgmann, S.; Schulte, B.; Jonas, D.; Serr, A.; et al. Spread of ampicillin/vancomycin-resistant enterococcus faecium of the epidemic-virulent clonal complex-17 carrying the genes esp and hyl in German hospitals. *Eur. J. Clin. Microbiol. Infect. Dis. Off. Publ. Eur. Soc. Clin. Microbiol.* **2005**, *24*, 815–825. [CrossRef] [PubMed]
44. Al-Ahmad, A.; Maier, J.; Follo, M.; Spitzmüller, B.; Wittmer, A.; Hellwig, E.; Hübner, J.; Jonas, D. Food-borne enterococci integrate into oral biofilm: An in vivo study. *J. Endod.* **2010**, *36*, 1812–1819. [CrossRef] [PubMed]
45. Comelli, E.M.; Guggenheim, B.; Stingele, F.; Neeser, J.R. Selection of dairy bacterial strains as probiotics for oral health. *Eur. J. Oral Sci.* **2002**, *110*, 218–224. [CrossRef] [PubMed]
46. Stamatova, I.; Kari, K.; Vladimirov, S.; Meurman, J.H. In vitro evaluation of yoghurt starter lactobacilli and lactobacillus rhamnosus gg adhesion to saliva-coated surfaces. *Oral Microbiol. Immunol.* **2009**, *24*, 218–223. [CrossRef]

47. Seerangaiyan, K.; Jüch, F.; Winkel, E.G. Tongue coating: Its characteristics and role in intra-oral halitosis and general health-a review. *J. Breath Res.* **2018**, *12*, 034001. [CrossRef]
48. Danser, M.M.; Gómez, S.M.; Van der Weijden, G.A. Tongue coating and tongue brushing: A literature review. *Int. J. Dent. Hyg.* **2003**, *1*, 151–158. [CrossRef]
49. Bernardi, S.; Karygianni, L.; Filippi, A.; Anderson, A.; Zurcher, A.; Hellwig, E.; Vach, K.; Macchiarelli, G.; Al-Ahmad, A. Combining culture and culture independent methods reveals new microbial composition of Halitosis patients' tongue biofilm. *Microbiol. Open* **2020**, *9*, e958. [CrossRef]
50. Michalek, S.M.; Hirasawa, M.; Kiyono, H.; Ochiai, K.; McGhee, J.R. Oral ecology and virulence of lactobacillus casei and streptococcus mutans in gnotobiotic rats. *Infect. Immun.* **1981**, *33*, 690–696. [CrossRef]
51. Näse, L.; Hatakka, K.; Savilahti, E.; Saxelin, M.; Pönkä, A.; Poussa, T.; Korpela, R.; Meurman, J.H. Effect of long-term consumption of a probiotic bacterium, lactobacillus rhamnosus gg, in milk on dental caries and caries risk in children. *Caries Res.* **2001**, *35*, 412–420. [CrossRef]
52. Stecksén-Blicks, C.; Sjöström, I.; Twetman, S. Effect of long-term consumption of milk supplemented with probiotic lactobacilli and fluoride on dental caries and general health in preschool children: A cluster-randomized study. *Caries Res.* **2009**, *43*, 374–381. [CrossRef] [PubMed]
53. Keller, M.K.; Hasslöf, P.; Stecksén-Blicks, C.; Twetman, S. Co-aggregation and growth inhibition of probiotic lactobacilli and clinical isolates of mutans streptococci: An in vitro study. *Acta Odontol. Scand.* **2011**, *69*, 263–268. [CrossRef] [PubMed]
54. Simark-Mattsson, C.; Emilson, C.G.; Håkansson, E.G.; Jacobsson, C.; Roos, K.; Holm, S. Lactobacillus-mediated interference of mutans streptococci in caries-free vs. Caries-active subjects. *Eur. J. Oral Sci.* **2007**, *115*, 308–314. [CrossRef] [PubMed]
55. Koliarakis, I.; Messaritakis, I.; Nikolouzakis, T.K.; Hamilos, G.; Souglakos, J.; Tsiaoussis, J. Oral Bacteria and Intestinal Dysbiosis in Colorectal Cancer. *Int. J. Mol. Sci.* **2019**, *20*, 4146. [CrossRef]

4

Th17 Cells and the IL-23/IL-17 Axis in the Pathogenesis of Periodontitis and Immune-Mediated Inflammatory Diseases

Kübra Bunte and Thomas Beikler *

Department of Periodontics, Preventive and Restorative Dentistry,
University Medical Centre Hamburg-Eppendorf, 20246 Hamburg, Germany
* Correspondence: t.beikler@uke.de

Abstract: Innate immunity represents the semi-specific first line of defense and provides the initial host response to tissue injury, trauma, and pathogens. Innate immunity activates the adaptive immunity, and both act highly regulated together to establish and maintain tissue homeostasis. Any dysregulation of this interaction can result in chronic inflammation and autoimmunity and is thought to be a major underlying cause in the initiation and progression of highly prevalent immune-mediated inflammatory diseases (IMIDs) such as psoriasis, rheumatoid arthritis, inflammatory bowel diseases among others, and periodontitis. Th1 and Th2 cells of the adaptive immune system are the major players in the pathogenesis of IMIDs. In addition, Th17 cells, their key cytokine IL-17, and IL-23 seem to play pivotal roles. This review aims to provide an overview of the current knowledge about the differentiation of Th17 cells and the role of the IL-17/IL-23 axis in the pathogenesis of IMIDs. Moreover, it aims to review the association of these IMIDs with periodontitis and briefly discusses the therapeutic potential of agents that modulate the IL-17/IL-23 axis.

Keywords: periodontitis; psoriasis; rheumatoid arthritis; Crohn's disease; ulcerative colitis; systemic lupus erythematosus; Sjögren syndrome; type 1 diabetes mellitus; cytokines; Th17 cells; interleukin-17; interleukin-23

---

1. Introduction

Innate immunity represents the semi-specific first line of defense for all primitive and complex multicellular organisms and provides the initial acute inflammatory reaction to tissue injury, trauma, or pathogens [1]. Innate immunity is a rather unspecific and immediate reaction that recruits immune cells to the injury or infection site through various cytokines (e.g., prostaglandins, tumor necrosis factor (TNF), interleukin (IL)-1β, and others). Moreover, it promotes phagocytosis, and activates the complement and adaptive immune system [2]. In contrast to the innate immune system, the activation of the adaptive immune system results in an antigen specific host response that is mediated by T and B cells. It usually requires more time than the innate immune system to react since it turns progenitor cells into regulatory and effector cells with distinct functions, such as (i) self and non-self-antigen recognition, (ii) enhanced elimination of pathogens or infected cells, and (iii) development of immune memory [3].

The innate and adaptive immunity interaction represents a complex system. They are equally required to establish and maintain health and tissue homeostasis and both comprise cellular and humoral immunity components. Humoral immunity refers to antigen-specific antibody production to neutralize toxins and pathogens, mediation of allergic reactions and autoimmunity, generation of immune memory cells, and stimulation of cytokine secretion; whereas, cellular immunity eradicates pathogens by macrophages or natural killer cells, eliminates intracellular bacteria via induction of cytotoxic T-cell-mediated apoptosis, and stimulates tissue cells, such as fibroblasts, to secrete cytokines that further modulate innate and adaptive immune system responses [4]. The inflammation triggered by pathogens, tissue injury, or trauma is typically self-limiting and results in tissue repair and reestablishment of tissue homeostasis following elimination of the cause. However, an alteration of the regular immune response may result in persistence of the acute inflammation, its transition into chronic inflammation, and could even induce autoimmune reactions in susceptible individuals. This altered inflammatory response is believed to be a major underlying cause in the initiation and progression of disorders, such as immune-mediated inflammatory diseases (IMIDs) [5].

IMIDs are the definition of a group of seemingly unrelated diseases that share common inflammatory pathways and are triggered by or result in the dysregulation of innate and adaptive immune system functions [6]. The definitive etiology is still unclear; however, genetic susceptibility and environmental factors such as infection and trauma may initiate these conditions, that include, but are not limited to, psoriasis, rheumatoid arthritis, inflammatory bowel diseases, systemic lupus erythematosus, Sjögren syndrome, and type 1 diabetes [7,8]. Any organ system may be inflicted, and individuals may encounter a considerable reduction in quality of life, significant morbidity, and reduced lifespan [6].

Initiated and perpetuated by a dysbiotic oral microbiome, periodontitis is the most common inflammatory disease of tooth supporting tissues, with a high prevalence of up to 70% among the world's dentate adults [9,10]. The host immune and inflammatory responses disrupted by a dysbiotic microbiome are considered to be the main cause for the initiation, establishment, and progression of periodontal inflammation and tissue breakdown [11]. If left untreated, periodontitis results in progressive periodontal attachment and alveolar bone loss, which subsequently results in tooth loss. Co-existence of an IMID with another systemic inflammatory/autoimmune disease or periodontitis is not uncommon, e.g., 20–30% of patients with psoriasis will eventually develop psoriatic arthritis (PsA) [12]. Although the pathogenesis of IMIDs is not yet entirely understood and elucidated and a causative bidirectional relationship between IMIDs and periodontitis has not been proven yet, the comorbidities indicate the involvement of a dysbalanced inflammatory cytokine network in the disease processes [13–15].

As mentioned before, cytokines and antigen presentation attract and activate adaptive immune system cells. In this regard, $CD4^+$ helper T cells are pivotal players [16]. $CD4^+$ helper T cells differentiate into regulatory and effector T cell subsets i.e., Th1, Th2, Th17, follicular helper T (Tfh) cells, and regulatory T cells (Tregs), following activation. Until the discovery of other cell lineages, Th1 and Th2 were thought to be the only cells differentiating from progenitor $CD4^+$ helper T cells [17]. In this classical Th1/Th2 paradigm, Th1 cells mainly produce interleukin(IL)-2 and interferon gamma (IFN-γ) and are involved in cellular immunity [18]. Th2 cells are mainly responsible for humoral immunity via the activation of B cells, mast cells, and production of immunoglobulin E, and primarily produce IL-4, IL-5, and IL-13 [19]. The first findings that indicated the existence of a novel effector population of $CD4^+$ helper T cells were provided by an animal model of multiple sclerosis (experimental autoimmune encephalitis, EAE) [20]. According to the Th1/Th2 paradigm, it was initially hypothesized that IL-12 and, hence, Th1 cells and IFNγ were playing the central role in this inflammatory disease; however, it was demonstrated that functional Th1 pathways downregulate the onset and progression of EAE in IFNγ- and IL-12-deficient mice [21–23]. Later it was demonstrated that indeed IL-23, and not IL-12, was involved in the EAE pathogenesis [24]. This was further substantiated when the transfer of IL-17 producing T cells to healthy mice was sufficient to induce EAE [25]. In addition, IL-23-deficient animals were shown to be unable to recruit IL-17 producing T cells [26]. These and other studies led to the identification of a novel $CD4^+$ helper T cell subset named T helper 17 (Th17) cell lineage that was characterized by IL-17 production, a cytokine that Th1 and Th2 are not able to produce [17,27].

The Th1/Th2 paradigm provided a framework for understanding the pathogenesis of several conditions, such as psoriasis, rheumatoid arthritis, inflammatory bowel diseases, and periodontitis. However, the identification of Th17 cells as a distinct lineage of $CD4^+$ helper T cells has greatly expanded the understanding of autoimmunity and inflammation and filled in some of the missing gaps in host immunity that could not be fully explained by the Th1/Th2. Although there is still much to be elucidated, this review aims to provide an overview of the current knowledge about the Th17 cell lineage, the role of its key cytokine IL-17, the IL-17/IL-23 axis in health and disease, and strategies that target IL-17 related pathways. Understanding the similar mechanisms that drive the pathogenesis of these diseases will support an interdisciplinary approach between medical doctors and dentists, and thus allow proper screening, prevention, and early treatment.

2. Differentiation and Regulation of Th17 Cells

The polarization of progenitor $CD4^+$ helper T cells involves specific signal transduction mechanisms, distinct transcription factors, and local cytokine profiles for each T helper cell lineage (Figure 1). For instance, the differentiation of IFNγ producing Th1 cells is induced by IL-12 (a heterodimer consisting of a p35 and a p40 subunit) and by activation of the transcription factor STAT4 (Figure 1d) [28]. Also, IFNγ stimulates STAT1 and T-bet (a downstream transcription factor) expression in $CD4^+$ helper T cells, which in turn upregulates Th1 specific gene expression (Figure 1a) [28]. Th2 cell differentiation is, however, mainly driven by IL-4. IL-4 increases STAT6 and GATA-3 expression; thus, upregulates of Th2 differentiation (Figure 1b) [29]. The differentiation of Th1 and Th2 is mutually antagonistic, primarily due to the antagonism of IFNγ and IL-4 on molecular and cellular levels [30].

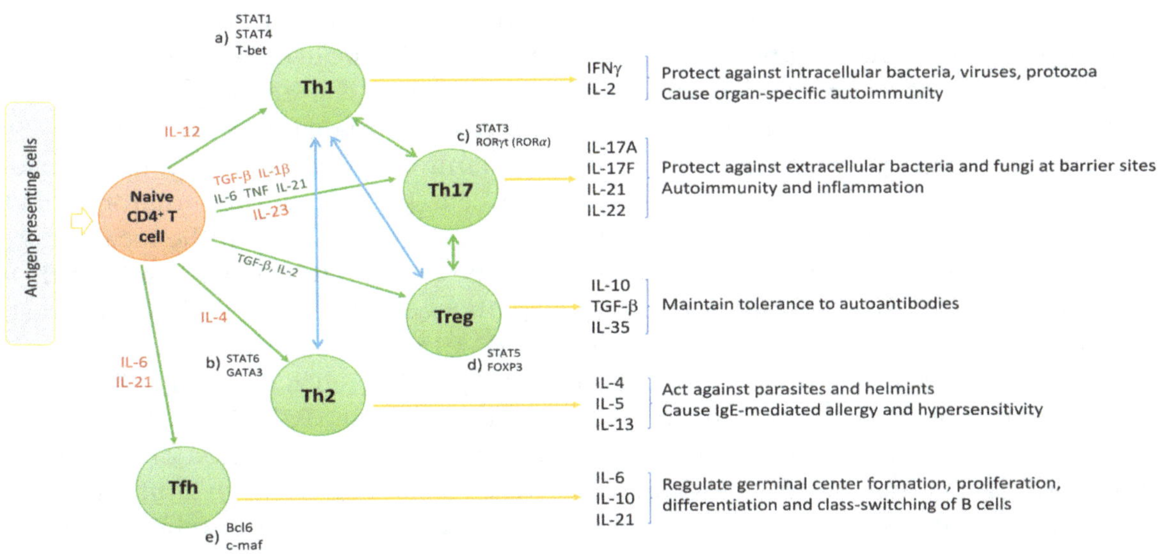

Figure 1. Differentiation of naïve $CD4^+$ cells into Th1, Th2, Th17, regulatory T cells (Treg), and follicular helper T (Tfh) cells. IL-12 leads to Th1-, IL-4 leads to Th2-, TGFβ leads to Treg-differentiation. Th17 cells differentiation is initiated by IL-1β, TGFβ, and further stimulated by TNF, IL-6, and IL-21; Th17 cells are maintained and expanded by IL-23. The transcription factors that governs Th cell subset differentiation are different, (**a**) STAT1, STAT4, and T-bet drive Th1; (**b**) STAT6 and GATA3 drive Th2; (**c**) STAT3 and RORγt (RORα, in the absence of RORγt) manage Th17 cell; (**d**) FOXP3 and STAT5 govern Treg cell differentiation; and (**e**) Bcl6 and c-maf are the regulators of Tfh cells differentiation.

Distinct from the differentiation of Th1 and Th2 cell lineages, Th17 cell differentiation is induced by STAT3 and retinoid acid related-orphan nuclear receptor γt (RORγt) that work synergistically with one another (Figure 1c) [31]. Similar to Th1/Th2 cell interaction, Tregs and Th17 cells are also maintained in an equilibrium. The transcription factor forkhead box P3 (FOXP3) is the negative regulator of RORγt and maintains the tolerance of the organism to self-antigens by inducing the differentiation of Tregs via STAT6 and downregulating differentiation of Th17 cells (Figure 1d) [32]. However, the Treg/Th17 balance is shifted in favor of Th17 in the presence of proinflammatory cytokines. In this regard, transforming growth factor beta (TGFβ) independently initiates the differentiation of Tregs from naïve $CD4^+$ helper T cells by activating FOXP3; whereas, it induces the differentiation of Th17 cells in the presence of IL-6 in mice and IL-1β in humans (Figure 1c,d) [33,34]. Exposure to TGFβ/IL-1β and IL-6 results in inhibition of FOXP3 and activation of RORγt, thus initiating the differentiation cascade of Th17 cells [35]. Furthermore, TNF and IL-1β can synergistically increase IL-6 production and contribute to further Th17 cell differentiation [36]. Following activation, RORγt promotes the expression of IL-17 and IL-23 receptor (IL-23R) [37]. In the absence of RORγt, RORα has been shown to stimulate IL-17 expression [38]. IL-23 is produced by antigen-presenting cells, such as dendritic cells and monocytes/macrophages upon activation and initiates signaling by binding to IL-23R, which in return increases the expression of RORγt and IL-17 via STAT3 (Figures 1c and 2) [39]. However, IL-23 is not able to induce Th17 cell development from naïve CD4+ helper T cells alone by itself, because IL-23R is expressed only after the differentiation of a naïve $CD4^+$ helper T cell into a Th17 cell is initiated [17]. This suggests that the role of IL-23 is rather to be seen in the maintenance, expansion, and survival of Th17 cells than in the initiation of their differentiation. IL-23 is able to maintain and expand Th17 cell populations through a positive feedback loop that upregulates IL-17, RORγt, along with TNF, IL-1β, and IL-6 [40]. In addition, IL-21 was also demonstrated to amplify Th17 cell differentiation in cooperation with TGFβ in an IL-6-independent manner through its feedback function on developing Th17 cells [31,41].

Some other general transcription factors, such as basic leucine zipper transcription factor ATF-like (BATF) and interferon regulatory factor 4 (IRF4), are also involved in the differentiation of naïve CD4+ helper T cells [42,43]. As such, IRF4 deficient mice were shown to have decreased levels of RORγt and increased levels of FOXP3 [44]. These non-nuclear transcription factors are, however, broadly expressed in both health and disease. Therefore, STAT3-induced RORγt is suggested to be the key transcriptional factor involved in Th17 differentiation. This was also supported by the finding that RORγt ($Rorc^{-/-}$) deficient CD4+ helper T cells failed to differentiate into Th17 [45].

Th17 cells are typically involved in vigorous proinflammatory responses, yet they also remain in the tissues, such as skin and mucosas as quiescent cells [46]. The inflammatory functions of Th17 cells depends on the different combinations of expressed cytokines in the local environment. For instance, Th17 cells were demonstrated to produce the anti-inflammatory cytokine IL-10 when stimulated with IFNα/β, thus downregulating their pathogenic functions [47]. In contrast to that, IL-23 was shown to reduce the expression levels of IL-10 in developing Th17 cells and induce pro-inflammatory Th17 cells that produce IL-17 [48]. Moreover, different subsets of TGF have also been demonstrated to induce distinct functions in Th17 cells. For instance, TGFβ1-and-IL-6-induced Th17 cells were unable to cause EAE in the absence of IL-23, whereas TGFβ3-induced Th17 cells presented highly pathogenic functions [49]. Moreover, Th-cells, especially Th17 cells, exhibit high phenotypic and functional plasticity, which means that they can transdifferentiate into other T cell subsets in different inflammatory settings [50]. As mentioned, the involvement of IL-6 during early stages of TGFβ-induced Treg differentiation can convert Treg cells into pathogenic Th17 cells [51]. Mature Th17 cells can furthermore be transformed by IL-6 into IFNγ producing Th1 cells [52]. In conclusion, differentiation and regulation of Th17 cells is mediated by a complex cytokine and transcription factor network, which may result in both pathologic and non-pathologic effector functions in inflammatory and autoimmune diseases.

3. Th17/IL-17 in Immunoprotection and Immunopathology

IL-17 is the key cytokine produced by Th17 cells and exerts versatile functions. The IL-17 receptor (IL-17R) lacks a homologous structure to other proteins; therefore, IL-17 cytokines are classified as a distinct family [53]. The IL-17 family consists of six ligands, IL-17A to IL-17F, that share similar structures and can exist as homodimers or form heterodimers, such as IL17A/F. IL-17A and IL-17F (henceforth referred to as IL-17) are produced by Th17 cells. They present 50% of structural homology and their intracellular signal transduction is dependent on the presence of the receptor heterodimer complex formed by the subunits IL-17 receptor A (IL-17RA) and IL-17 receptor C (IL-17RC) [54]. IL-17 receptor is expressed on a broad range of cells, including osteoblasts, endothelial cells, epithelial cells, fibroblast-like synoviocytes, chrondrocytes, fibroblasts, keratinocytes, and macrophages (Figure 2) [40,55–57]. Although IL-17 is predominantly produced by Th17 cells, it can also be expressed by natural killer T (NKT) cells, γδ T cells, lymphoid tissue inducer cells, neutrophils, and group 3 innate lymphoid cells (ILC3s) (Figure 2) [58,59]. Moreover, Th17 cells not only produce IL-17, but also IL-21, IL-22, IFNγ, and TNF and can express CCR6, i.e., the receptor of chemokine (C-C motif) ligand 20 (CCL20) that directs IL-17 producing cells to the epithelial barrier sites [60]. IL-17-producing cells accumulate at mucosal surfaces of the oral cavity, gastrointestinal tract, lungs, vagina, and skin epithelium, and regulate protective immunity against extracellular pathogens (especially Gram-negative bacteria and fungi) by maintaining barrier integrity, promoting antimicrobial factors, and activating granulopoiesis [31,59]. Furthermore, the Th17-cytokine IL-22 was shown to contribute to IL-17-induced protective functions by enhancing the production of antimicrobial peptides and recruiting neutrophils [61]. Therefore, the disruption of IL-17 production or signaling can increase the susceptibility to bacterial and fungal infections. In this context, IL-17 receptor deficiency is associated with mortality in mice due to the inability to recruit neutrophils when being infected with *Klebsiella pneumoniae* [62]. Moreover, genetic defects in IL-17 immunity, such as in STAT3 (manifested as hyper-IgE syndrome), result in recurrent and persistent Candida spp. infections; e.g., chronic mucocutaneous candidiasis [63]. Direct IL-17 inhibition with monoclonal antibodies in patients with psoriasis or psoriatic arthritis has been shown to increase the risk of candida infections; similarly, the reactivation of latent tuberculosis infection was observed in patients treated with TNF-inhibitors [64,65]. Th17 cells are also regularly maintained in the gingival tissues, suggesting a protective role in the oral barrier; however, the mechanism that maintains these cells in the tissue is yet to be clarified [66]. Interestingly, IL-17R lacking mice are shown to be more susceptible to *Porphyromonas gingivalis (Pg)*-induced bone loss, suggesting a protective role of IL-17 in bone remodeling and homeostasis [67]. Although IL-17 may exert protective functions, several clinical human studies indicate that excessive production of IL-17 is associated with periodontitis, as well as psoriasis, rheumatoid arthritis, and other IMIDs [52,68].

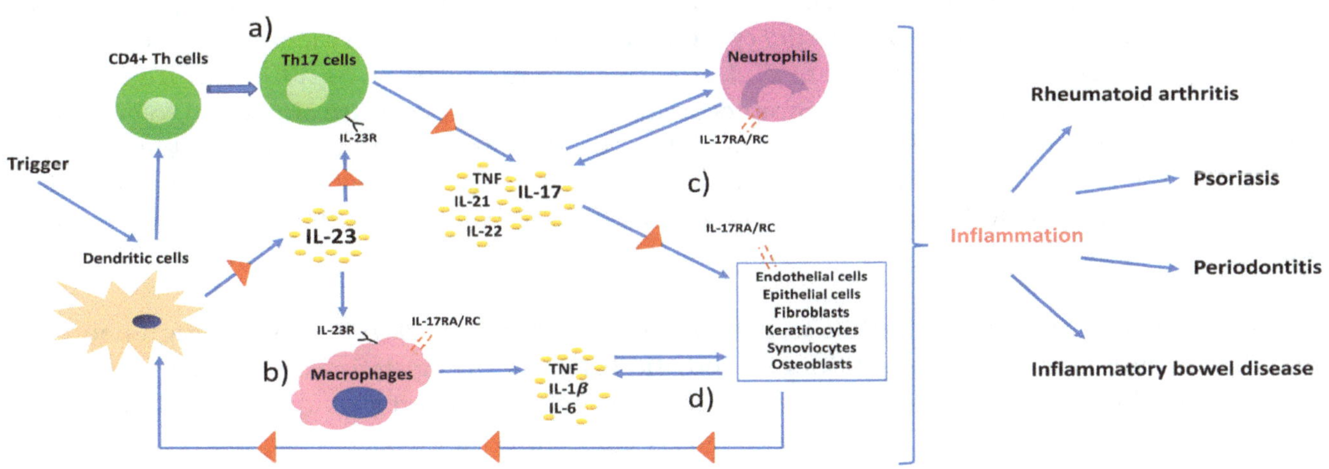

Figure 2. A pathophysiology model of immune-mediated inflammatory diseases. Dendritic cells (DCs) are triggered by a stimulus, such as environmental stress or infection, present the antigen that leads to differentiation of CD4$^+$ helper T cells, and release IL-23. IL-23 stimulates the production of proinflammatory cytokines, such as TNF, IL-1β, and IL-17 from (**a**) Th17 cells, and IL-6 from (**b**) macrophages and DCs. (**c**) IL-17 interacts with IL-17RA/RC complex on receptor carrying cells. These cells further produce inflammatory mediators that regulate functionality of DCs and create a self-sustaining feedback loop via IL-23 (**d**).

IL-17 by itself is a weak inducer of inflammation; its potent inflammatory effects are derived from its synergistic functions with other cytokines and its ability to recruit and maintain inflammatory cells, such as neutrophils. Moreover, IL-17 eases the access of these cells to tissues through regulating the expression of chemokine (C-X-C motif) ligands (CXCL1, CXCL2, CXCL5, CXCL8), CCL20, IL-1β, MMPs, PGE2, and granulocyte- and granulocyte-macrophage colony-stimulating factors (G-CSF and GM-CSF) [51,59]. GM-CSF and G-CSF are the primary regulators of granulopoiesis and neutrophil release from the bone marrow. Its upregulation by IL-17 can lead to excessive activation and mobilization of neutrophils and production of chemokines that increase neutrophil diapedesis, which in return intensifies tissue damage. In addition to that, IL-17 works synergistically with other inflammatory cytokines, such as IL-1β, to increase CCL20 production from human gingival fibroblasts and stimulates further recruitment of Th17 cells; hence, IL-17 production [52]. Typically, neutrophils are found in inflamed periodontal tissues, but infiltration of activated Th17 cells can also be observed in inflamed sites [69,70]. This explains the upregulation of IL-17 in gingival crevicular fluid, bone, and gingiva of periodontitis patients [71–73]. In addition to the locally increased production of IL-17, the serum levels of IL-17 were also detected to be up to nine-fold higher in periodontitis patients compared to healthy controls [74]. Moreover, RORγt encoding gene (*Rorc*) expression levels were reported to be significantly higher in periodontal tissues of patients with periodontitis compared to healthy controls [75]. At last, the presence of T cell populations that can produce IL-17 in both, health and disease, demonstrates the versatile role of this cytokine.

3.1. IL-17 Dependent Processes in Psoriasis and Association with Periodontitis

Characterized by abnormal and rapid keratinocyte differentiation and thickened epidermis, psoriasis is an immune-mediated inflammatory skin disorder that affects 0.1–3% of the general population [76]. Although psoriasis is manifested in 90% of the cases in a skin plaque form called "psoriasis vulgaris", it can also manifest itself in guttate, pustular, and erythrodermic subtypes, as well as in psoriatic arthritis [77,78]. Psoriasis is also associated with other systemic conditions such as hypertension, atherosclerosis, and diabetes [79,80]. The definitive etiology of psoriatic diseases is not clear yet; however, genetic, epigenetic, and environmental factors seem to contribute to the atypical activation of the innate and adaptive immune system resulting in disease onset, progression, and comorbidities [81,82]. Streptococcal peptidoglycan was also suggested to be involved in the pathogenesis of psoriasis; however, whether the skin microbiota is significant as a primary cause or a contributing factor remains to be elucidated [83]. Psoriasis has been primarily considered a Th1-mediated disease, today it is known that the IL-23/IL-17 axis governs the accelerated progress of inflammation [84,85].

Briefly, IL-17 attracts neutrophils to the epidermis of psoriatic skin lesions through neutrophil chemoattractants and recruits additional dendritic cells via upregulation of CCL20 release from keratinocytes (Figure 3a). The dendritic cells release TNF and IL-1β and activate further differentiation of Th17 cells, and thus increased IL-17 production. IL-17 disrupts the integrity of the skin barrier through downregulation of filaggrin and adhesion molecule expression from keratinocytes, and further induces keratinocyte hyperproliferation (Figure 3a) [86]. The disease severity correlates with the numbers of IL-17 producing T cells in psoriatic lesions and their ability to increase keratinocyte proliferation and IL-17 production [87,88]. In addition, IL-22 aggravates psoriasis lesions in synergy with IL-17, although it exerts protective functions in non-psoriatic skin (Figure 3a) [89]. Also, the expression of RORγt, IL-1β, IL-6, and IL-23 was reported to be increased in psoriatic skin lesions compared to the non-psoriatic skin of patients and healthy volunteers; whereas the levels of anti-inflammatory cytokines, i.e., IL-4 and IL-10, were found to be decreased [14,86]. Besides the local changes TNF, IFNγ, IL-2, IL-17, and IL-22 levels were found to be increased in serum of psoriasis patients [14]. Increased levels of TNF, IL-1β, and IL-22 augment the inflammatory effects of IL-17 by enhancing the expression of TNF receptors, suggesting a synergistic interplay between these cytokines in psoriasis pathogenesis [90].

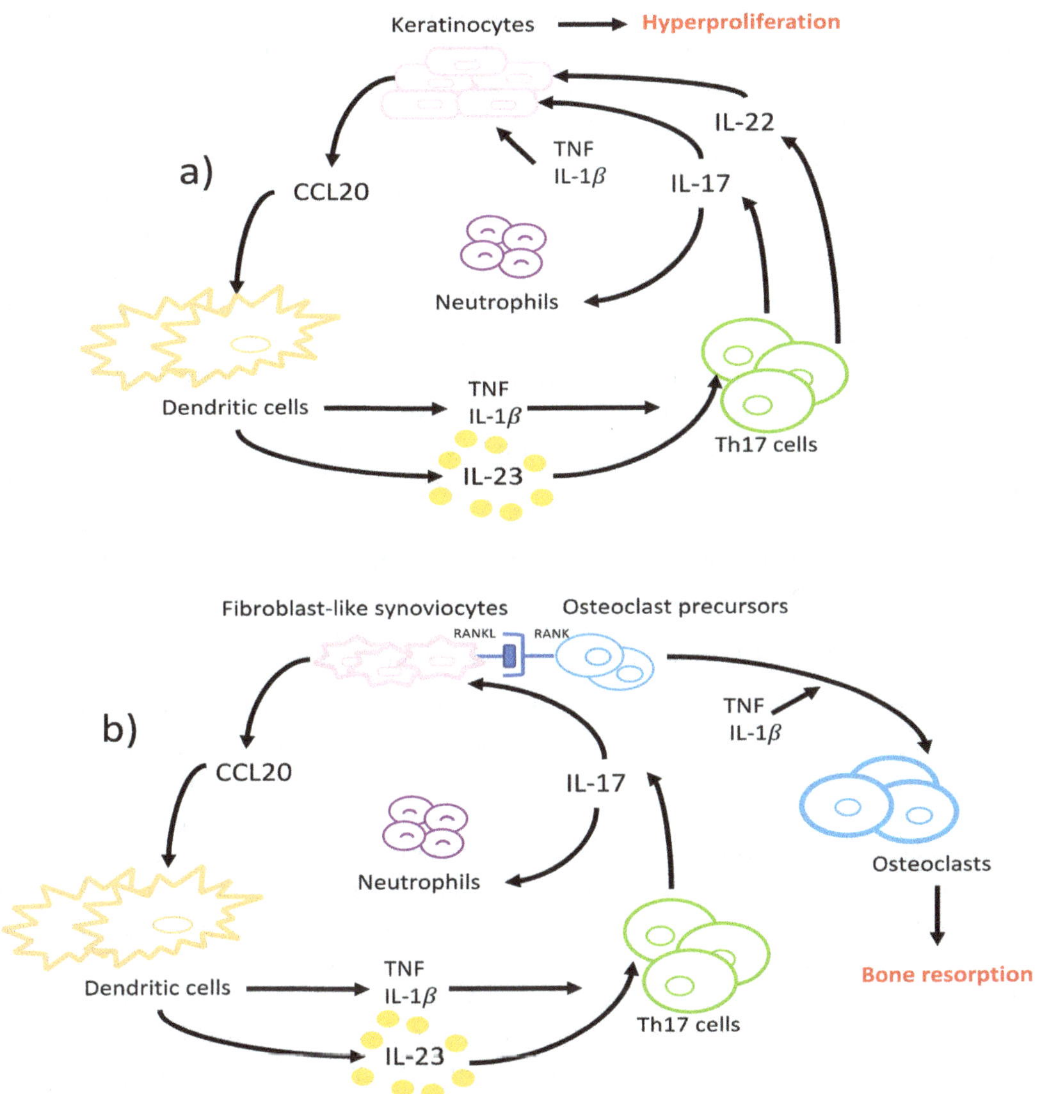

Figure 3. A simplified model of Th17 cells and the cytokines involved in the pathogenesis of (**a**) psoriasis and (**b**) rheumatoid arthritis. This figure can also be interpreted as a model of pathogenesis of gingival, periodontal, and oral mucosal inflammatory diseases, where cells such as gingival fibroblasts, keratinocytes, and epithelial cells are involved.

The role of a dysbiotic skin microbiota is controversially discussed in the pathogenesis of psoriasis. In periodontitis, however, a dysbiotic oral microbiome is known to contribute to the disease onset and progression [11]. Interestingly, it has recently been suggested that IL-17 creates a shift towards a highly pathologic bacterial environment, hence aggravating the periodontal inflammation like a vicious circle [91]. In addition, IL-23-dependent IL-17 production led to bacterial overgrowth, as demonstrated in leukocyte adhesion deficient (LAD) I periodontal phenotype mice and its inhibition reduced the bacterial overgrowth, which linked overexpression of IL-17 to microbial dysbiosis in periodontitis [92]. LAD1 is an immunodeficiency caused by a genetic mutation that results in defective neutrophil adhesion and tissue transmigration and is characterized by recurrent skin infections, oral ulcers, severe periodontal inflammation, and bone loss [93]. Although severe periodontitis in LAD1 was solely attributed to the lack of neutrophil surveillance in gingival and periodontal tissues, recent findings demonstrate that the excessive inflammatory response, mediated by IL-17, contributes to its manifestation [93,94].

Many retrospective and case-control studies have reported an association between psoriatic diseases, mainly psoriasis vulgaris and psoriatic arthritis, and periodontal disease [95–97]. A large

5-year follow-up cohort study indicated that in psoriasis patients (psoriasis subtypes not specified), chronic periodontitis showed an incidence rate of 1.88 per 1000 patient-years compared to 1.22 in the control group [98]. In accordance with these results, a longitudinal cohort study conducted in the Danish population retrospectively screened more than 5 million subjects to assess the risk for the development of periodontitis after the diagnosis of mild and severe psoriasis, and/or psoriatic arthritis [99]. Following adjustment for age, sex, co-morbidities, and smoking, the results demonstrated an increased risk for periodontitis among patients with psoriatic diseases, with the highest risk found in patients with psoriatic arthritis (risk ratio of 1.66, 2.24 and 3.48 for mild psoriasis, severe psoriasis and psoriatic arthritis, respectively). Moreover, the severity of periodontitis has been shown to be correlated with psoriasis severity [100]. Both diseases share common risk factors, i.e., smoking, obesity, and these risk factors can independently contribute to disease manifestation and severity. The risk for periodontitis was increased by six-fold in smoking psoriasis subjects compared to non-smoking psoriasis subjects [101]. Also, a significant correlation between periodontitis and psoriasis was reported after adjustment for smoking [102]. Although none of these studies could demonstrate a bidirectional causal relationship, regular periodontal screening seems to be reasonable in individuals with psoriatic diseases, since the risk for periodontitis is increased, especially in the presence of shared risk factors that negatively influence both diseases.

3.2. IL-17 Dependent Processes in Rheumatoid Arthritis and Association with Periodontitis

Rheumatoid arthritis (RA) is a chronic inflammatory and autoimmune disease of the joints, characterized by the presence of rheumatic factor and anti-citrullinated protein antibodies (ACPAs) and persistent symmetrical and erosive polyarthritis, which results in progressive articular bone and cartilage destruction [103]. The prevalence is 0.5–1% among adults, and women are affected two to three times more frequently than men [55]. The development of rheumatoid arthritis is also considered to be of genetic, epigenetic, and environmental origin [104]. HLA-DR1 and HLA-DR4-positive individuals are reported to be at significantly higher risk for manifesting ACPA-positive RA, although only about 67% of the rheumatoid arthritis patients are ACPA-positive in the early stages [105,106]. Synovitis, the inflammation of the synovial membrane in joints, causes the clinical signs and symptoms of RA. Similar to psoriasis, an interactive and complex network of immune system cells and cytokines are involved in RA pathogenesis. ACPA establishes an abnormal immune response over time that promotes inflammation, and the synovial membrane becomes highly vascularized and infiltrated with fibroblasts, macrophages, T- and B- cells, plasma cells, mast cells, dendritic cells, and neutrophils [107]. Increased TNF in the synovial fluid induces IL-1β production, T- and B-cell activation, and a cascade of inflammatory reactions that is mainly led by dendritic- and Th17-cells, that eventually leads to articular bone and cartilage destruction (Figure 3b) [57]. In the RA-affected synovium, IL-17, IL-1β, and TNF act together to induce the chemotaxis of T cells and immature dendritic cells. This results in an upregulated CCL20 production in synoviocytes and an overall increased concentration of proinflammatory cytokines in the synovial tissues [108]. The role of IL-17 in rheumatoid arthritis was clearly demonstrated when long-term intra-articular administration of IL-17 in mice resulted in rheumatoid arthritis key features like inflammation, articular bone, and cartilage destruction [109]. Furthermore, several animal models of rheumatoid arthritis reported a reduced incidence, severity, and even resistance to disease upon the induction of IL-17 deficiency [110–112].

In addition to the inflammatory effects of IL-17, the osteoclastogenic character of IL-17 puts it in the focus of interest in bone-destructing diseases. The information regarding the effects of IL-17 on bone metabolism mainly originates from studies conducted on rheumatoid arthritis; however, several studies also report its effects on periodontal bone destruction. As mentioned before, dendritic cells that are present in the synovial fluid increase the release of TNF, IL-1β, IL-6, and IL-23 and stimulate Th17-cell differentiation, and thus IL-17 production in rheumatoid arthritis joints [55]. IL-17 disturbs the bone homeostasis by inducing osteoclastogenesis, which results in extensive and rapid bone destruction [113]. This is initiated by the increase of the receptor activator of nuclear factor kappa-B ligand (RANKL) expression on fibroblasts and osteoblasts by IL-17. RANKL interacts with the receptor activator of nuclear factor kappa-B (RANK) on dendritic cells and osteoclasts and activates synovial macrophages to secrete IL-1β and TNF—both are known to induce osteoclastogenesis [114]. Similarly to the mechanism in RA, IL-17 induces RANKL expression by stimulating MMP-1, MMP-3, IL-6, and IL-8 secretion from human gingival fibroblasts and TNF release from macrophages in periodontal tissues [115]. IL-17 levels are shown to be positively correlated to RANKL expression levels in periodontal ligament cells [116,117]. Furthermore, upregulated TNF and IL-17 can synergistically lead to further stimulation of the fibroblasts and epithelial cells to secrete IL-6, IL-8, PGE2, and the neutrophil chemoattractants; thus, intensifying the inflammation [35]. Independently from IL-17, IL-22 was also demonstrated to increase synovial inflammation in rheumatoid arthritis joints and clinical attachment loss in periodontitis patients, similarly to its proinflammatory function in psoriasis [118–120].

The fact that periodontitis is reported to be twice as frequent and severe in rheumatoid arthritis patients compared to healthy controls indicates the correlated inflammatory processes in rheumatoid arthritis and periodontitis [121]. Accordingly, IL-17 levels were found to be increased in the gingival crevicular fluid of rheumatoid arthritis patients, further contributing to the inflammatory response in the gingival sulcus and the severity of periodontal inflammation [121,122]. Several links between rheumatoid arthritis and periodontitis have been suggested. One of the most striking ones is the citrullinated peptides production induced by *P. gingivalis*. Citrullinated peptides are considered to break tolerance and induce ACPA production in RA [123]. *P. gingivalis* is currently the only bacteria that is known to produce peptidyl arginine deiminase (PAD), an enzyme that leads to citrullination of the human and bacterial proteins [124]. In addition, the antibody titer against *P. gingivalis* was significantly increased in RA-patients, further supporting the role of this periodontal pathogen not only in periodontitis, but also in RA pathogenesis [125].

3.3. IL-17 Dependent Processes in Inflammatory Bowel Diseases and Association with Periodontitis

Inflammatory bowel diseases (IBD) are chronic inflammatory conditions of the gastrointestinal system and consist of ulcerative colitis (UC) and Crohn's disease (CD). Ulcerative colitis is characterized by the chronic mucosal inflammation of the colon that manifests itself with abdominal pain, haematochezia, and diarrhoea [126,127]. In Crohn's disease, however, any part of the gastrointestinal tract can be afflicted. This disease can typically be associated with extra-gastrointestinal symptoms such as anaemia, arthritis, skin rashes, oral lesions, and eye inflammations [128,129]. Although the etiology of IBDs remains largely unclear, a dysbiotic intestinal microbiome and risk factors, such as smoking and diet, were suggested to contribute to the disease onset via activation of inflammatory pathways that results in the disruption of the epithelial barrier integrity in genetically susceptible individuals [130]. The involvement of IL-23 and IL-17 in IBD is well documented; however, the different functions of IL-17 in IBD are still controversially discussed in the literature [131,132]. On the one hand, IL-17 deficient or anti-IL-17 treated mice exhibited severe epithelial damage in the colon, indicating a protective function of IL-17 [133]. This is further substantiated when inactivation of IL-17 resulted in a milder course of disease in an animal model of UC [134]. On the other hand, high IL-23 receptor and IL-17 mRNA expression levels were detected in intestinal mucosa samples of patients with active UC and CD [135,136]. Furthermore, many other studies reported increased levels of IL-17 in the intestinal mucosa and serum of active UC and CD patients [137,138].

Oral manifestations and implications of inflammatory bowel diseases are reported in a varying range from 0,5% to 37% among diseased individuals; they may appear as the first signs of the disease, especially in children, and include edema, mucogingivitis, oral ulcers, and hyperplastic lesions among others [139–141]. Involvement of upper regions of gastrointestinal tract and extra-gastrointestinal symptoms predict a more severe phenotype of the disease and may present with comorbidities due to the increased risk of systemic involvement [142]. Caries and periodontitis prevalence are reported to be often higher in individuals with CD and UC [143]. In a large nationwide cohort study, the prevalence of periodontitis was reported to be higher in patients with CD, with a hazard ratio of 1.36 (95% CI

= 1.25–1.48) compared to the control group [144]. Similarly, a meta-analysis of cross-sectional studies, including a total of 1297 subjects, reported a significantly higher prevalence of periodontitis as well as a worse decayed-missing-filled-teeth index in patients with CD and UC compared to non-IBD individuals [145]. Interestingly, worse clinical periodontal parameters were observed among smokers with UC compared to smokers with CD [143]. Unfortunately, studies regarding the effect of periodontal inflammation on CD or UC currently remain deficient [146].

3.4. IL-17 Dependent Processes in Other Immune-Mediated Inflammatory Diseases and Association with Periodontitis

IL-17 also plays an important role in the pathogenesis of other IMIDs, such as Sjögren syndrome, systemic lupus erythematosus, and type 1 diabetes, among others. Sjögren syndrome is an autoimmune disease characterized by diffuse lymphocyte infiltration into exocrine glands that results primarily in xerostomia and ocular dryness, known as "sicca symptoms" [147]. Extra-glandular tissues and organs, such as skin, lungs, nervous system, kidneys, and the gastrointestinal tract are also affected by Sjögren syndrome in at least 30% of patients, classifying it as a systemic disease [148]. Sjögren syndrome can appear independently of other conditions as a primary disease (primary Sjögren syndrome) or manifest itself secondarily as a late complication with sicca symptoms (secondary Sjögren syndrome) in the presence of other systemic conditions, such as rheumatoid arthritis, systemic lupus erythematosus, or scleroderma [149,150]. In Sjögren syndrome affected tissues, several subsets of B and T cells can be identified, predominantly consisting of CD4+ T helper cell subtypes, such as Th1, Th17, and Tfh cells [151]. The interaction between epithelial cells, dendritic cells, and B and T cells results in an increased production of Tfh and Th17 cells, which intensifies the inflammation and increases autoantibody production [152]. Tfh cells govern the ectopic germinal center formation in salivary glands and potentiate the production of autoantibodies from B cells, whereas Th17 cells secrete IL-17 and IL-22 and stimulate inflammation [153,154]. Increased levels of IL-17 in plasma of patients with primary Sjögren syndrome, as well as an abundant presence of IL-1β, TGF-β, IL-6, and IL-23 in tissues affected by the disease, demonstrate the significance of Th17 cells and IL-17 in the disease pathogenesis [155–157]. Non-surgical periodontal therapy was demonstrated to improve the salivary flow rate and decrease the subjective disease activity index in primary Sjögren syndrome patients with periodontitis [158]. However, despite this finding and common IL-17-dependent pathways in periodontitis and Sjögren syndrome, a significant association between both diseases remains to be confirmed [159,160].

Systemic lupus erythematosus (SLE) is a connective-tissue disorder characterized by T cell abnormalities and production of a wide array of autoantibodies directed against double-stranded (ds) DNA. It affects multiple tissues and organs, often causing glomerulonephritis, arthritis, and blood cell abnormalities [161]. The interaction of Th17 cells, Tfh cells, extrafollicular T helper cells (eTfh, a Tfh cell analogue $CD4^+$ subpopulation), Tregs, $CD8^+$ cells, B cell subsets, and innate immune system cells results in a reduced IL-2- and an increased IL-17-production, as well as increased antibody-production from B cells [161–163]. Since IL-17, IL-6, and IL-33 were found to be significantly elevated in the saliva of SLE/periodontitis subjects compared to periodontitis-only subjects, this systemic imbalance of cytokines may have an impact on periodontal tissues [164]. However, the long-term corticosteroid therapy may also have resulted in the observed periodontal damage [164]. In a nation-wide retrospective population-based study, the history of periodontitis was associated with an increased risk of SLE; however, the common risk factors, such as smoking status, were not adjusted [165]. Conversely, periodontal treatment in SLE/periodontitis subjects was reported to significantly improve the responsiveness of SLE patients to the immunosuppressive therapy compared to the control group [166].

The autoimmune destruction of insulin-producing β cells in the Langerhans islets of pancreas results in type 1 diabetes, which is characterized by an insufficient insulin production leading to persistent or recurrent hyperglycemia [167]. Often diagnosed in childhood, type 1 diabetes causes lifelong dependence on insulin, as well as an increased risk of cardiovascular disease, neuropathy, nephropathy, and other autoimmune and inflammatory conditions such as rheumatoid arthritis [168]. $CD4^+$ cells, especially Tregs, and CD8+ cells, autoantibody-producing B cells, and innate immune cells are involved in the disease pathogenesis [167]. IFNγ, produced by the infiltrated T cells, is a major cytokine involved in the destruction of the β cell islets; however, IL-17 was also demonstrated to play a role, when its neutralization prevented further disease development in 10-week old non-obese diabetic mice by reducing peri-islet T cell infiltration [169]. Also, increased secretion and expression of IL-17 and IL-22 were demonstrated to contribute to the disease development in type 1 diabetic children [170]. Impaired IL-2 functions that affect Treg functions lead to increased production of IL-17 and contributes to disease development in an animal model of type 1 diabetes [171]. Uncontrolled diabetes has been proven to be a predisposing risk factor for the onset and progression of periodontitis [172]. Conversely, the presence of periodontitis is suggested to affect the insulin metabolism by increasing the circulatory levels of proinflammatory cytokines [173]. Eventually, the treatment of periodontal disease has been shown to improve glycemic control, further substantiating the existing bidirectional relationship between diabetes and periodontal disease [174].

It is noteworthy to mention that the role of IL-17 has also been demonstrated in other IMIDs, such as ankylosing spondylitis, multiple sclerosis, Behcet disease, or scleroderma, in which aberrant immune and inflammatory responses also result in disease manifestation via similar mechanisms [175–178]. Unfortunately, conflicting data exists on the association of periodontitis and multiple sclerosis. In this regard, a large case control study found that no association between periodontitis and multiple sclerosis was seen between the groups after adjustment of covariates [179]. On the other hand, previous diagnosis of periodontitis was reported to be higher among female multiple sclerosis patients after adjustment of risk factors (odds ratio = 2.08; 95% CI, 1.49–2.95) [180]. In patients with scleroderma and periodontitis, a higher number of missing teeth and more clinical attachment loss were reported compared to patients with periodontitis only [181]. An association between Behcet disease severity and worse periodontal disease parameters (clinical attachment loss, bleeding on probing, and pocket probing depth) was also demonstrated in a cross-sectional study [182].

Based on the multiple interactions between genetic and environmental factors and aberrant immunological responses, multiple associations may exist between immune mediated inflammatory diseases and periodontitis. However, whether these association are causative and mutual needs to be further investigated. The findings of this research will expand the knowledge about the pathogenesis of IMIDs and periodontitis, and may help to improve the prevention, diagnosis, and the treatment of their systemic and oral complications.

4. Th17/IL-17 as Targets in the Management of IMIDs and Its Implications on Periodontal Inflammation

The treatment of immune-mediated inflammatory diseases is traditionally based on the use of glucocorticoids, non-steroidal anti-inflammatory drugs (NSAIDs), and disease-modifying antirheumatic drugs (DMARDs), such as methotrexate (MTX). They are proven to be effective against clinical signs and symptoms and are prescribed as the first-line therapy. However, intolerance, ineffectiveness, and severe adverse effects created the need for developing alternative therapies. Hence, in the early 1990s, monoclonal antibodies (mAbs) and fusion proteins, referred to as biologics or biological agents, were introduced. Biologics are a group of immunosuppressive drugs and are produced from a single clone of plasma B cells by modifying the Fc domain structures of its immunoglobulins. Initially, mAbs were only of murine origin and exhibited a reduced affinity due to the variability of the interaction of murine Fc with human Fc receptors, as well as caused the development of human anti-mouse antibodies [183–185]. To overcome these drawbacks, mAbs are nowadays bioengineered via recombinant techniques to produce chimeric, humanized, and fully human mAbs [186].

Biologics revolutionized the treatment of a wide range of immune-mediated inflammatory diseases, including but not limited to psoriasis, rheumatoid and psoriatic arthritis, ankylosing spondylitis, and inflammatory bowel diseases (Table 1). The first biologics that were introduced in the market were the TNF antagonists (Table 1). TNF antagonists act by inhibiting the binding of TNF to its receptor [186]. There are currently five TNF antagonists available, i.e., etanercept, infliximab, adalimumab, certolizumab, and golimumab. Besides others, TNF antagonists reduce IL-17 controlled inflammatory pathways (Figure 3a,b), and thus, slow down joint destruction in rheumatoid arthritis, reduce psoriatic lesions, as well as resolve chronic intestinal inflammation and ulcerations in IBD [183,187,188]. Etanercept, a TNF receptor-2 and IgG1-Fc fusion protein, reduces infiltration of polymorphonuclear cells into gingival tissues and improves periodontitis parameters in a murine model of experimental periodontitis [189]. In contrast to these anti-inflammatory functions, TNF antagonists interestingly can also cause the appearance of psoriasis-like lesions in 5–10% of treated patients, named as 'paradoxical psoriasis' [129,190]. Paradoxical psoriasis is suggested to be a side effect of all TNF antagonists, irrespective of the type and dosage, and usually disappears upon discontinuation [190,191]. In addition to paradoxical psoriasis, TNF inhibition was reported to increase susceptibility to bacterial infections [192]. The pharmacokinetic and pharmacodynamic properties differ among TNF antagonists as a result of their different molecular structures and mode of administration. Therefore, their effects show a considerable variability among individuals and diseases. Several reports indicate that in case of an ineffective response or intolerance to a specific TNF antagonist, the treatment can be continued with another TNF antagonist or replaced by a different biological drug, such as an IL-17 inhibitor [183,193]. It is noteworthy to mention that periodontitis is associated with an increased risk of etanercept discontinuation with an hazard ratio of 1.27 (95% CI, 1.01–1.60) in anti-TNF-naïve rheumatoid arthritis patients if they have been diagnosed with periodontitis within 5 years prior to or during etanercept treatment [194].

Table 1. Target cytokines involved in IL-17 pathways and approved inhibitors in the management of immune-mediated inflammatory diseases.

Targeted Cytokine	Drug	Indicated Conditions
TNF	Etanercept	Psoriasis, RA, PsA
	Infliximab	Psoriasis, RA, PsA, ankylosing spondylitis (AS), Crohn's disease (CD), ulcerative colitis
	Adalimumab	Psoriasis, RA, PsA, AS, CD, uveitis, hidradenitis suppurativa
	Certolizumab	Psoriasis, RA, PsA, AS, CD,
	Golimumab	RA, PsA, CD, ulcerative colitis, AS
IL-1	Anakinra	RA
IL-6	Tocilizumab	RA
IL-12/23	Ustenikumab	Psoriasis, PsA, CD
IL-23	Guselkumab	Psoriasis
	Tildrakizumab	Psoriasis
IL-17	Secukinumab (IL-17A)	Psoriasis, RA, PsA, CD, asthma, AS, uveitis, multiple sclerosis
	Ixekizumab (IL-17A)	Psoriasis, RA
	Brodalumab (IL-17RA)	Psoriasis, PsA, RA, Crohn's disease, asthma

Due to the synergistic effects of IL-17 and TNF in inflammation, diseases that are treated with TNF antagonists can also be managed with mAbs that target IL-17 or the IL-23/IL-17 axis [195]. Moreover, the inhibition of both TNF and IL-17 was shown to be more effective compared to TNF or IL-17 inhibition alone [196]. The first introduced anti-IL-17 drug was secukinumab, a human IgG1k monoclonal antibody, which acts by binding directly to IL-17A and inhibits its action (Figure 4b). Ixekizumab is a slightly different antibody that is developed from IgG4k, with affinity only to the IL-17A homodimer and IL-17A/F heterodimer of the IL-17 family (Figure 4c). Similarly to secukinumab, ixekizumab inhibits the IL-17 action by binding directly to this cytokine. Brodalumab, a human IgG2k mAb and the first anti-IL-17 receptor agent, inhibits the action of IL-17 by binding to the IL-17 receptor (Figure 4a) [197]. Phase II and III clinical studies proved IL-17 inhibitors as safe and efficient for the treatment of psoriasis, rheumatoid arthritis, and inflammatory bowel disease [198–201]. In psoriasis, however, the efficacy of ixekizumab was shown to be significantly superior when compared to etanercept and ustenikumab (IL-12/23 mAb) [202,203].

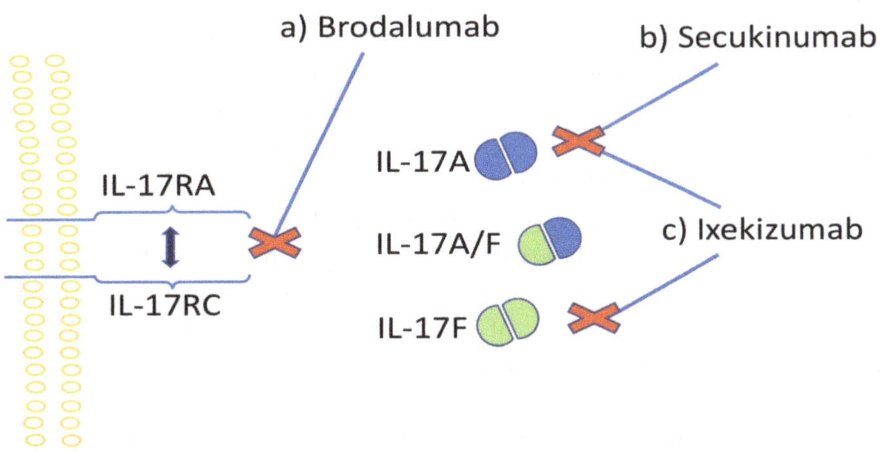

Figure 4. IL-17 cytokine inhibitors; (**a**) brodalumab, with affinity to IL-17RA/RC receptor complex, (**b**) secukinumab, with affinity to IL-17A, and (**c**) ixekizumab, with affinity to both IL-17A and IL-17F, interrupt the intracellular signaling by inhibiting the interaction between IL-17 and its receptor.

Comparative reviews on anti-IL-17 drugs reported that all three drugs were well-tolerated in patients with moderate-to-severe psoriasis; however, adverse effects, such as respiratory tract infections, were reported more frequently for ixekizumab, and it was withdrawn in some cases due to its toxicity [204,205]. A meta-analysis on efficacy of anti-IL-17 drugs on rheumatoid arthritis showed that secukinumab and ixekizumab were more effective compared to placebo; however, an increased risk of infection in the test group has also been reported [206]. Low levels of IL-17 in the synovium, heterogeneity in expression patterns of IL-17 and its receptors were shown to reduce anti-IL-17 drug effect in animal model studies, which could be the explanation to the insufficient efficacy in some patients [207].

Since the maintenance and expansion of Th17 cells are IL-23-dependent, the inhibition of IL-23 can also reduce IL-17 production and accomplish a clinical improvement. Ustekinumab is a human IgG1k monoclonal antibody that binds to the p-40 subunits of both IL-23 and IL-12 and interferes with the binding to their receptors. Long-term, multicenter, placebo-controlled phase III studies demonstrate the safety, efficacy, and superiority of ustekinumab to etanercept in patients with moderate to severe psoriasis [208–210]. However, an increased risk for neoplasia during IL-12/23 inhibitor use was reported in animal studies, which was attributed to IL-12 involvement in tumor surveillance [211,212]. Ustenikumab has also been demonstrated to reduce inflammatory responses in a patient with leukocyte adhesion deficiency type 1 (LAD1) periodontitis without serious adverse effects already after 3 weeks of treatment [213]. In addition to IL-12/IL-23 inhibitors, drugs such as guselkumab and tildrakizumab were developed to target the unique p19 subunit of IL-23 (Figure 1d,e). As expected, Th17-cell infiltration was decreased in psoriasis patients while anti-inflammatory IL-10 expression from Th1-cells was increased following the administration of IL-23 inhibitors [214,215].

As mentioned before, an increased risk of infections, especially by *Candida* spp., is often reported among patients that use these biologics over a prolonged time. Nevertheless, it is noteworthy to mention that overexpression of inflammatory cytokines may also increase infection risk, as periodontal pathogens were suggested to thrive in a highly proinflammatory cytokine environment [59].

5. Conclusions

IL-17 plays an important role in inflammatory events that lead to the manifestation of psoriasis, rheumatoid arthritis, inflammatory bowel disease, and periodontitis. Although much remains to be clarified regarding its protective and pathologic functions, the current knowledge suggests its role as a potent proinflammatory mediator and bridge between innate and adaptive immune responses. Comorbid periodontitis is often observed in patients diagnosed with an immune-mediated inflammatory disease. Although a bidirectional causal relationship is yet to be confirmed, regular screenings, preventive measures, and early treatment could reduce the burden of periodontitis in these patients, and vice versa. Many clinical randomized controlled trials prove the efficacy of cytokine inhibitors that manipulate IL-17 and related pathways in the management of psoriasis, rheumatoid arthritis, and inflammatory bowel disease. Unfortunately, reports regarding the therapeutic effects of cytokine inhibitors on gingival, periodontal, and oral mucocutaneous diseases are scant, which could be due to their restricted indication for severe systemic conditions, high costs, and adverse effects. However, further clinical research on the effects of biologics on gingival, periodontal, and oral tissues is needed to further elucidate the role of Th17-cells and the IL-23/IL-17 axis in the pathogenesis of periodontitis and its potential association with IMIDs.

Author Contributions: Conceptualization and resources, K.B. and T.B.; Investigation, K.B.; Writing—Original Draft Preparation, Review and Editing, K.B.; Writing—Review and Editing, T.B.

Acknowledgments: This research did not receive any specific grant from funding agencies in the public, commercial, or not-for-profit sectors.

References

1. Riera Romo, M.; Perez-Martinez, D.; Castillo Ferrer, C. Innate immunity in vertebrates: An overview. *Immunology* **2016**, *148*, 125–139. [CrossRef] [PubMed]
2. Rubartelli, A.; Lotze, M.T. Inside, outside, upside down: Damage-associated molecular-pattern molecules (DAMPs) and redox. *Trends Immunol.* **2007**, *28*, 429–436. [CrossRef] [PubMed]
3. Janeway, C.A., Jr. How the immune system works to protect the host from infection: A personal view. *Proc. Natl. Acad. Sci. USA* **2001**, *98*, 7461–7468. [CrossRef] [PubMed]
4. Nicholson, L.B. The immune system. *Essays Biochem.* **2016**, *60*, 275–301. [CrossRef] [PubMed]
5. Feghali, C.A.; Wright, T.M. Cytokines in acute and chronic inflammation. *Front. Biosci.* **1997**, *2*, d12–d26. [PubMed]
6. Kuek, A.; Hazleman, B.L.; Ostor, A.J. Immune-mediated inflammatory diseases (IMIDs) and biologic therapy: A medical revolution. *Postgrad. Med. J.* **2007**, *83*, 251–260. [CrossRef] [PubMed]
7. Martin, J.C.; Baeten, D.L.; Josien, R. Emerging role of IL-17 and Th17 cells in systemic lupus erythematosus. *Clin. Immunol.* **2014**, *154*, 1–12. [CrossRef]
8. McGinley, A.M.; Edwards, S.C.; Raverdeau, M.; Mills, K.H.G. Th17cells, gammadelta T cells and their interplay in EAE and multiple sclerosis. *J. Autoimmun.* **2018**, *87*, 97–108. [CrossRef]
9. Beikler, T.; Flemmig, T.F. Oral biofilm-associated diseases: Trends and implications for quality of life, systemic health and expenditures. *Periodontology* **2011**, *55*, 87–103. [CrossRef]
10. Demmer, R.T.; Papapanou, P.N. Epidemiologic patterns of chronic and aggressive periodontitis. *Periodontology* **2010**, *53*, 28–44. [CrossRef]
11. Cekici, A.; Kantarci, A.; Hasturk, H.; Van Dyke, T.E. Inflammatory and immune pathways in the pathogenesis of periodontal disease. *Periodontology* **2014**, *64*, 57–80. [CrossRef] [PubMed]
12. Krueger, J.G.; Bowcock, A. Psoriasis pathophysiology: Current concepts of pathogenesis. *Ann. Rheum. Dis.* **2005**, *64*, ii30–ii36. [CrossRef] [PubMed]
13. Wu, J.J.; Nguyen, T.U.; Poon, K.Y.; Herrinton, L.J. The association of psoriasis with autoimmune diseases. *J. Am. Acad. Derm.* **2012**, *67*, 924–930. [CrossRef] [PubMed]

14. Tan, Y.; Qi, Q.; Lu, C.; Niu, X.; Bai, Y.; Jiang, C.; Wang, Y.; Zhou, Y.; Lu, A.; Xiao, C. Cytokine Imbalance as a Common Mechanism in Both Psoriasis and Rheumatoid Arthritis. *Mediat. Inflamm.* **2017**, *2017*, 2405291. [CrossRef] [PubMed]
15. Thilagar, S.; Theyagarajan, R.; Sudhakar, U.; Suresh, S.; Saketharaman, P.; Ahamed, N. Comparison of serum tumor necrosis factor-alpha levels in rheumatoid arthritis individuals with and without chronic periodontitis: A biochemical study. *J. Indian Soc. Periodontol.* **2018**, *22*, 116–121. [CrossRef]
16. Hirahara, K.; Nakayama, T. CD4+ T-cell subsets in inflammatory diseases: Beyond the Th1/Th2 paradigm. *Int. Immunol.* **2016**, *28*, 163–171. [CrossRef]
17. Zhu, J.; Yamane, H.; Paul, W.E. Differentiation of effector CD4 T cell populations. *Annu. Rev. Immunol.* **2010**, *28*, 445–489. [CrossRef]
18. Romagnani, S. T-cell subsets (Th1 versus Th2). *Ann. Allergy Asthma Immunol.* **2000**, *85*, 9–18. [CrossRef]
19. Romagnani, S. Th1/Th2 cells. *Inflamm. Bowel Dis.* **1999**, *5*, 285–294. [CrossRef]
20. Cua, D.J.; Sherlock, J.; Chen, Y.; Murphy, C.A.; Joyce, B.; Seymour, B.; Lucian, L.; To, W.; Kwan, S.; Churakova, T.; et al. Interleukin-23 rather than interleukin-12 is the critical cytokine for autoimmune inflammation of the brain. *Nature* **2003**, *421*, 744–748. [CrossRef]
21. Chu, C.Q.; Wittmer, S.; Dalton, D.K. Failure to suppress the expansion of the activated CD4 T cell population in interferon gamma-deficient mice leads to exacerbation of experimental autoimmune encephalomyelitis. *J. Exp. Med.* **2000**, *192*, 123–128. [CrossRef] [PubMed]
22. Ferber, I.A.; Brocke, S.; Taylor-Edwards, C.; Ridgway, W.; Dinisco, C.; Steinman, L.; Dalton, D.; Fathman, C.G. Mice with a disrupted IFN-gamma gene are susceptible to the induction of experimental autoimmune encephalomyelitis (EAE). *J. Immunol.* **1996**, *156*, 5–7. [PubMed]
23. Zhang, G.X.; Gran, B.; Yu, S.; Li, J.; Siglienti, I.; Chen, X.; Kamoun, M.; Rostami, A. Induction of experimental autoimmune encephalomyelitis in IL-12 receptor-beta 2-deficient mice: IL-12 responsiveness is not required in the pathogenesis of inflammatory demyelination in the central nervous system. *J. Immunol.* **2003**, *170*, 2153–2160. [CrossRef] [PubMed]
24. Oppmann, B.; Lesley, R.; Blom, B.; Timans, J.C.; Xu, Y.; Hunte, B.; Vega, F.; Yu, N.; Wang, J.; Singh, K.; et al. Novel p19 protein engages IL-12p40 to form a cytokine, IL-23, with biological activities similar as well as distinct from IL-12. *Immunity* **2000**, *13*, 715–725. [CrossRef]
25. Langrish, C.L.; Chen, Y.; Blumenschein, W.M.; Mattson, J.; Basham, B.; Sedgwick, J.D.; McClanahan, T.; Kastelein, R.A.; Cua, D.J. IL-23 drives a pathogenic T cell population that induces autoimmune inflammation. *J. Exp. Med.* **2005**, *201*, 233–240. [CrossRef] [PubMed]
26. Murphy, C.A.; Langrish, C.L.; Chen, Y.; Blumenschein, W.; McClanahan, T.; Kastelein, R.A.; Sedgwick, J.D.; Cua, D.J. Divergent pro- and antiinflammatory roles for IL-23 and IL-12 in joint autoimmune inflammation. *J. Exp. Med.* **2003**, *198*, 1951–1957. [CrossRef] [PubMed]
27. Harrington, L.E.; Hatton, R.D.; Mangan, P.R.; Turner, H.; Murphy, T.L.; Murphy, K.M.; Weaver, C.T. Interleukin 17-producing CD4+ effector T cells develop via a lineage distinct from the T helper type 1 and 2 lineages. *Nat. Immunol.* **2005**, *6*, 1123–1132. [CrossRef]
28. Zhang, Y.; Zhang, Y.; Gu, W.; Sun, B. TH1/TH2 cell differentiation and molecular signals. *Adv. Exp. Med. Biol.* **2014**, *841*, 15–44.
29. Elo, L.L.; Jarvenpaa, H.; Tuomela, S.; Raghav, S.; Ahlfors, H.; Laurila, K.; Gupta, B.; Lund, R.J.; Tahvanainen, J.; Hawkins, R.D.; et al. Genome-wide profiling of interleukin-4 and STAT6 transcription factor regulation of human Th2 cell programming. *Immunity* **2010**, *32*, 852–862. [CrossRef]
30. Gaffen, S.L.; Hajishengallis, G. A new inflammatory cytokine on the block: Re-thinking periodontal disease and the Th1/Th2 paradigm in the context of Th17 cells and IL-17. *J. Dent. Res.* **2008**, *87*, 817–828. [CrossRef]
31. Yang, J.; Sundrud, M.S.; Skepner, J.; Yamagata, T. Targeting Th17 cells in autoimmune diseases. *Trends Pharm. Sci.* **2014**, *35*, 493–500. [CrossRef] [PubMed]
32. Fasching, P.; Stradner, M.; Graninger, W.; Dejaco, C.; Fessler, J. Therapeutic Potential of Targeting the Th17/Treg Axis in Autoimmune Disorders. *Molecules* **2017**, *22*, 134. [CrossRef] [PubMed]
33. Veldhoen, M.; Hocking, R.J.; Atkins, C.J.; Locksley, R.M.; Stockinger, B. TGFbeta in the context of an inflammatory cytokine milieu supports de novo differentiation of IL-17-producing T cells. *Immunity* **2006**, *24*, 179–189. [CrossRef] [PubMed]

34. Ichiyama, K.; Yoshida, H.; Wakabayashi, Y.; Chinen, T.; Saeki, K.; Nakaya, M.; Takaesu, G.; Hori, S.; Yoshimura, A.; Kobayashi, T. Foxp3 inhibits RORgammat-mediated IL-17A mRNA transcription through direct interaction with RORgammat. *J. Biol. Chem.* **2008**, *283*, 17003–17008. [CrossRef] [PubMed]
35. Wang, M.; Tian, T.; Yu, S.; He, N.; Ma, D. Th17 and Treg cells in bone related diseases. *Clin. Dev. Immunol.* **2013**, *2013*, 203705. [CrossRef] [PubMed]
36. Ruddy, M.J.; Wong, G.C.; Liu, X.K.; Yamamoto, H.; Kasayama, S.; Kirkwood, K.L.; Gaffen, S.L. Functional cooperation between interleukin-17 and tumor necrosis factor-alpha is mediated by CCAAT/enhancer-binding protein family members. *J. Biol. Chem.* **2004**, *279*, 2559–2567. [CrossRef] [PubMed]
37. Khan, D.; Ansar Ahmed, S. Regulation of IL-17 in autoimmune diseases by transcriptional factors and microRNAs. *Front. Genet.* **2015**, *6*, 236. [CrossRef] [PubMed]
38. Yang, X.O.; Pappu, B.P.; Nurieva, R.; Akimzhanov, A.; Kang, H.S.; Chung, Y.; Ma, L.; Shah, B.; Panopoulos, A.D.; Schluns, K.S.; et al. T helper 17 lineage differentiation is programmed by orphan nuclear receptors ROR alpha and ROR gamma. *Immunity* **2008**, *28*, 29–39. [CrossRef] [PubMed]
39. Gooderham, M.J.; Papp, K.A.; Lynde, C.W. Shifting the focus—the primary role of IL-23 in psoriasis and other inflammatory disorders. *J. Eur. Acad. Derm. Venereol.* **2018**, *32*, 1111–1119. [CrossRef]
40. Iwakura, Y.; Ishigame, H. The IL-23/IL-17 axis in inflammation. *J. Clin. Investig.* **2006**, *116*, 1218–1222. [CrossRef]
41. Korn, T.; Bettelli, E.; Gao, W.; Awasthi, A.; Jager, A.; Strom, T.B.; Oukka, M.; Kuchroo, V.K. IL-21 initiates an alternative pathway to induce proinflammatory T(H)17 cells. *Nature* **2007**, *448*, 484–487. [CrossRef] [PubMed]
42. Ciofani, M.; Madar, A.; Galan, C.; Sellars, M.; Mace, K.; Pauli, F.; Agarwal, A.; Huang, W.; Parkhurst, C.N.; Muratet, M.; et al. A validated regulatory network for Th17 cell specification. *Cell* **2012**, *151*, 289–303. [CrossRef] [PubMed]
43. Bystrom, J.; Taher, T.E.; Muhyaddin, M.S.; Clanchy, F.I.; Mangat, P.; Jawad, A.S.; Williams, R.O.; Mageed, R.A. Harnessing the Therapeutic Potential of Th17 Cells. *Mediat. Inflamm.* **2015**, *2015*, 205156. [CrossRef] [PubMed]
44. Brustle, A.; Heink, S.; Huber, M.; Rosenplanter, C.; Stadelmann, C.; Yu, P.; Arpaia, E.; Mak, T.W.; Kamradt, T.; Lohoff, M. The development of inflammatory T(H)-17 cells requires interferon-regulatory factor 4. *Nat. Immunol.* **2007**, *8*, 958–966. [CrossRef] [PubMed]
45. Ivanov, I.I.; McKenzie, B.S.; Zhou, L.; Tadokoro, C.E.; Lepelley, A.; Lafaille, J.J.; Cua, D.J.; Littman, D.R. The orphan nuclear receptor RORgammat directs the differentiation program of proinflammatory IL-17+ T helper cells. *Cell* **2006**, *126*, 1121–1133. [CrossRef] [PubMed]
46. Kryczek, I.; Zhao, E.; Liu, Y.; Wang, Y.; Vatan, L.; Szeliga, W.; Moyer, J.; Klimczak, A.; Lange, A.; Zou, W. Human TH17 cells are long-lived effector memory cells. *Sci. Transl. Med.* **2011**, *3*, 104ra100. [CrossRef]
47. Guo, B. IL-10 Modulates Th17 Pathogenicity during Autoimmune Diseases. *J. Clin. Cell. Immunol.* **2016**, 7. [CrossRef]
48. McGeachy, M.J.; Bak-Jensen, K.S.; Chen, Y.; Tato, C.M.; Blumenschein, W.; McClanahan, T.; Cua, D.J. TGF-beta and IL-6 drive the production of IL-17 and IL-10 by T cells and restrain T(H)-17 cell-mediated pathology. *Nat. Immunol.* **2007**, *8*, 1390–1397. [CrossRef]
49. Lee, Y.; Awasthi, A.; Yosef, N.; Quintana, F.J.; Xiao, S.; Peters, A.; Wu, C.; Kleinewietfeld, M.; Kunder, S.; Hafler, D.A.; et al. Induction and molecular signature of pathogenic TH17 cells. *Nat. Immunol.* **2012**, *13*, 991–999. [CrossRef]
50. Hirota, K.; Duarte, J.H.; Veldhoen, M.; Hornsby, E.; Li, Y.; Cua, D.J.; Ahlfors, H.; Wilhelm, C.; Tolaini, M.; Menzel, U.; et al. Fate mapping of IL-17-producing T cells in inflammatory responses. *Nat. Immunol.* **2011**, *12*, 255–263. [CrossRef]
51. Veldhoen, M. Interleukin 17 is a chief orchestrator of immunity. *Nat. Immunol.* **2017**, *18*, 612–621. [CrossRef] [PubMed]
52. Zenobia, C.; Hajishengallis, G. Basic biology and role of interleukin-17 in immunity and inflammation. *Periodontology* **2015**, *69*, 142–159. [CrossRef]
53. Gaffen, S.L. Life before seventeen: Cloning of the IL-17 receptor. *J. Immunol.* **2011**, *187*, 4389–4391. [CrossRef] [PubMed]
54. Pappu, R.; Ramirez-Carrozzi, V.; Sambandam, A. The interleukin-17 cytokine family: Critical players in host defence and inflammatory diseases. *Immunology* **2011**, *134*, 8–16. [CrossRef] [PubMed]

55. Sharif, K.; Sharif, A.; Jumah, F.; Oskouian, R.; Tubbs, R.S. Rheumatoid arthritis in review: Clinical, anatomical, cellular and molecular points of view. *Clin. Anat.* **2018**, *31*, 216–223. [CrossRef] [PubMed]
56. Mitra, A.; Raychaudhuri, S.K.; Raychaudhuri, S.P. IL-17 and IL-17R: An auspicious therapeutic target for psoriatic disease. *Actas Dermosifiliogr.* **2014**, *105*, 21–33. [CrossRef]
57. Ganesan, R.; Rasool, M. Fibroblast-like synoviocytes-dependent effector molecules as a critical mediator for rheumatoid arthritis: Current status and future directions. *Int. Rev. Immunol.* **2017**, *36*, 20–30. [CrossRef]
58. Matsuzaki, G.; Umemura, M. Interleukin-17 family cytokines in protective immunity against infections: Role of hematopoietic cell-derived and non-hematopoietic cell-derived interleukin-17s. *Microbiol. Immunol.* **2018**, *62*, 1–13. [CrossRef]
59. Abusleme, L.; Moutsopoulos, N.M. IL-17: Overview and role in oral immunity and microbiome. *Oral Dis.* **2017**, *23*, 854–865. [CrossRef]
60. Bedoya, S.K.; Lam, B.; Lau, K.; Larkin, J. Th17 cells in immunity and autoimmunity. *Clin. Dev. Immunol.* **2013**, *2013*, 986789. [CrossRef]
61. Valeri, M.; Raffatellu, M. Cytokines IL-17 and IL-22 in the host response to infection. *Pathog. Dis.* **2016**, *74*, ftw111. [CrossRef] [PubMed]
62. Ye, P.; Rodriguez, F.H.; Kanaly, S.; Stocking, K.L.; Schurr, J.; Schwarzenberger, P.; Oliver, P.; Huang, W.; Zhang, P.; Zhang, J.; et al. Requirement of interleukin 17 receptor signaling for lung CXC chemokine and granulocyte colony-stimulating factor expression, neutrophil recruitment, and host defense. *J. Exp. Med.* **2001**, *194*, 519–527. [CrossRef] [PubMed]
63. Ling, Y.; Puel, A. IL-17 and infections. *Actas Dermosifiliogr.* **2014**, *105*, 34–40. [CrossRef]
64. Saunte, D.M.; Mrowietz, U.; Puig, L.; Zachariae, C. Candida infections in patients with psoriasis and psoriatic arthritis treated with interleukin-17 inhibitors and their practical management. *Br. J. Derm.* **2017**, *177*, 47–62. [CrossRef] [PubMed]
65. Souto, A.; Maneiro, J.R.; Salgado, E.; Carmona, L.; Gomez-Reino, J.J. Risk of tuberculosis in patients with chronic immune-mediated inflammatory diseases treated with biologics and tofacitinib: A systematic review and meta-analysis of randomized controlled trials and long-term extension studies. *Rheumatology* **2014**, *53*, 1872–1885. [CrossRef] [PubMed]
66. Dutzan, N.; Abusleme, L.; Bridgeman, H.; Greenwell-Wild, T.; Zangerle-Murray, T.; Fife, M.E.; Bouladoux, N.; Linley, H.; Brenchley, L.; Wemyss, K.; et al. On-going Mechanical Damage from Mastication Drives Homeostatic Th17 Cell Responses at the Oral Barrier. *Immunity* **2017**, *46*, 133–147. [CrossRef] [PubMed]
67. Yu, J.J.; Ruddy, M.J.; Wong, G.C.; Sfintescu, C.; Baker, P.J.; Smith, J.B.; Evans, R.T.; Gaffen, S.L. An essential role for IL-17 in preventing pathogen-initiated bone destruction: Recruitment of neutrophils to inflamed bone requires IL-17 receptor-dependent signals. *Blood* **2007**, *109*, 3794–3802. [CrossRef]
68. Awang, R.A.; Lappin, D.F.; MacPherson, A.; Riggio, M.; Robertson, D.; Hodge, P.; Ramage, G.; Culshaw, S.; Preshaw, P.M.; Taylor, J.; et al. Clinical associations between IL-17 family cytokines and periodontitis and potential differential roles for IL-17A and IL-17E in periodontal immunity. *Inflamm. Res.* **2014**, *63*, 1001–1012. [CrossRef]
69. Ito, H.; Honda, T.; Domon, H.; Oda, T.; Okui, T.; Amanuma, R.; Nakajima, T.; Yamazaki, K. Gene expression analysis of the CD4+ T-cell clones derived from gingival tissues of periodontitis patients. *Oral Microbiol Immunol.* **2005**, *20*, 382–386. [CrossRef]
70. Cheng, W.C.; Hughes, F.J.; Taams, L.S. The presence, function and regulation of IL-17 and Th17 cells in periodontitis. *J. Clin. Periodontol.* **2014**, *41*, 541–549. [CrossRef]
71. Cardoso, C.R.; Garlet, G.P.; Crippa, G.E.; Rosa, A.L.; Junior, W.M.; Rossi, M.A.; Silva, J.S. Evidence of the presence of T helper type 17 cells in chronic lesions of human periodontal disease. *Oral Microbiol. Immunol.* **2009**, *24*, 1–6. [CrossRef] [PubMed]
72. Vernal, R.; Dutzan, N.; Chaparro, A.; Puente, J.; Antonieta Valenzuela, M.; Gamonal, J. Levels of interleukin-17 in gingival crevicular fluid and in supernatants of cellular cultures of gingival tissue from patients with chronic periodontitis. *J. Clin. Periodontol.* **2005**, *32*, 383–389. [CrossRef] [PubMed]
73. Adibrad, M.; Deyhimi, P.; Ganjalikhani Hakemi, M.; Behfarnia, P.; Shahabuei, M.; Rafiee, L. Signs of the presence of Th17 cells in chronic periodontal disease. *J. Periodontal Res.* **2012**, *47*, 525–531. [CrossRef] [PubMed]
74. Schenkein, H.A.; Koertge, T.E.; Brooks, C.N.; Sabatini, R.; Purkall, D.E.; Tew, J.G. IL-17 in sera from patients with aggressive periodontitis. *J. Dent. Res.* **2010**, *89*, 943–947. [CrossRef] [PubMed]

75. Behfarnia, P.; Birang, R.; Pishva, S.S.; Hakemi, M.G.; Khorasani, M.M. Expression levels of th-2 and th-17 characteristic genes in healthy tissue versus periodontitis. *J. Dent.* **2013**, *10*, 23–31.
76. Furue, K.; Ito, T.; Tsuji, G.; Kadono, T.; Nakahara, T.; Furue, M. Autoimmunity and autoimmune co-morbidities in psoriasis. *Immunology* **2018**, *154*, 21–27. [CrossRef]
77. Raychaudhuri, S.K.; Maverakis, E.; Raychaudhuri, S.P. Diagnosis and classification of psoriasis. *Autoimmun. Rev.* **2014**, *13*, 490–495. [CrossRef]
78. Boehncke, W.H.; Schon, M.P. Psoriasis. *Lancet* **2015**, *386*, 983–994. [CrossRef]
79. Takeshita, J.; Grewal, S.; Langan, S.M.; Mehta, N.N.; Ogdie, A.; Van Voorhees, A.S.; Gelfand, J.M. Psoriasis and comorbid diseases: Epidemiology. *J. Am. Acad. Derm.* **2017**, *76*, 377–390. [CrossRef]
80. Stuart, P.E.; Nair, R.P.; Tsoi, L.C.; Tejasvi, T.; Das, S.; Kang, H.M.; Ellinghaus, E.; Chandran, V.; Callis-Duffin, K.; Ike, R.; et al. Genome-wide association analysis of psoriatic arthritis and cutaneous psoriasis reveals differences in their genetic architecture. *Am. J. Hum. Genet.* **2015**, *97*, 816–836. [CrossRef]
81. Gudjonsson, J.E.; Krueger, G. A role for epigenetics in psoriasis: Methylated Cytosine-Guanine sites differentiate lesional from nonlesional skin and from normal skin. *J. Investig. Derm.* **2012**, *132*, 506–508. [CrossRef] [PubMed]
82. Nibali, L.; Henderson, B.; Sadiq, S.T.; Donos, N. Genetic dysbiosis: The role of microbial insults in chronic inflammatory diseases. *J. Oral Microbiol.* **2014**, *6*, 22962. [CrossRef]
83. Fry, L.; Baker, B.S.; Powles, A.V.; Engstrand, L. Psoriasis is not an autoimmune disease? *Exp. Derm.* **2015**, *24*, 241–244. [CrossRef] [PubMed]
84. Mease, P.J. Inhibition of interleukin-17, interleukin-23 and the TH17 cell pathway in the treatment of psoriatic arthritis and psoriasis. *Curr. Opin. Rheumatol.* **2015**, *27*, 127–133. [CrossRef] [PubMed]
85. Chhabra, S.; Narang, T.; Joshi, N.; Goel, S.; Sawatkar, G.; Saikia, B.; Dogra, S.; Bansal, F.; Minz, R. Circulating T-helper 17 cells and associated cytokines in psoriasis. *Clin. Exp. Derm.* **2016**, *41*, 806–810. [CrossRef] [PubMed]
86. Raychaudhuri, S.K.; Saxena, A.; Raychaudhuri, S.P. Role of IL-17 in the pathogenesis of psoriatic arthritis and axial spondyloarthritis. *Clin. Rheumatol.* **2015**, *34*, 1019–1023. [CrossRef] [PubMed]
87. Di Cesare, A.; Di Meglio, P.; Nestle, F.O. The IL-23/Th17 axis in the immunopathogenesis of psoriasis. *J. Investig. Derm.* **2009**, *129*, 1339–1350. [CrossRef] [PubMed]
88. Grine, L.; Dejager, L.; Libert, C.; Vandenbroucke, R.E. An inflammatory triangle in psoriasis: TNF, type I IFNs and IL-17. *Cytokine Growth Factor Rev.* **2015**, *26*, 25–33. [CrossRef]
89. Ekman, A.K.; Bivik Eding, C.; Rundquist, I.; Enerback, C. IL-17 and IL-22 promote keratinocyte stemness in the germinative compartment in psoriasis. *J. Investig. Derm.* **2019**, *139*, 1564–1573. [CrossRef]
90. Chabaud, M.; Fossiez, F.; Taupin, J.L.; Miossec, P. Enhancing effect of IL-17 on IL-1-induced IL-6 and leukemia inhibitory factor production by rheumatoid arthritis synoviocytes and its regulation by Th2 cytokines. *J. Immunol.* **1998**, *161*, 409–414.
91. Graves, D.T.; Correa, J.D.; Silva, T.A. The Oral Microbiota Is Modified by Systemic Diseases. *J. Dent. Res.* **2019**, *98*, 148–156. [CrossRef] [PubMed]
92. Hajishengallis, G.; Moutsopoulos, N.M. Role of bacteria in leukocyte adhesion deficiency-associated periodontitis. *Microb. Pathog.* **2016**, *94*, 21–26. [CrossRef] [PubMed]
93. Moutsopoulos, N.M.; Konkel, J.; Sarmadi, M.; Eskan, M.A.; Wild, T.; Dutzan, N.; Abusleme, L.; Zenobia, C.; Hosur, K.B.; Abe, T.; et al. Defective neutrophil recruitment in leukocyte adhesion deficiency type I disease causes local IL-17-driven inflammatory bone loss. *Sci. Transl. Med.* **2014**, *6*, 229ra40. [CrossRef] [PubMed]
94. Hajishengallis, G.; Moutsopoulos, N.M. Etiology of leukocyte adhesion deficiency-associated periodontitis revisited: Not a raging infection but a raging inflammatory response. *Expert Rev. Clin. Immunol.* **2014**, *10*, 973–975. [CrossRef] [PubMed]
95. Su, N.Y.; Huang, J.Y.; Hu, C.J.; Yu, H.C.; Chang, Y.C. Increased risk of periodontitis in patients with psoriatic disease: A nationwide population-based retrospective cohort study. *PeerJ* **2017**, *5*, e4064.
96. Mendes, V.S.; Cota, L.O.M.; Costa, A.A.; Oliveira, A.; Costa, F.O. Periodontitis as another comorbidity associated with psoriasis: A case-control study. *J. Periodontol.* **2018**, *90*, 358–366. [CrossRef] [PubMed]
97. Lazaridou, E.; Tsikrikoni, A.; Fotiadou, C.; Kyrmanidou, E.; Vakirlis, E.; Giannopoulou, C.; Apalla, Z.; Ioannides, D. Association of chronic plaque psoriasis and severe periodontitis: A hospital based case-control study. *J. Eur. Acad. Derm. Venereol.* **2013**, *27*, 967–972. [CrossRef]

98. Keller, J.J.; Lin, H.C. The effects of chronic periodontitis and its treatment on the subsequent risk of psoriasis. *Br. J. Derm.* **2012**, *167*, 1338–1344. [CrossRef]
99. Egeberg, A.; Mallbris, L.; Gislason, G.; Hansen, P.R.; Mrowietz, U. Risk of periodontitis in patients with psoriasis and psoriatic arthritis. *J. Eur. Acad. Derm. Venereol.* **2017**, *31*, 288–293. [CrossRef]
100. Sharma, A.; Raman, A.; Pradeep, A.R. Association of chronic periodontitis and psoriasis: Periodontal status with severity of psoriasis. *Oral Dis.* **2015**, *21*, 314–319. [CrossRef]
101. Gheorghita, D.; Antal, M.A.; Nagy, K.; Kertesz, A.; Braunitzer, G. Smoking and Psoriasis as Synergistic Risk Factors in Periodontal disease. *Fogorv. Szle.* **2016**, *109*, 119–124.
102. Antal, M.; Braunitzer, G.; Mattheos, N.; Gyulai, R.; Nagy, K. Smoking as a permissive factor of periodontal disease in psoriasis. *PloS ONE* **2014**, *9*, e92333. [CrossRef] [PubMed]
103. Hueber, W.; Tomooka, B.H.; Zhao, X.; Kidd, B.A.; Drijfhout, J.W.; Fries, J.F.; van Venrooij, W.J.; Metzger, A.L.; Genovese, M.C.; Robinson, W.H. Proteomic analysis of secreted proteins in early rheumatoid arthritis: Anti-citrulline autoreactivity is associated with up regulation of proinflammatory cytokines. *Ann. Rheum. Dis.* **2007**, *66*, 712–719. [CrossRef] [PubMed]
104. Viatte, S.; Plant, D.; Raychaudhuri, S. Genetics and epigenetics of rheumatoid arthritis. *Nat. Rev. Rheumatol.* **2013**, *9*, 141–153. [CrossRef] [PubMed]
105. Guo, Q.; Wang, Y.; Xu, D.; Nossent, J.; Pavlos, N.J.; Xu, J. Rheumatoid arthritis: Pathological mechanisms and modern pharmacologic therapies. *Bone Res.* **2018**, *6*, 15. [CrossRef] [PubMed]
106. Veale, D.J.; Orr, C.; Fearon, U. Cellular and molecular perspectives in rheumatoid arthritis. *Semin. Immunopathol.* **2017**, *39*, 343–354. [CrossRef] [PubMed]
107. Firestein, G.S.; McInnes, I.B. Immunopathogenesis of Rheumatoid Arthritis. *Immunity* **2017**, *46*, 183–196. [CrossRef]
108. Hirota, K.; Yoshitomi, H.; Hashimoto, M.; Maeda, S.; Teradaira, S.; Sugimoto, N.; Yamaguchi, T.; Nomura, T.; Ito, H.; Nakamura, T.; et al. Preferential recruitment of CCR6-expressing Th17 cells to inflamed joints via CCL20 in rheumatoid arthritis and its animal model. *J. Exp. Med.* **2007**, *204*, 2803–2812. [CrossRef]
109. Lubberts, E.; Joosten, L.A.; van de Loo, F.A.; Schwarzenberger, P.; Kolls, J.; van den Berg, W.B. Overexpression of IL-17 in the knee joint of collagen type II immunized mice promotes collagen arthritis and aggravates joint destruction. *Inflamm. Res.* **2002**, *51*, 102–104. [CrossRef]
110. Nakae, S.; Nambu, A.; Sudo, K.; Iwakura, Y. Suppression of immune induction of collagen-induced arthritis in IL-17-deficient mice. *J. Immunol.* **2003**, *171*, 6173–6177. [CrossRef]
111. Hirota, K.; Hashimoto, M.; Yoshitomi, H.; Tanaka, S.; Nomura, T.; Yamaguchi, T.; Iwakura, Y.; Sakaguchi, N.; Sakaguchi, S. T cell self-reactivity forms a cytokine milieu for spontaneous development of IL-17+ Th cells that cause autoimmune arthritis. *J. Exp. Med.* **2007**, *204*, 41–47. [CrossRef] [PubMed]
112. Jaller Char, J.J.; Jaller, J.A.; Waibel, J.S.; Bhanusali, D.G.; Bhanusali, N. The Role of IL-17 in the Human Immune System and Its Blockage as a Treatment of Rheumatoid Arthritis, Ankylosing Spondylitis, and Psoriatic Arthritis. *J. Drugs Derm.* **2018**, *17*, 539–542.
113. Sato, K.; Suematsu, A.; Okamoto, K.; Yamaguchi, A.; Morishita, Y.; Kadono, Y.; Tanaka, S.; Kodama, T.; Akira, S.; Iwakura, Y.; et al. Th17 functions as an osteoclastogenic helper T cell subset that links T cell activation and bone destruction. *J. Exp. Med.* **2006**, *203*, 2673–2682. [CrossRef] [PubMed]
114. Kurebayashi, Y.; Nagai, S.; Ikejiri, A.; Koyasu, S. Recent advances in understanding the molecular mechanisms of the development and function of Th17 cells. *Genes Cells* **2013**, *18*, 247–265. [CrossRef] [PubMed]
115. Beklen, A.; Ainola, M.; Hukkanen, M.; Gurgan, C.; Sorsa, T.; Konttinen, Y.T. MMPs, IL-1, and TNF are regulated by IL-17 in periodontitis. *J. Dent. Res.* **2007**, *86*, 347–351. [CrossRef] [PubMed]
116. Dutzan, N.; Gamonal, J.; Silva, A.; Sanz, M.; Vernal, R. Over-expression of forkhead box P3 and its association with receptor activator of nuclear factor-kappa B ligand, interleukin (IL)-17, IL-10 and transforming growth factor-beta during the progression of chronic periodontitis. *J. Clin. Periodontol.* **2009**, *36*, 396–403. [CrossRef] [PubMed]
117. Lin, D.; Li, L.; Sun, Y.; Wang, W.; Wang, X.; Ye, Y.; Chen, X.; Xu, Y. IL-17 regulates the expressions of RANKL and OPG in human periodontal ligament cells via TRAF6/TBK1-JNK/NF-kappaB pathways. *Immunology* **2014**, *3*, 472–485.
118. Van Hamburg, J.P.; Corneth, O.B.; Paulissen, S.M.; Davelaar, N.; Asmawidjaja, P.S.; Mus, A.M.; Lubberts, E. IL-17/Th17 mediated synovial inflammation is IL-22 independent. *Ann. Rheum. Dis.* **2013**, *72*, 1700–1707. [CrossRef]

119. Miyazaki, Y.; Nakayamada, S.; Kubo, S.; Nakano, K.; Iwata, S.; Miyagawa, I.; Ma, X.; Trimova, G.; Sakata, K.; Tanaka, Y. Th22 Cells Promote Osteoclast Differentiation via Production of IL-22 in Rheumatoid Arthritis. *Front. Immunol.* **2018**, *9*, 2901. [CrossRef]
120. Diaz-Zuniga, J.; Melgar-Rodriguez, S.; Rojas, L.; Alvarez, C.; Monasterio, G.; Carvajal, P.; Vernal, R. Increased levels of the T-helper 22-associated cytokine (interleukin-22) and transcription factor (aryl hydrocarbon receptor) in patients with periodontitis are associated with osteoclast resorptive activity and severity of the disease. *J. Periodontal Res.* **2017**, *52*, 893–902.
121. De Pablo, P.; Dietrich, T.; McAlindon, T.E. Association of periodontal disease and tooth loss with rheumatoid arthritis in the US population. *J. Rheumatol.* **2008**, *35*, 70–76. [PubMed]
122. Gumus, P.; Buduneli, E.; Biyikoglu, B.; Aksu, K.; Sarac, F.; Nile, C.; Lappin, D.; Buduneli, N. Gingival crevicular fluid, serum levels of receptor activator of nuclear factor-kappaB ligand, osteoprotegerin, and interleukin-17 in patients with rheumatoid arthritis and osteoporosis and with periodontal disease. *J. Periodontol.* **2013**, *84*, 1627–1637. [PubMed]
123. Correa, M.G.; Sacchetti, S.B.; Ribeiro, F.V.; Pimentel, S.P.; Casarin, R.C.; Cirano, F.R.; Casati, M.Z. Periodontitis increases rheumatic factor serum levels and citrullinated proteins in gingival tissues and alter cytokine balance in arthritic rats. *PLoS ONE* **2017**, *12*, e0174442. [CrossRef] [PubMed]
124. Arunachalam, L.T. Autoimmune correlation of rheumatoid arthritis and periodontitis. *J. Indian Soc. Periodontol.* **2014**, *18*, 666–669. [CrossRef] [PubMed]
125. Mikuls, T.R.; Payne, J.B.; Reinhardt, R.A.; Thiele, G.M.; Maziarz, E.; Cannella, A.C.; Holers, V.M.; Kuhn, K.A.; O'Dell, J.R. Antibody responses to Porphyromonas gingivalis (P. gingivalis) in subjects with rheumatoid arthritis and periodontitis. *Int. Immunopharmacol.* **2009**, *9*, 38–42. [CrossRef] [PubMed]
126. Ordas, I.; Eckmann, L.; Talamini, M.; Baumgart, D.C.; Sandborn, W.J. Ulcerative colitis. *Lancet* **2012**, *380*, 1606–1619. [CrossRef]
127. Adams, S.M.; Bornemann, P.H. Ulcerative colitis. *Am. Fam. Physician* **2013**, *87*, 699–705.
128. Baumgart, D.C.; Sandborn, W.J. Crohn's disease. *Lancet* **2012**, *380*, 1590–1605. [CrossRef]
129. Iida, T.; Hida, T.; Matsuura, M.; Uhara, H.; Nakase, H. Current clinical issue of skin lesions in patients with inflammatory bowel disease. *Clin. J. Gastroenterol.* **2019**, *5*, 1–10. [CrossRef]
130. Zhang, Y.Z.; Li, Y.Y. Inflammatory bowel disease: Pathogenesis. *World J. Gastroenterol.* **2014**, *20*, 91–99. [CrossRef]
131. Siakavellas, S.I.; Bamias, G. Role of the IL-23/IL-17 axis in Crohn's disease. *Discov. Med.* **2012**, *14*, 253–262. [PubMed]
132. Kobayashi, T.; Okamoto, S.; Hisamatsu, T.; Kamada, N.; Chinen, H.; Saito, R.; Kitazume, M.T.; Nakazawa, A.; Sugita, A.; Koganei, K.; et al. IL23 differentially regulates the Th1/Th17 balance in ulcerative colitis and Crohn's disease. *Gut* **2008**, *57*, 1682–1689. [CrossRef]
133. Ogawa, A.; Andoh, A.; Araki, Y.; Bamba, T.; Fujiyama, Y. Neutralization of interleukin-17 aggravates dextran sulfate sodium-induced colitis in mice. *Clin. Immunol.* **2004**, *110*, 55–62. [CrossRef] [PubMed]
134. Ito, R.; Kita, M.; Shin-Ya, M.; Kishida, T.; Urano, A.; Takada, R.; Sakagami, J.; Imanishi, J.; Iwakura, Y.; Okanoue, T.; et al. Involvement of IL-17A in the pathogenesis of DSS-induced colitis in mice. *Biochem. Biophys. Res. Commun.* **2008**, *377*, 12–16. [CrossRef] [PubMed]
135. Sugihara, T.; Kobori, A.; Imaeda, H.; Tsujikawa, T.; Amagase, K.; Takeuchi, K.; Fujiyama, Y.; Andoh, A. The increased mucosal mRNA expressions of complement C3 and interleukin-17 in inflammatory bowel disease. *Clin. Exp. Immunol.* **2010**, *160*, 386–393. [CrossRef] [PubMed]
136. Song, L.; Zhou, R.; Huang, S.; Zhou, F.; Xu, S.; Wang, W.; Yi, F.; Wang, X.; Xia, B. High intestinal and systemic levels of interleukin-23/T-helper 17 pathway in Chinese patients with inflammatory bowel disease. *Mediat. Inflamm.* **2013**, *2013*, 425915. [CrossRef] [PubMed]
137. Fujino, S.; Andoh, A.; Bamba, S.; Ogawa, A.; Hata, K.; Araki, Y.; Bamba, T.; Fujiyama, Y. Increased expression of interleukin 17 in inflammatory bowel disease. *Gut* **2003**, *52*, 65–70. [CrossRef] [PubMed]
138. Seiderer, J.; Elben, I.; Diegelmann, J.; Glas, J.; Stallhofer, J.; Tillack, C.; Pfennig, S.; Jurgens, M.; Schmechel, S.; Konrad, A.; et al. Role of the novel Th17 cytokine IL-17F in inflammatory bowel disease (IBD): Upregulated colonic IL-17F expression in active Crohn's disease and analysis of the IL17F p.His161Arg polymorphism in IBD. *Inflamm. Bowel Dis.* **2008**, *14*, 437–445. [CrossRef]
139. Chi, A.C.; Neville, B.W.; Krayer, J.W.; Gonsalves, W.C. Oral manifestations of systemic disease. *Am. Fam. Physician* **2010**, *82*, 1381–1388.

140. Eckel, A.; Lee, D.; Deutsch, G.; Maxin, A.; Oda, D. Oral manifestations as the first presenting sign of Crohn's disease in a pediatric patient. *J. Clin. Exp. Dent.* **2017**, *9*, e934–e938. [CrossRef]
141. Tan, C.X.; Brand, H.S.; de Boer, N.K.; Forouzanfar, T. Gastrointestinal diseases and their oro-dental manifestations: Part 1: Crohn's disease. *Br. Dent. J.* **2016**, *221*, 794–799. [CrossRef] [PubMed]
142. Feuerstein, J.D.; Cheifetz, A.S. Crohn Disease: epidemiology, diagnosis, and management. *Mayo Clin. Proc.* **2017**, *92*, 1088–1103. [CrossRef] [PubMed]
143. Brito, F.; de Barros, F.C.; Zaltman, C.; Carvalho, A.T.; Carneiro, A.J.; Fischer, R.G.; Gustafsson, A.; Figueredo, C.M. Prevalence of periodontitis and DMFT index in patients with Crohn's disease and ulcerative colitis. *J. Clin. Periodontol.* **2008**, *35*, 555–560. [CrossRef] [PubMed]
144. Chi, Y.C.; Chen, J.L.; Wang, L.H.; Chang, K.; Wu, C.L.; Lin, S.Y.; Keller, J.J.; Bai, C.H. Increased risk of periodontitis among patients with Crohn's disease: A population-based matched-cohort study. *Int. J. Colorectal Dis.* **2018**, *33*, 1437–1444. [CrossRef] [PubMed]
145. Papageorgiou, S.N.; Hagner, M.; Nogueira, A.V.; Franke, A.; Jager, A.; Deschner, J. Inflammatory bowel disease and oral health: Systematic review and a meta-analysis. *J. Clin. Periodontol.* **2017**, *44*, 382–393. [CrossRef] [PubMed]
146. Lira-Junior, R.; Figueredo, C.M. Periodontal and inflammatory bowel diseases: Is there evidence of complex pathogenic interactions? *World J. Gastroenterol.* **2016**, *22*, 7963–7972. [CrossRef] [PubMed]
147. Fox, R.I. Sjogren's syndrome. *Lancet* **2005**, *366*, 321–331. [CrossRef]
148. Brito-Zeron, P.; Ramos-Casals, M. Advances in the understanding and treatment of systemic complications in Sjogren's syndrome. *Curr. Opin. Rheumatol.* **2014**, *26*, 520–527. [CrossRef] [PubMed]
149. Carsons, S.E.; Patel, B.C. Sjogren Syndrome. In *StatPearls*; StatPearls Publishing LLC.: Treasure Island, FL, USA, 2019.
150. Bowman, S.J. Primary Sjogren's syndrome. *Lupus* **2018**, *27*, 32–35. [CrossRef] [PubMed]
151. Saito, M.; Otsuka, K.; Ushio, A.; Yamada, A.; Arakaki, R.; Kudo, Y.; Ishimaru, N. Unique Phenotypes and Functions of Follicular Helper T Cells and Regulatory T Cells in Sjogren's Syndrome. *Curr. Rheumatol. Rev.* **2018**, *14*, 239–245. [CrossRef] [PubMed]
152. Hillen, M.R.; Ververs, F.A.; Kruize, A.A.; Van Roon, J.A. Dendritic cells, T-cells and epithelial cells: A crucial interplay in immunopathology of primary Sjogren's syndrome. *Expert Rev. Clin. Immunol.* **2014**, *10*, 521–531. [CrossRef] [PubMed]
153. Matsui, K.; Sano, H. T Helper 17 Cells in Primary Sjogren's Syndrome. *J. Clin. Med.* **2017**, 65. [CrossRef] [PubMed]
154. Weinstein, J.S.; Herman, E.I.; Lainez, B.; Licona-Limon, P.; Esplugues, E.; Flavell, R.; Craft, J. TFH cells progressively differentiate to regulate the germinal center response. *Nat. Immunol.* **2016**, *17*, 1197–1205. [CrossRef] [PubMed]
155. Katsifis, G.E.; Rekka, S.; Moutsopoulos, N.M.; Pillemer, S.; Wahl, S.M. Systemic and local interleukin-17 and linked cytokines associated with Sjogren's syndrome immunopathogenesis. *Am. J. Pathol.* **2009**, *175*, 1167–1177. [CrossRef] [PubMed]
156. Kwok, S.K.; Cho, M.L.; Her, Y.M.; Oh, H.J.; Park, M.K.; Lee, S.Y.; Woo, Y.J.; Ju, J.H.; Park, K.S.; Kim, H.Y.; et al. TLR2 ligation induces the production of IL-23/IL-17 via IL-6, STAT3 and NF-kB pathway in patients with primary Sjogren's syndrome. *Arthritis Res.* **2012**, *14*, R64. [CrossRef] [PubMed]
157. Pollard, R.P.; Abdulahad, W.H.; Bootsma, H.; Meiners, P.M.; Spijkervet, F.K.; Huitema, M.G.; Burgerhof, J.G.; Vissink, A.; Kroese, F.G. Predominantly proinflammatory cytokines decrease after B cell depletion therapy in patients with primary Sjogren's syndrome. *Ann. Rheum. Dis.* **2013**, *72*, 2048–2050. [CrossRef] [PubMed]
158. Ambrosio, L.M.; Rovai, E.S.; Franca, B.N.; Balzarini, D.A.; Abreu, I.S.; Lopes, S.B.; Nunes, T.B.; Lourenco, S.V.; Pasoto, S.G.; Saraiva, L.; et al. Effects of periodontal treatment on primary sjogren's syndrome symptoms. *Braz. Oral Res.* **2017**, *31*, e8. [CrossRef]
159. Lugonja, B.; Yeo, L.; Milward, M.R.; Smith, D.; Dietrich, T.; Chapple, I.L.; Rauz, S.; Williams, G.P.; Barone, F.; de Pablo, P.; et al. Periodontitis prevalence and serum antibody reactivity to periodontal bacteria in primary Sjogren's syndrome: A pilot study. *J. Clin. Periodontol.* **2016**, *43*, 26–33. [CrossRef]
160. De Goes Soares, L.; Rocha, R.L.; Bagordakis, E.; Galvao, E.L.; Douglas-de-Oliveira, D.W.; Falci, S.G.M. Relationship between sjogren syndrome and periodontal status: A systematic review. *Oral Surg. Oral Med. Oral Pathol. Oral Radiol.* **2018**, *125*, 223–231. [CrossRef]

161. Koga, T.; Ichinose, K.; Tsokos, G.C. T cells and IL-17 in lupus nephritis. *Clin. Immunol.* **2017**, *185*, 95–99. [CrossRef]
162. Kluger, M.A.; Nosko, A.; Ramcke, T.; Goerke, B.; Meyer, M.C.; Wegscheid, C.; Luig, M.; Tiegs, G.; Stahl, R.A.; Steinmetz, O.M. RORgammat expression in Tregs promotes systemic lupus erythematosus via IL-17 secretion, alteration of Treg phenotype and suppression of Th2 responses. *Clin. Exp. Immunol.* **2017**, *188*, 63–78. [CrossRef] [PubMed]
163. Moulton, V.R.; Suarez-Fueyo, A.; Meidan, E.; Li, H.; Mizui, M.; Tsokos, G.C. Pathogenesis of Human Systemic Lupus Erythematosus: A Cellular Perspective. *Trends Mol. Med.* **2017**, *23*, 615–635. [CrossRef] [PubMed]
164. Mendonca, S.M.S.; Correa, J.D.; Souza, A.F.; Travassos, D.V.; Calderaro, D.C.; Rocha, N.P.; Vieira, E.L.M.; Teixeira, A.L.; Ferreira, G.A.; Silva, T.A. Immunological signatures in saliva of systemic lupus erythematosus patients: Influence of periodontal condition. *Clin. Exp. Rheumatol.* **2019**, *37*, 208–214. [PubMed]
165. Wu, Y.D.; Lin, C.H.; Chao, W.C.; Liao, T.L.; Chen, D.Y.; Chen, H.H. Association between a history of periodontitis and the risk of systemic lupus erythematosus in Taiwan: A nationwide, population-based, case-control study. *PLoS ONE* **2017**, *12*, e0187075. [CrossRef] [PubMed]
166. Fabbri, C.; Fuller, R.; Bonfa, E.; Guedes, L.K.; D'Alleva, P.S.; Borba, E.F. Periodontitis treatment improves systemic lupus erythematosus response to immunosuppressive therapy. *Clin. Rheumatol.* **2014**, *33*, 505–509. [CrossRef] [PubMed]
167. Bluestone, J.A.; Herold, K.; Eisenbarth, G. Genetics, pathogenesis and clinical interventions in type 1 diabetes. *Nature* **2010**, *464*, 1293–1300. [CrossRef]
168. Wu, Y.L.; Ding, Y.P.; Gao, J.; Tanaka, Y.; Zhang, W. Risk factors and primary prevention trials for type 1 diabetes. *Int. J. Biol. Sci.* **2013**, *9*, 666–679. [CrossRef]
169. Emamaullee, J.A.; Davis, J.; Merani, S.; Toso, C.; Elliott, J.F.; Thiesen, A.; Shapiro, A.M. Inhibition of Th17 cells regulates autoimmune diabetes in NOD mice. *Diabetes* **2009**, *58*, 1302–1311. [CrossRef]
170. Honkanen, J.; Nieminen, J.K.; Gao, R.; Luopajarvi, K.; Salo, H.M.; Ilonen, J.; Knip, M.; Otonkoski, T.; Vaarala, O. IL-17 immunity in human type 1 diabetes. *J. Immunol.* **2010**, *185*, 1959–1967. [CrossRef]
171. Marwaha, A.K.; Panagiotopoulos, C.; Biggs, C.M.; Staiger, S.; Del Bel, K.L.; Hirschfeld, A.F.; Priatel, J.J.; Turvey, S.E.; Tan, R. Pre-diagnostic genotyping identifies T1D subjects with impaired Treg IL-2 signaling and an elevated proportion of FOXP3(+)IL-17(+) cells. *Genes Immun.* **2017**, *18*, 15–21. [CrossRef]
172. Novotna, M.; Podzimek, S.; Broukal, Z.; Lencova, E.; Duskova, J. Periodontal Diseases and Dental Caries in Children with Type 1 Diabetes Mellitus. *Mediat. Inflamm.* **2015**, *2015*, 379626. [CrossRef] [PubMed]
173. Preshaw, P.M.; Alba, A.L.; Herrera, D.; Jepsen, S.; Konstantinidis, A.; Makrilakis, K.; Taylor, R. Periodontitis and diabetes: A two-way relationship. *Diabetologia* **2012**, *55*, 21–31. [CrossRef] [PubMed]
174. Simpson, T.C.; Weldon, J.C.; Worthington, H.V.; Needleman, I.; Wild, S.H.; Moles, D.R.; Stevenson, B.; Furness, S.; Iheozor-Ejiofor, Z. Treatment of periodontal disease for glycaemic control in people with diabetes mellitus. *Cochrane Database Syst. Rev.* **2015**, *11*, Cd004714. [CrossRef] [PubMed]
175. Emmi, G.; Silvestri, E.; Bella, C.D.; Grassi, A.; Benagiano, M.; Cianchi, F.; Squatrito, D.; Cantarini, L.; Emmi, L.; Selmi, C.; et al. Cytotoxic Th1 and Th17 cells infiltrate the intestinal mucosa of Behcet patients and exhibit high levels of TNF-alpha in early phases of the disease. *Medicine* **2016**, *95*, e5516. [CrossRef] [PubMed]
176. Lei, L.; Zhao, C.; Qin, F.; He, Z.Y.; Wang, X.; Zhong, X.N. Th17 cells and IL-17 promote the skin and lung inflammation and fibrosis process in a bleomycin-induced murine model of systemic sclerosis. *Clin. Exp. Rheumatol.* **2016**, *34*, 14–22. [PubMed]
177. Jethwa, H.; Bowness, P. The interleukin (IL)-23/IL-17 axis in ankylosing spondylitis: New advances and potentials for treatment. *Clin. Exp. Immunol.* **2016**, *183*, 30–36. [CrossRef] [PubMed]
178. Li, Y.F.; Zhang, S.X.; Ma, X.W.; Xue, Y.L.; Gao, C.; Li, X.Y. Levels of peripheral Th17 cells and serum Th17-related cytokines in patients with multiple sclerosis: A meta-analysis. *Mult. Scler. Relat. Disord.* **2017**, *18*, 20–25. [CrossRef]
179. Gustavsen, M.W.; Celius, E.G.; Moen, S.M.; Bjolgerud, A.; Berg-Hansen, P.; Nygaard, G.O.; Sandvik, L.; Lie, B.A.; Harbo, H.F. No association between multiple sclerosis and periodontitis after adjusting for smoking habits. *Eur. J. Neurol.* **2015**, *22*, 588–590. [CrossRef]
180. Sheu, J.J.; Lin, H.C. Association between multiple sclerosis and chronic periodontitis: A population-based pilot study. *Eur. J. Neurol.* **2013**, *20*, 1053–1059. [CrossRef]

181. Isola, G.; Williams, R.C.; Lo Gullo, A.; Ramaglia, L.; Matarese, M.; Iorio-Siciliano, V.; Cosio, C.; Matarese, G. Risk association between scleroderma disease characteristics, periodontitis, and tooth loss. *Clin. Rheumatol.* **2017**, *36*, 2733–2741. [CrossRef]
182. Habibagahi, Z.; Khorshidi, H.; Hekmati, S. Periodontal health status among patients with Behcet's Disease. *Scientifica* **2016**, *2016*, 7506041. [CrossRef] [PubMed]
183. Ma, X.; Xu, S. TNF inhibitor therapy for rheumatoid arthritis. *Biomed. Rep.* **2013**, *1*, 177–184. [CrossRef] [PubMed]
184. Kalden, J.R.; Schulze-Koops, H. Immunogenicity and loss of response to TNF inhibitors: Implications for rheumatoid arthritis treatment. *Nat. Rev. Rheumatol.* **2017**, *13*, 707–718. [CrossRef] [PubMed]
185. Nissim, A.; Chernajovsky, Y. Historical development of monoclonal antibody therapeutics. *Handb. Exp. Pharmacol.* **2008**, *181*, 3–18.
186. Breedveld, F.C. Therapeutic monoclonal antibodies. *Lancet* **2000**, *355*, 735–740. [CrossRef]
187. Levin, A.D.; Wildenberg, M.E.; van den Brink, G.R. Mechanism of Action of Anti-TNF Therapy in Inflammatory Bowel Disease. *J. Crohn's Colitis* **2016**, *10*, 989–997. [CrossRef] [PubMed]
188. Yost, J.; Gudjonsson, J.E. The role of TNF inhibitors in psoriasis therapy: New implications for associated comorbidities. *F1000 Med. Rep.* **2009**, *1*. [CrossRef]
189. Di Paola, R.; Mazzon, E.; Muia, C.; Crisafulli, C.; Terrana, D.; Greco, S.; Britti, D.; Santori, D.; Oteri, G.; Cordasco, G.; et al. Effects of etanercept, a tumour necrosis factor-alpha antagonist, in an experimental model of periodontitis in rats. *Br. J. Pharmacol.* **2007**, *150*, 286–297. [CrossRef]
190. Mylonas, A.; Conrad, C. Psoriasis: Classical vs. Paradoxical. The Yin-Yang of TNF and Type I Interferon. *Front. Immunol.* **2018**, *9*, 2746. [CrossRef]
191. Brown, G.; Wang, E.; Leon, A.; Huynh, M.; Wehner, M.; Matro, R.; Linos, E.; Liao, W.; Haemel, A. Tumor necrosis factor-alpha inhibitor-induced psoriasis: Systematic review of clinical features, histopathological findings, and management experience. *J. Am. Acad. Derm.* **2017**, *76*, 334–341. [CrossRef]
192. Segaert, S.; Hermans, C. Clinical Signs, Pathophysiology and Management of Cutaneous Side Effects of Anti-Tumor Necrosis Factor Agents. *Am. J. Clin. Dermatol.* **2017**, *18*, 771–787. [CrossRef] [PubMed]
193. Blanco, F.J.; Moricke, R.; Dokoupilova, E.; Codding, C.; Neal, J.; Andersson, M.; Rohrer, S.; Richards, H. Secukinumab in Active Rheumatoid Arthritis: A Phase III Randomized, Double-Blind, Active Comparator- and Placebo-Controlled Study. *Arthritis Rheumatol.* **2017**, *69*, 1144–1153. [CrossRef] [PubMed]
194. Chen, H.H.; Chen, D.Y.; Lai, K.L.; Chen, Y.M.; Chou, Y.J.; Chou, P.; Lin, C.H.; Huang, N. Periodontitis and etanercept discontinuation risk in anti-tumor necrosis factor-naive rheumatoid arthritis patients: A nationwide population-based cohort study. *J. Clin. Rheumatol.* **2013**, *19*, 432–438. [CrossRef] [PubMed]
195. Miossec, P. Diseases that may benefit from manipulating the Th17 pathway. *Eur. J. Immunol.* **2009**, *39*, 667–669. [CrossRef] [PubMed]
196. Alzabin, S.; Abraham, S.M.; Taher, T.E.; Palfreeman, A.; Hull, D.; McNamee, K.; Jawad, A.; Pathan, E.; Kinderlerer, A.; Taylor, P.C.; et al. Incomplete response of inflammatory arthritis to TNFalpha blockade is associated with the Th17 pathway. *Ann. Rheum. Dis.* **2012**, *71*, 1741–1748. [CrossRef]
197. Beck, K.M.; Koo, J. Brodalumab for the treatment of plaque psoriasis: Up-to-date. *Expert Opin. Biol. Ther.* **2019**, *19*, 287–292. [CrossRef]
198. Genovese, M.C.; Durez, P.; Richards, H.B.; Supronik, J.; Dokoupilova, E.; Mazurov, V.; Aelion, J.A.; Lee, S.H.; Codding, C.E.; Kellner, H.; et al. Efficacy and safety of secukinumab in patients with rheumatoid arthritis: A phase II, dose-finding, double-blind, randomised, placebo controlled study. *Ann. Rheum. Dis.* **2013**, *72*, 863–869. [CrossRef]
199. Genovese, M.C.; Braun, D.K.; Erickson, J.S.; Berclaz, P.Y.; Banerjee, S.; Heffernan, M.P.; Carlier, H. Safety and Efficacy of Open-label Subcutaneous Ixekizumab Treatment for 48 Weeks in a Phase II Study in Biologic-naive and TNF-IR Patients with Rheumatoid Arthritis. *J. Rheumatol.* **2016**, *43*, 289–297. [CrossRef]
200. Leonardi, C.; Matheson, R.; Zachariae, C.; Cameron, G.; Li, L.; Edson-Heredia, E.; Braun, D.; Banerjee, S. Anti-interleukin-17 monoclonal antibody ixekizumab in chronic plaque psoriasis. *N. Engl. J. Med.* **2012**, *366*, 1190–1199. [CrossRef]
201. Hueber, W.; Patel, D.D.; Dryja, T.; Wright, A.M.; Koroleva, I.; Bruin, G.; Antoni, C.; Draelos, Z.; Gold, M.H.; Durez, P.; et al. Effects of AIN457, a fully human antibody to interleukin-17A, on psoriasis, rheumatoid arthritis, and uveitis. *Sci. Transl. Med.* **2010**, *2*, 52ra72. [CrossRef]

202. Shelton, S.K.; Bai, S.R.; Jordan, J.K.; Sheehan, A.H. Ixekizumab: A Review of Its Use for the Management of Moderate to Severe Plaque Psoriasis. *Ann. Pharmacother.* **2019**, *53*, 276–284. [CrossRef] [PubMed]
203. Blauvelt, A.; Lomaga, M.; Burge, R.; Zhu, B.; Shen, W.; Shrom, D.; Dossenbach, M.; Pinter, A. Greater Cumulative Benefits from Ixekizumab versus Ustekinumab Treatment over 52 Weeks for Patients with Moderate-to-Severe Psoriasis in a Randomized, Double-Blinded Phase 3b Clinical Trial. *J. Dermatol. Treat.* **2019**, 1–21. [CrossRef] [PubMed]
204. Amin, M.; Darji, K.; No, D.J.; Bhutani, T.; Wu, J.J. Review of IL-17 inhibitors for psoriasis. *J. Dermatol. Treat.* **2017**, 1–6. [CrossRef] [PubMed]
205. Bilal, J.; Berlinberg, A.; Bhattacharjee, S.; Trost, J.; Riaz, I.B.; Kurtzman, D.J.B. A systematic review and meta-analysis of the efficacy and safety of the interleukin (IL)-12/23 and IL-17 inhibitors ustekinumab, secukinumab, ixekizumab, brodalumab, guselkumab and tildrakizumab for the treatment of moderate to severe plaque psoriasis. *J. Dermatol. Treat.* **2018**, *29*, 569–578. [CrossRef] [PubMed]
206. Kunwar, S.; Dahal, K.; Sharma, S. Anti-IL-17 therapy in treatment of rheumatoid arthritis: A systematic literature review and meta-analysis of randomized controlled trials. *Rheumatol. Int.* **2016**, *36*, 1065–1075. [CrossRef] [PubMed]
207. Van Baarsen, L.G.; Lebre, M.C.; van der Coelen, D.; Aarrass, S.; Tang, M.W.; Ramwadhdoebe, T.H.; Gerlag, D.M.; Tak, P.P. Heterogeneous expression pattern of interleukin 17A (IL-17A), IL-17F and their receptors in synovium of rheumatoid arthritis, psoriatic arthritis and osteoarthritis: Possible explanation for nonresponse to anti-IL-17 therapy? *Arthritis Res. Ther.* **2014**, *16*, 426. [CrossRef] [PubMed]
208. Griffiths, C.E.; Strober, B.E.; van de Kerkhof, P.; Ho, V.; Fidelus-Gort, R.; Yeilding, N.; Guzzo, C.; Xia, Y.; Zhou, B.; Li, S.; et al. Comparison of ustekinumab and etanercept for moderate-to-severe psoriasis. *N. Engl. J. Med.* **2010**, *362*, 118–128. [CrossRef] [PubMed]
209. Leonardi, C.L.; Kimball, A.B.; Papp, K.A.; Yeilding, N.; Guzzo, C.; Wang, Y.; Li, S.; Dooley, L.T.; Gordon, K.B. Efficacy and safety of ustekinumab, a human interleukin-12/23 monoclonal antibody, in patients with psoriasis: 76-week results from a randomised, double-blind, placebo-controlled trial (PHOENIX 1). *Lancet* **2008**, *371*, 1665–1674. [CrossRef]
210. Papp, K.A.; Langley, R.G.; Lebwohl, M.; Krueger, G.G.; Szapary, P.; Yeilding, N.; Guzzo, C.; Hsu, M.C.; Wang, Y.; Li, S.; et al. Efficacy and safety of ustekinumab, a human interleukin-12/23 monoclonal antibody, in patients with psoriasis: 52-week results from a randomised, double-blind, placebo-controlled trial (PHOENIX 2). *Lancet* **2008**, *371*, 1675–1684. [CrossRef]
211. Ghosh, S.; Gensler, L.S.; Yang, Z.; Gasink, C.; Chakravarty, S.D.; Farahi, K.; Ramachandran, P.; Ott, E.; Strober, B.E. Ustekinumab Safety in Psoriasis, Psoriatic Arthritis, and Crohn's Disease: An Integrated Analysis of Phase II/III Clinical Development Programs. *Drug Saf.* **2019**, *42*, 751–768. [CrossRef]
212. Ustekinumab: New drug. Suspicion of carcinogenicity: Too great a risk for psoriasis patients. *Prescrire Int.* **2009**, *18*, 202–204.
213. Moutsopoulos, N.M.; Zerbe, C.S.; Wild, T.; Dutzan, N.; Brenchley, L.; DiPasquale, G.; Uzel, G.; Axelrod, K.C.; Lisco, A.; Notarangelo, L.D.; et al. Interleukin-12 and Interleukin-23 Blockade in Leukocyte Adhesion Deficiency Type 1. *N. Engl. J. Med.* **2017**, *376*, 1141–1146. [CrossRef] [PubMed]
214. Machado, A.; Torres, T. Guselkumab for the Treatment of Psoriasis. *Biodrugs Clin. Immunother. Biopharm. Gene Ther.* **2018**, *32*, 119–128. [CrossRef] [PubMed]
215. Kolli, S.S.; Gabros, S.D.; Pona, A.; Cline, A.; Feldman, S.R. Tildrakizumab: A Review of Phase II and III Clinical Trials. *Ann. Pharmacother.* **2019**, *53*, 413–418. [CrossRef] [PubMed]

5

Recent Progress of Basic Studies of Natural Products and their Dental Application

Hiroshi Sakagami [1,*], Taihei Watanabe [2], Tomonori Hoshino [2], Naoto Suda [3], Kazumasa Mori [4], Toshikazu Yasui [5], Naoki Yamauchi [6], Harutsugu Kashiwagi [7], Tsuneaki Gomi [8], Takaaki Oizumi [9], Junko Nagai [10], Yoshihiro Uesawa [10], Koichi Takao [11] and Yoshiaki Sugita [11]

1 Meikai University Research Institute of Odontology (M-RIO), 1-1 Keyakidai, Sakado, Saitama 350-0283, Japan
2 Division of Pediatric Dentistry, Meikai University School of Dentistry, 1-1 Keyakidai, Sakado, Saitama 350-0283, Japan; taiheidental10627@gmail.com (T.W.); thoshino1@dent.meikai.ac.jp (T.H.)
3 Division of Orthodontics, Meikai University School of Dentistry, 1-1 Keyakidai, Sakado, Saitama 350-0283, Japan; n-suda@dent.meikai.ac.jp
4 Division of First Oral and Maxillofacial Surgery, Meikai University School of Dentistry, 1-1 Keyakidai, Sakado, Saitama 350-0283, Japan; kazu-mori@dent.meikai.ac.jp
5 Division of Oral Health, Meikai University School of Dentistry, 1-1 Keyakidai, Sakado, Saitama 350-0283, Japan; yasui@dent.meikai.ac.jp
6 Masuko Memorial Hospital, 35-28 Takehashi-cho, Nakamura-ku, Nagoya 453-8566, Japan; yamauchi@masuko.or.jp
7 Ecopale Co., Ltd., 885 Minamiisshiki, Nagaizumi-cho, Suntou-gun, Shizuoka 411-0932, Japan; ecopale@fujibamboogarden.com
8 Gomi clinic, 1-10-12 Hyakunin-cho, Shinjuku-ku, Tokyo 169-0073, Japan; fwkz9633@mb.infoweb.ne.jp
9 Daiwa Biological Research Institute Co., Ltd., 3-2-1 Sakado, Takatsu-ku, Kawasaki, Kanagawa 213-0012, Japan; takaakio@daiwaseibutsu.co.jp
10 Department of Medical Molecular Informatics, Meiji Pharmaceutical University, 2-522-1 Noshio, Kiyose, Tokyo 204-8588, Japan, nagai-j@my-pharm.ac.jp (J.N.); uesawa@my-pharm.ac.jp (Y.U.)
11 Department of Pharmaceutical Sciences, Faculty of Pharmacy and Pharmaceutical Sciences, Josai University, Sakado, Saitama 350-0295, Japan; ktakao@josai.ac.jp (K.T.); sugita@josai.ac.jp (Y.S.)
* Correspondence: sakagami@dent.meikai.ac.jp

Abstract: The present article reviews the research progress of three major polyphenols (tannins, flavonoids and lignin carbohydrate complexes), chromone (backbone structure of flavonoids) and herbal extracts. Chemical modified chromone derivatives showed highly specific toxicity against human oral squamous cell carcinoma cell lines, with much lower toxicity against human oral keratinocytes, as compared with various anticancer drugs. QSAR analysis suggests the possible correlation between their tumor-specificity and three-dimensional molecular shape. Condensed tannins in the tea extracts inactivated the glucosyltransferase enzymes, involved in the biofilm formation. Lignin-carbohydrate complexes (prepared by alkaline extraction and acid-precipitation) and crude alkaline extract of the leaves of *Sasa* species (SE, available as an over-the-counter drug) showed much higher anti-HIV activity, than tannins, flavonoids and Japanese traditional medicine (Kampo). Long-term treatment with SE and several Kampo medicines showed an anti-inflammatory and anti-oxidant effects in small size of clinical trials. Although the anti-periodontitis activity of synthetic angiotensin II blockers has been suggested in many papers, natural angiotensin II blockers has not yet been tested for their possible anti-periodontitis activity. There should be still many unknown substances that are useful for treating the oral diseases in the natural kingdom.

Keywords: polyphenol; chromone; lignin-carbohydrate complex; alkaline extract; Kampo medicine; glucosyltransferase; angiotensin II blocker; QSAR analysis; oral diseases; dental application

1. Introduction

The etiology of stomatitis is largely unclear [1]. However, oral inflammation such as stomatitis are considered to be triggered or aggravated by various factors including bacterial and viral infections, nutritional deficiencies, declined immune functions, allergic reactions, radiotherapy, stress, cigarettes, diseases and genetic backgrounds [1,2]. Applications of topical steroids, transdermal patches, vitamins, throat lozenges, mouth washes and cryotherapy are sometimes not effective for the treatment of stomatitis and therefore exploration of new-type of treatment are necessary [3]. In this sense, natural products having broader spectrum of biological activities are potential candidates as alternative medicine for oral diseases.

Polyphenols in the natural kingdom are defined as substances that possess an aromatic ring bearing one or more hydroxyl substituents and roughly classified into tannins, flavonoids and lignin-carbohydrate complexes (LCC) (Figure 1) [4].

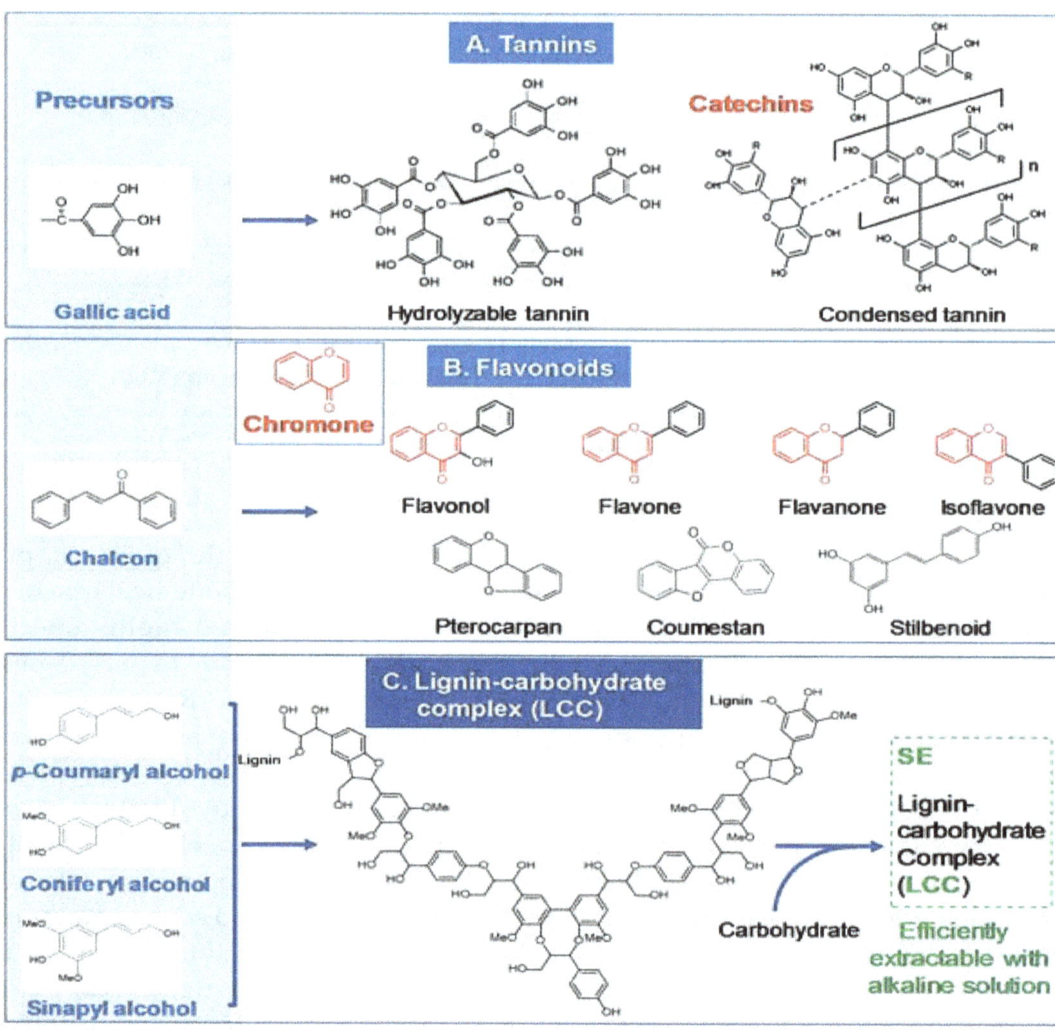

Figure 1. Three major polyphenols, that is tannins (**A**), flavonoids with or with backbone structure of chromone (**B**) and lignin-carbohydrate complex (LCC) (**C**), in the natural kingdom. Cited and modified from Reference [4] with permission.

Tannins are further classified into hydrolysable tannins (in which a polyalcohol is esterified with a galloyl, hexahydroxydiphenoyl, valoneoyl or dehydrohexahydroxydiphenoyl group) and condensed tannins (composed of catechin, epicatechin or their analogs) (Figure 1A) [5].

Flavonoids, synthesized from chalcones [6], are classified into flavonols, flavones, flavanones and isoflavones (that contain the chromone structure in the molecule), pterocarpan and coumestan (Figure 1B). Due to the recent development of separation technology [7,8], chemical structures and biological functions of thousands of tannins and flavonoids have been elucidated.

Lignin is formed by dehydrogenative polymerization of *p*-coumaryl, *p*-conifery and sinapyl alcohols and forms a complex with some polysaccharides (Figure 1C). Lignin-carbohydrate complex (LCC) has amorphous structure with very high molecular weight, thus making it difficult to determine the complete chemical structure, although it shows prominent anti-HIV activity [9]. Since LCC can be prepared by alkaline solution and acid-precipitation, it was not surprising that alkaline extract of the leaves of *Sasa* species (*Sasa* sp.) (SE) described later contains significant amount of LCC and shows several over-lapped biological activities with LCC.

It is generally accepted that improvement of oral functions by periodontal treatment [10], insertion of dentures and implants [11], oral hygiene [12], nutrition [13] and fluoride treatment [14] elevates the general health and quality of life [10,11]. Orally administered products directly contact the oral tissues or cells where they may exert their effects very fast, without being metabolizing and excretion [15], if they have a chance to bind to the target molecules or pattern-recognition receptors such as TLR2 (Toll-like receptor 2), TLR4, Dectin-1 (receptor for glucan) and Dectin-2 (receptor for LCC or mannan) in keratinocytes, macrophages, monocytes and dendritic cells [16]. This article reviews the recent progress of three major polyphenols (tannins, flavonoids and LCCs), chromone (backbone structure of flavonoids) and herbal extracts, glucosyltransferase inhibitor and angiotensin II blocker on dental diseases.

2. Chromone Derivatives as New Type of Anticancer Candidate

2.1. Most of Anticancer Drugs Show Severe Keratinocyte Toxicity

Development of anticancer drugs is shifting from classical anti-cancer drugs to molecular targeted therapeutic agents. However, the incidence of complete response in gastroesophageal cancer patients treated with targeted agents has been reported to be 2.0%, only 0.3 increase from the control arms [17]. ErbB receptor-targeting inhibitors failed to show any significant differences on overall response rate, clinical benefit rate and overall survival, with the increased risk of serious adverse events [18]. Likewise, cyclin-dependent kinase inhibitor combined with chemotherapy slightly increased the mean progression-free survival but also stimulated the senescence-associated (SA) marker expression (assessed by the accumulation of by SA β-galactosidase in the lysosome) by yet unknown mechanism [19]. This points out another unfavorable effect of targeted therapy, the resolution of which we have to find urgently.

Administration of anticancer agents has been reported to induce skin toxicity [20–26]. This prompted us to re-evaluate the cytotoxicity and tumor-specificity of anticancer drugs. We demonstrated for the first time that classical anticancer drugs (doxorubicin, daunorubicin, etoposide, mitomycin C, methotrexate, 5-fluorouracil, melphalan) and molecular targeted therapeutic drug (gefinitib) are highly toxic to epithelial normal cells (keratinocytes) as well as human oral squamous cell carcinoma (OSCC) cell lines. Tumor specificity (TS), determined with human normal oral epithelial cells *vs* OSCC cells (TS_E = 0.1 to 1.5) was usually one to two-orders lower than TS, determined with mesenchymal normal cells *vs* OSCC cells (TS_M = 3.8 to 92.9) [27] (Exp. 1, Table 1).

Also, doxorubicin induced apoptosis characterized by chromatin condensation, nuclear fragmentation and loss of cell surface microvilli) (A) and caspase-3 activation (cleavage of PARP and pro-caspase-3) (B) in human oral keratinocytes [27] (Figure 2). This urged us to survey many natural products which show lower keratinocyte toxicity.

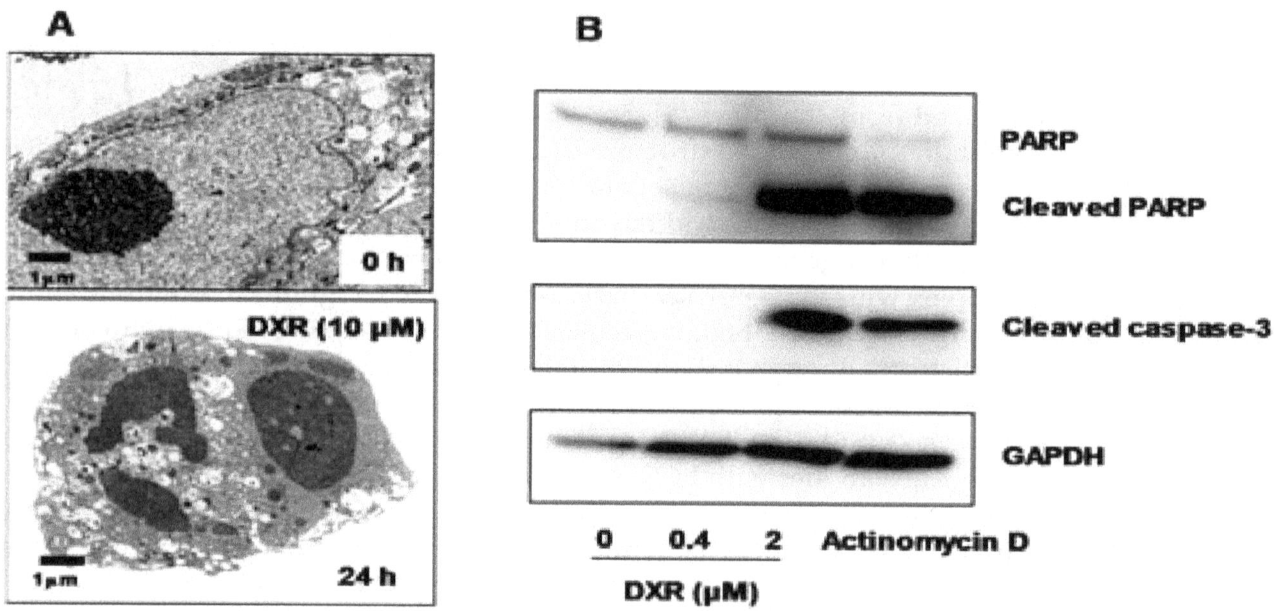

Figure 2. Doxorubicin induced apoptosis in human oral keratinocyte, demonstrated by transmission electron (**A**) and western blot analysis (**B**). Cited from Reference [27] with permission.

2.2. Limitations of Apoptosis-Oriented Research

Many studies have reported the apoptosis-inducing activity of tannins and flavonoids but have not tested for their toxicity to normal cells or tumor selectivity. We reevaluated the antitumor effect of various groups of natural products, based on the TS values determined as shown in the insert of Figure 3. As expected, anticancer drugs showed excellent tumor-specificity (TS_M, determined by the ratio of mean CC_{50} for human normal oral mesenchymal cells to that for human OSCC cell lines, indicated by red color). We found that one among14 poly-herbal formula extracts (supplied by Himalaya drug company) showed excellent tumor-specificity [28]. The active principle (s) are yet to be determined. It was surprising that the tumor selectivity of flavonoids, procyanidins, macrocyclic ellagitannins, hydrolysable tannins, catechins and gallic acid, which has been reported to induce apoptosis, was surprisingly low (TS_M = 1 to 5) (green color), as compared with anticancer agents. Similarly, antioxidants (vitamin C, chlorogenic acid, curcumin), ketones (α,β-unsaturated ketones, α-hydroxyketones, β-diketones, trifluoromethylketones, zulenequinones) and amides (pheylpropanoid amides, piperic acid amides, oleoylamides) showed lower TS_M values. On the other hand, the tumor selectivity of eight chromone derivatives (A–H) described later was relatively high (yellow color) (Figure 3).

2.3. Synthesis of Chromone Derivatives Having High Tumor-Specificity and Low Keratinocyte Toxicity

Chromone (4*H*-1-benzopyran-4-one) is a backbone structure of flavonols, flavones, flavanones and isoflavones [29] (Figure 1B). We synthesized eight classes of chromones derivatives (total 134 compounds): 3-styrylchromones (15 compounds) [30,31] (containing compound A), 3-benzylidenechromanones (17 compounds) [32] (containing compound B), 3-styryl-2*H*-chromenes (16 compounds) [33] (containing compound C), 2-azolylchromones (24 compounds) [34] (containing compound D), 3-(*N*-cyclicamino)chromones (15 compounds) [35] (containing compound E), 2-(*N*-cyclicamino)chromones (15 compounds) [36] (containing compound F), furo[2,3-*b*]chromones (12 compounds) [37] (containing compound G) and pyrano[4,3-*b*]chromones (20 compounds) [38] (containing compound H). The eight compounds that produced the highest TS value in each group are listed in Figure 4.

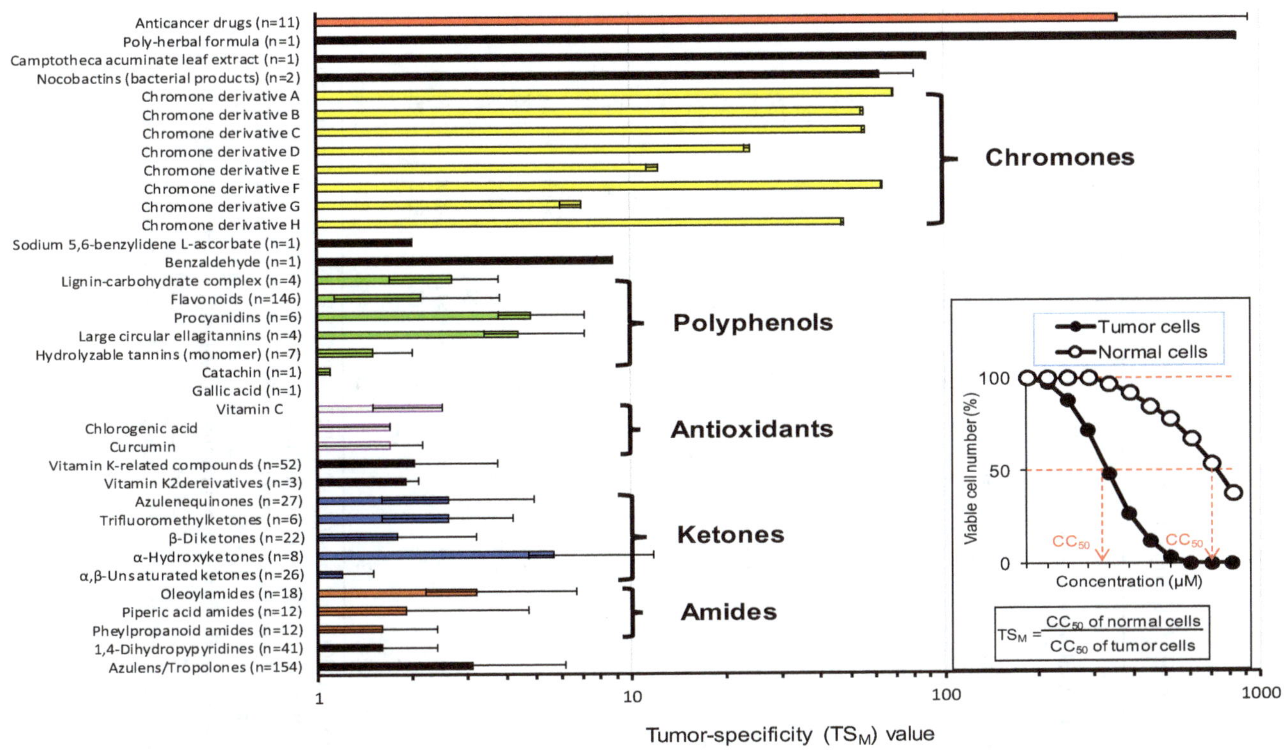

Figure 3. Chromone derivatives showed higher tumor-specificity (TS_M) value than most of the polyphenols. TS_M was determined by the following equation: TS_M = (mean CC_{50} for human OSCC cell lines/mean CC_{50} for human normal oral mesenchymal cells. Tumor and normal cells in the insert represent human OSCC cell lines and human normal oral mesenchymal cells. Data of chromones [30,32–38] and other compounds [4] were cited with permission. n, number of compounds tested.

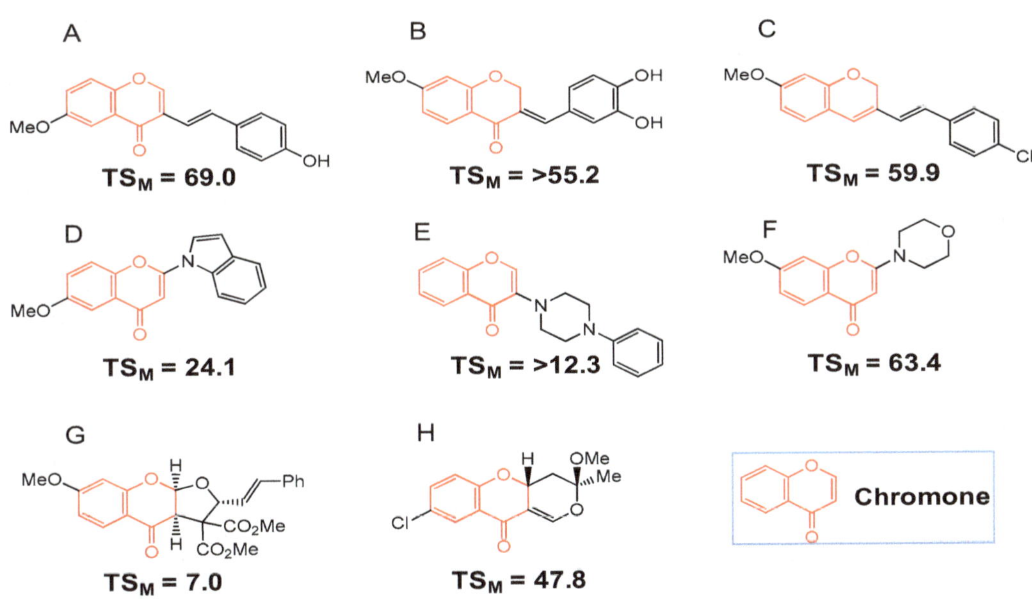

Figure 4. Compounds that showed the highest tumor-specificity (TS_M) values (determined with human OSCC and human oral mesenchymal cell) in eight groups of chromone derivatives. Structure and TS_M values of (**A**) that belongs to 3-styrylchromones [30], (**B**) that belongs to 3-benzylidenechromanones [32], (**C**) that belongs to 3-styryl-2*H*-chromenes [33], (**D**) that belongs to 2-azolylchromones [34], (**E**) that belongs to 3-(*N*-cyclicamino)chromones [35], (**F**) that belongs to 2-(*N*-cyclicamino)chromones [36], (**G**) that belongs to furo[2,3-*b*]chromones [37] and (**H**) that belongs to pyrano[4,3-*b*]chromones [38] were cited with permission.

Table 1. Comparison of keratinocyte toxicity between popular anticancer drugs (Exp. 1) and chromone derivatives (Exp. 2).

Compounds	CC_{50} (μM)												TS_M	TS_E	
	Human Oral Squamous Cell Carcinoma					Human Oral Normal Cells							Mes	Epi	
						Mesenchymal Cells				Epithelial Cells			vs	vs	
	Ca9-22	HSC-2	HSC-3	HSC-4	mean	HGF	HPLF	HPC	mean	HOK	HGEP	mean	OSCC	OSCC	Ref.
					(A)				(B)			(C)	(B/A)	(C/A)	
Exp. 1 Anticancer drugs:															
CPT	<0.06	<0.06	<0.06	<0.06	<0.06	200	10	146	119	0.3	3.9	2.1	**>1853**	**>33**	[27]
SN-38	<0.06	<0.06	<0.06	<0.06	<0.06	143	29	16	63	<0.075	1.5	<0.77	**>979**	**<12**	[27]
DXR	0.13	0.06	0.09	0.06	0.09	7.3	1.3	9.3	6.0	0.1	0.2	0.1	**69.9**	**1.7**	[27]
DNR	0.27	0.07	0.13	0.09	0.14	4.9	10.0	8.2	7.7	<0.004	0.4	<0.21	**54.6**	**<1.5**	[27]
ETP	11.3	3.0	2.7	2.5	4.9	351	500	500	450	1.8	3.2	2.5	**92.9**	**0.5**	[27]
MMC	3.97	0.36	0.14	0.78	1.31	22	65	34	40	0.10	0.28	0.19	**30.8**	**0.1**	[27]
MTX	9.0	0.2	<0.13	<0.13	<2.35	>400	>400	>400	>400	1000	<0.13	500	**>170**	**>212**	[27]
5-FU	15.3	100.3	186.3	92.7	98.7	1000	1000	1000	1000	11.7	14.2	12.9	**>10**	**0.1**	[27]
DOC	<0.03	<0.03	<0.03	<0.03	<0.03	70	100	91	87	0.12	0.03	0.08	**>2708**	**>2.4**	[27]
MEL	114.0	29.0	18.3	19.0	45.1	153	197	170	173	13.5	18.7	16.1	**3.8**	**0.4**	[27]
Gefitinib	18.0	22.3	15.7	13.7	17.4	58	68	83	70	3.5	4.1	3.8	**4.0**	**0.2**	[27]
Exp. 2 Chromone derivatives:															
A	2.1	1.0	3.6	1.2	2.0	67	74	272	138	19	>800	>410	**69.0**	**>205**	[30]
B	3.2	11.3			7.3	>400	>400		>400	3.8	3.3	3.6	**>55.2**	**0.5**	[32]
C	3.5	1.5	5.5	8.3	4.7	400	41	400	280	>400	>400	>400	**59.9**	**>85.1**	[33]
D	1.6	1.3			1.5	36	35		36				**24.1**		[34]
E	46.0	20.0	36.7	26.3	32.3	390	>400	>400	>397	>400		>400	**>12.3**	**>12.4**	[36]
F	9.1	6.0	3.7	3.1	5.5	244	>400	>400	>348	356		355.7	**63.4**	**65.2**	[35]
G	13.8		27.7	70.1	37.2	185	273	324	261				**7.0**		[37]
H	4.7	5.3			5.0	247	233		240	20		20	**47.8**	**4.1**	[38]

The mean of 50% cytotoxic concentration (CC_{50}) of each test compound for human oral squamous cell carcinoma (OSCC) cell lines (Ca9-22, HSC-2, HSC-3, HSC-4) (A) and human normal oral mesenchymal cells (human gingival fibroblast HGF, human periodontal ligament fibroblast HPLF, human pulp cell HPC) (B) and human normal oral epithelial cells (HOK, HGEP) (C) were determined after incubation for 48 h with various concentrations of them. Tumor-specificity (TS) for mesenchymal normal cells *vs* OSCC cells (TS_M) and that for epithelial normal cells *vs* OSCC (TS_E) was determined by the following equation: $TS_M = B/A$, $TS_E = C/A$. Structures of A–H (Exp. 2) that showed the highest tumor-specificity in each group are shown in Figure 4. A, (*E*)-3-(4-hydroxystyryl)-6-methoxy-4*H*-chromen-4-one; B, (3*E*)-2,3-dihydro-3-[(3,4-dihydroxyphenyl)methylene]-7-methoxy-4*H*-1-benzopyran-4-one; C, (*E*)-3-(4-cholorostyryl)-7-methoxy-2*H*-chromene; D, 2-(1*H*-indol-1-yl)-6-methoxy-4*H*-1-benzopyran-4-one; E, 2-(4-phenyl-1-piperazinyl)-4*H*-1-benzopyran-4-one; F, 7-methoxy-2-(4-morpholinyl)-4*H*-1-benzopyran-4-one; G, (2*R*,3*aR*,9*aR*)-rac-3*a*,9*a*-dihydro-7-methoxy-4-oxo-2-(2-phenylethenyl)-4*H*-furo[2,3-*b*][1]benzopyran-3,3(2*H*)-dicarboxylic acid 3,3-dimethyl ester; H, 8-chloro-4,4a-dihydro-3-methoxy-3-methyl-3*H*,10*H*-pyrano[4,3-*b*][1]benzopyran-10-one.

All compounds showed much higher cytotoxicity against human oral squamous cell carcinoma (OSCC) cell lines (Ca9-22, HSC-2, HSC-3, HSC-4) than against human normal oral mesenchymal cells (gingival fibroblast HGF, periodontal ligament fibroblast HPLF, pulp cell HPC). These compounds except for 3-benzylidenechromanones were 2.6~2000-fold less cytotoxic to human oral keratinocytes as compared with doxorubicin (Exp. 2, Table 1). We reported that 3-styrylchromones [30] and azolylchromones [34] induced apoptosis (caspase-3 activation) in human OSCC cell line. On the contrary, 7-methoxy-2-(4-morpholinyl)-4*H*-1-benzopyran-4-one, the most active compound among fifteen 2-(*N*-cyclicamino)chromone derivatives (structure depicted in Figure 4F) showed an excellent tumor-specificity (TS = 63.4) (Figure 5A), low keratinocyte toxicity (Table 1, Exp. 2), without induction of apoptosis in human OSCC cell line (HSC-2), as evidenced by the lack of caspase-3 activation (cleavage of PARP and procaspase-3) (Figure 5B) nor of the accumulation of subG_1 population (Figure 5C).

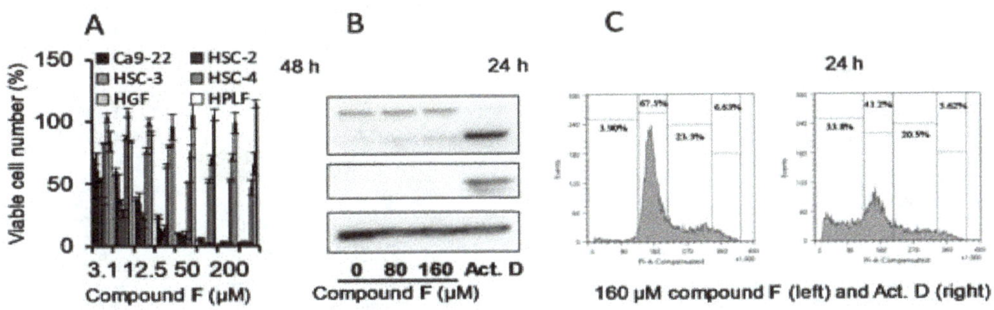

Figure 5. 7-Methoxy-2-(4-morpholinyl)-4*H*-1-benzopyran-4-one (Compound F, Figure 4F) showed higher cytotoxicity against human OSCC cell lines as compared with normal oral mesenchymal cells (**A**), without induction of caspase-3 activation (**B**) nor producing subG_1 cell population (**C**). Actinomycin (Act. D) (1 μM) was used as positive control. Cited from Reference [35] with permission.

In order to perform the QSAR analysis with each group of compounds, the 3D structure of each chemical structure was optimized by CORINA Classic (Molecular Networks GmbH, Nürnberg, Germany) with forcefield calculations (amber-10: EHT) in Molecular Operating Environment (MOE) version 2018.0101 (Chemical Computing Group Inc., Quebec, Canada). Approximately 3000 chemical descriptors were analyzed for their correlation with cytotoxicity against tumor cells (**T**) and normal cells (**N**) and tumor-specificity (**T–N**), suggesting that molecular shape is the most important determinant for tumor-specificity (Table 2). For example, we have reported previously that **T–N** of 3-styrylchromones can be estimated by diameter (largest value in the distance matrix defined by the elements Dij), vsurf_DD23 and R3 OH (n = 15, R^2 = 0.764, Q^2 = 0.570, s = 0.308) (right), according to the following equation: **T–N** = 0.607(± 0.169)diameter − 0.121 (± 0.035)vsurf_DD23 + 1.11 (± 0.235)R3OH − 7.17 (± 2.26) [30]. QSAR analysis can be applied to estimate the most potent chemical structures. By repeating the process of synthesis of the estimated structure and reconfirmation of its activity, more active compounds with defied structure will be manufactured.

Table 2. Top six chemical descriptors that showed the highest correlation to cytotoxicity to tumor cells (**T**) or normal cells (**N**) or tumor-specificity (**T–N**). Descriptors are explained in the footnote. Pink, molecular size; yellow, 3D shape; orange, topological shape; blue, electrostatic; green, lipophilicity.

	Category	Number of Descriptors Searched	T	N	T-N	Ref.
A	3-Styrylchromones		OMe at R1 OH at R3	vsurf_DD23 G1u	OH at R3 vsurf_DD23 G2u	[30]
B	3-Benzylidenechromanones	3134	RDF095i RDF095u RDF095e vsurf_IW6 vsurf_ID7 vsurf_ID1	Mor03v Mor03m Mor09m G1u Mor03p R3m+	Mor3m Mor03v SpMAD_AEA(dm) vsurf_HB7 R3m+ Mor25v	[32]

Table 2. *Cont.*

	Category	Number of Descriptors Searched	T	N	T-N	Ref.
C	3-Styryl-2*H*-chromenes	330	chi1v	std_dim2	std_dim3	[33]
			KierFlex	E_tor	BCUT_SLOGP_1	
			KierA1	E_oop	vsurf_D4	
			SMR_VSA7	std_dim3	vsurf_R	
			KierA3	vsurf_A	vsurf_D5	
			Weight	BCUT_SMR_1	E-oop	
D	2-Azolylchromones	3062	G3m	SpMin8_Bh(s)	Kp	[34]
			G3e	Q_RPC-	P1p	
			G3v	G3s	Mor32i	
			Gm	G3e	P2p	
			G3p	G3m	Mor32u	
			G3s	Gm	CATS2D_02_LL	
E	3-(*N*-Cyclicamino)chromones	3096	RDF075v	Mor28s	CATS3D_12_LL	[36]
			RDF075p	CATS3D_02_A	VE3sign_G	
			Mor06s	CATS2D_02_A	J_D/Dt	
			SpMAD_AEA(dm)	Inflammat-80	FCASA-	
			RDF090p	Depressant-80	CATS3D_11_LL	
			E3m	TDB05i	Chi_G/D	
F	2-(*N*-Cyclicamino)chromones	3089	SpPosA_B(m)	Mor32u	Mor22m	[35]
			SpPosA_B(e)	Mor32e	GCUT_SLOGP_1	
			GCUT_SLOGF	VR2_G/D	Mor17v	
			Mor17v	JGI4	Mor17m	
			Mor17m	VR2_G		
			VE1sign_B(v)	SPH		
G	Furo[2,3-*b*]chromones	2820	b_double	rsynth	b_double	[37]
			SlogP_VSA2	b_double	SlogP_VSA2	
			rsynth	SlogP_VSA2	rsynth	
			std_dim3	std_dim3	std_dim3	
			E_str	E_str	b_rotR	
			dens	dens	E_str	
H	Pyrano[4,3-*b*]chromones	3072	R8s	R6v+	R8s	[38]
			J_G	R1s	HATS7i	
			RDF055s	R4v	HATS3i	
			R7s	J_G	HATS3u	
			HATS7s	R4p	HATS7u	
			RTs	R3v+	Mor10i	

b_double: Number of double bonds. Aromatic bonds are not considered to be double bonds. b_rotR: Fraction of rotatable bonds; CATS2D_02_AL: CATS2D Acceptor-lipophilic at lag 02; CATS2D_02_LL: CATS2D Lipophilic-Lipophilic at lag 02; CATS3D_02_AL: CATS3D Acceptor-lipophilic BIN 02 (2.000-3.000Å); CATS3D_11_LL: CATS3D lipophilic-lipophilic BIN 11 (11.000-12.000Å); CATS3D_12_LL: CATS3D Lipophilic-Lipophilic BIN 12 (12.000-13.000Å); Chi_G/D: Randic-like index from distance/distance matrix; chi1v: atomic valence connectivity index; dens: Mass density: molecular weight divided by van der Waal's volume; Depressant-80: Ghose-Viswanadhan-Wendoloski antidepressant-like index at 80%; E3m: 3rd component accessibility directional WHIM index/weighted by mass; E_oop: out-of-plane potential energy; E_str: Bond stretch potential energy; E_tor: torsion potential energy; FCASA-: Fractional CASA-(negative charge weighted surface area, ASA-times max { qi<0 }) calculated as CASA-/accessible surface area; GCUT_SLOGP_1: The GCUT descriptors using atomic contribution to logP (using the Wildman and Crippen SlogP method); Gm: total symmetry index/weighted by mass; G1u: (the first component symmetry directional WHIM index/unweighted encoding molecular symmetry that extracts the global symmetry information; G2u: (the second component symmetry directional WHIM index/unweighted encoding molecular symmetry that extracts the global symmetry information; G3e: 3rd component symmetry directional WHIM index/weighted by Sanderson electronegativity; G3m: 3rd component symmetry directional WHIM index/weighted by mass; G3p: 3rd component symmetry directional WHIM index/weighted by polarizability; G3s: 3rd component symmetry directional WHIM index/weighted by I-state; G3v: 3rd component symmetry directional WHIM index/weighted by van der Waals volume; HATS3i: Leverage-weighted autocorrelation of lag 3/weighted by ionization potential; HATS3u: Leverage-weighted autocorrelation of lag 3/unweighted; HATS7i: Leverage-weighted autocorrelation of lag 7/weighted by ionization potential; HATS7s: Leverage-weighted autocorrelation of lag 7/weighted by I-state; HATS7u: Leverage-weighted autocorrelation of lag 7/unweighted; Inflammat-80: Ghose-Viswanadhan-Wendoloski anti-inflammatory-like index at 80%; J_D/Dt: Balaban-like index from distance/detour matrix; J_G: Balaban-like index from geometrical matrix; JGI4: Mean topological charge index of order 4; KierA1: First alpha modified shape index; KierA3: Third alpha modified shape index; KierFlex: Kier molecular flexibility index; Kp: K global shape index/weighted by polarizability; Mor03m: signal 03/weighted by mass; Mor03p: signal 03/weighted by polarizability; Mor03v: signal 03/weighted by van der Waals volume; Mor06s: Signal 06/weighted by I-state; Mor09m: signal 09/weighted by mass; Mor10i: Signal 10/weighted by ionization potential; Mor17m: Signal 17/weighted by mass; Mor17v: Signal 17/weighted by van der Waals volume; Mor22m: Signal 22/weighted by mass; Mor25v: signal 25/weighted by van der Waals volume; Mor28s: Signal 28/weighted by I-state; Mor32e: Signal 32/weighted by Sanderson electronegativity; Mor32i: signal 32/weighted by ionization potential in 3D-MoRSE descriptors; Mor32u: signal 32/unweighted in 3D-MoRSE descriptors; OMe at R1: methoxy substitution at the 6-position on the chromone ring group; OH at R3: 4′-hydroxy substitution in the phenyl group of styryl moiety; P1p: 1st component shape directional WHIM index/weighted by polarizability; P2p: 2nd component shape directional WHIM index/weighted by polarizability;Q_RPC-: Relative negative partial charge: the smallest negative partial charge atom i divided by the sum of the negative partial charge atom i; RDF055s: Radial Distribution Function- 055/weighted by I-state; RDF075p: Radial distribution function-075/weighted by polarizability; RDF075v: Radial distribution function-075/weighted by van der Waal's volume RDF; RDF090p: Radial distribution function-090/weighted by polarizability;RDF095i: Radial Distribution Function - 095/weighted by ionization potential;

RDF095u: Radial Distribution Function - 095/unweighted; RDF095e: Radial Distribution Function - 095/weighted by Sanderson electronegativity; rsynth: The synthetic reasonableness or feasibility, of the chemical structure; RTs: R total index/weighted by I-state; R1s: R autocorrelation of lag 1/weighted by I-state; R3m+: R maximal autocorrelation of lag 3/weighted by mass; R3v+: R maximal autocorrelation of lag 3/weighted by van der Waals volume; R4p: R autocorrelation of lag 4/weighted by polarizability; R4v: R autocorrelation of lag 4/weighted by van der Waals volume; R6v+: R maximal autocorrelation of lag 6/weighted by van der Waals volume; R7s: R autocorrelation of lag 7/weighted by I-state; R8s: R autocorrelation of lag 8/weighted by I-state; SCUT_SLOGP_1: using atomic contribution to logP1; SCUt_SMR_1: using atomic contribution to molar refractivity1; SlogP_VSA2: Sum of approximate accessible van der Waal's surface area i such that logP for atom i is from −0.2 to 0; SMR_VSA7: sum of vi such that Ri > 0.56; SPH: Spherosity; SpMAD_AEA: Spectral mean absolute deviation from augmented edge adjacency matrix weighted by dipole moment edge adjacency indices; SpPosA_B(e): Normalized spectral positive sum from Burden matrix weighted by Sanderson electronegativity; SpPosA_B(m): Normalized spectral positive sum from Burden matrix weighted by mass; SpMin8_Bh(s): Smallest eigenvalue n. 8 of Burden matrix weighted by I-state; std_dim2, std_dim3: standard dimension 2 or 3 that depend on the structure connectivity and conformation; TDB05i: 3D Topological distance based descriptors-lag 5 weighted by ionization potential; VE1sign_B(v): Coefficient sum of the last eigenvector from Burden matrix weighted by van der Waals volume; VE3sign_G: logarithmic coefficient sum of the last eigenvector from geometrical matrix; VR2_G: Normalized Randic-like eigenvector-based index from geometrical matrix; VR2_G/D: Normalized Randic-like eigenvector-based index from distance/distance matrix; vsurf_A: amphiphilic moment; vsurf_D4: hydrophobic volume 4; vsurf_D5: hydrophobic volume 5; vsurf_DD23: the interaction with hydrophobic probe assumed surrounding the molecule; vsurf_HB7: H-bond donor capacity 7; vsurf_ID1: Hydrophobic interaction-energy moment 1; vsurf_IW6: Hydrophilic interaction-energy moment 6; vsurf_ID7: Hydrophobic interaction-energy moment 7; vsurf_R: surface rugosity; Weight: molecular weight.

Metabolomic analysis is powerful to determine the early event of cell death induction process. We have reported that compoun. A (which induced apoptosis) increased the intracellular levels of diethanolamine and CDP-choline and reduced that of choline, suggesting the down-regulation of the glycerophospholipid pathway [31]. It remains to be determined which metabolic pathway is first affected at early stages after treatment with compound F (which did not induce apoptosis).

3. Catechins as Inhibitors of Glucosyltransferase

3.1. Classification of Oral Streptococcal GTF Enzymes

Dental plaque is the oral biofilm that consists of bacteria themselves and bacterial metabolites. Glucan, polymer of glucose, is one of the metabolically-produced polysaccharides as the basic structures of the dental plaque and is produced from sucrose by glucosyltransferase enzymes (GTFs). Since dental plaque is a fertile ground of the pathogenic bacteria and virus that cause oral disease such as stomatitis, dental caries, gingivitis and periodontitis, glucan and/or GTFs are the pathogen of those diseases. These GTFs are produced mainly by streptococci in oral cavity [39,40].

Oral streptococcal GTFs (EC: 2.4.1.5) [41] are encoded by *gtf* genes, belong to the glycosyl hydrolase family 70 and basically catalyze the transfer of D-glucopyranosyl units from sucrose to acceptor molecules [42]. Biochemically, GTFs are classified into mainly 2 types according to their products, water-soluble glucan (WSG) and water-insoluble glucan (WIG), main components of oral biofilm. Especially in *Streptococcus mutans (S. mutans)*, GTFB, water-insoluble glucan synthesizing glucosyltransferase enzyme is one of virulence factors for dental caries, because water-insoluble glucan plays an important role in adhesion and establishment of *S. mutans* on tooth surface [43–45].

To clarify the ancestry of streptococcal GTFs, we investigated the distribution of GTFs among bacteria, such as *Lactobacillus*, *Leuconostoc* and *Lactococcus* and phylogenetically analyzed glycosyl hydrolase family 70 enzymes [46]. The sequences of glycosyl hydrolase family 70 proteins used in this study were obtained from GenBank at NCBI (http://www.ncbi.nlm.nih.gov/) with reference to Pfam (http://pfam.sanger.ac.uk/). Sequence alignment was performed using ClustalW software version 1.83 [47] (http://clustalw.ddbj.nig.ac.jp/index.php?, DNA Data Bank of Japan, Mishima, Japan). Multiple alignment files saved by ClustalW in Clustal format were converted to MEGA format with the MEGA version 5 software [48] (http://www.megasoftware.net/). Phylogenetic analysis was performed by the maximum parsimony methods using MEGA version 4.0 software. We analyzed 20 glucosyltransferases from *Streptococcus*; 2 glucosyltransferases, 9 dextran sucrases and 1 alternan sucrase from *Leuconostoc*; 10 glucan sucrases from *Lactobacillus*; and 1 glucosyltransferases from *Lactococcus*. PspA, glucosyltransferases from *Lactococcus* was defined as the convenient ancestor in this analysis (Figure 6) [46].

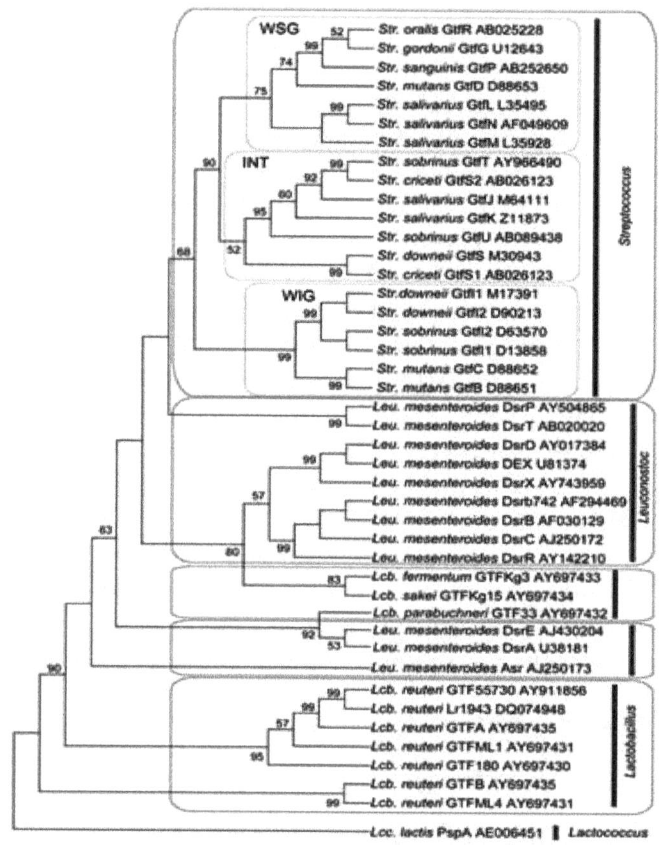

Figure 6. Phylogenetic analysis of glycosyl hydrolase family 70 enzymes by amino acid sequence. Cited from Reference [46] with permission.

The accession numbers in NCBI of these glycosyl hydrolases are provided after species and enzyme name in Figure 6. Here, we have shown that enzymes in the lower part of the phylogenetic tree synthesize glucans with various linkage types such as α-1,3; α-1,6; α-1,2; and α-1,4, while those in the upper part of the tree synthesize only water-soluble α-1,6-linked glucans. The phylogenetic tree would suggest that the streptococcal GTFs were derived from other lactic acid bacteria following their spread through the genera in the order of *Lactococcus*, *Lactobacillus*, *Leuconostoc* and *Streptococcus* and that the streptococcal GTF family can be phylogenetically classified into 3 clusters: the water-soluble glucan-synthesizing group (WSG), the water-insoluble glucan synthesizing group (WIG) and the intermediate group (INT).

A phylogenetic tree was constructed using the maximum parsimony (MP) method. The value on each branch is the estimated confidence limit (expressed as a percentage) for the position of the branches, as determined by bootstrap analysis. Only values exceeding 50% are shown. [46]

3.2. *Purification of GTF Enzymes*

Streptococcal GTFs can be divided into 2 types, WIG- and WIG- synthesizing GTFs by glucan product. Native WIG-synthesizing GTF, for example, GTFB and GTFC was purified from *S. mutans* MT8148, cultured in TTY medium [49,50]. The bacteria were collected by centrifugation and the cell-associated GTF (CA-GTF) was extracted by 8 M urea. The extract was precipitated by 60% saturated ammonium sulfate, applied to a DEAE Sepharose FF and eluted with a linear gradient of 0 to 1.0 M NaCl in the same buffer. Active fractions measured were concentrated by ammonium sulfate precipitation and then applied to a Bio-Scale CHT10-I column and then eluted with a 10 to 500 mM potassium phosphate buffer (KPB) linear gradient [51]. To select the GTFB and GTFC fractions, we carried out glucan synthesis assay [52], ELISA using anti-CA-GTF antibody, SDS-PAGE and Western blot using anti-GTF-I (GTFB) monoclonal antibody and anti-GTF-SI (GTFC) monoclonal antibody (Figure 7) [49].

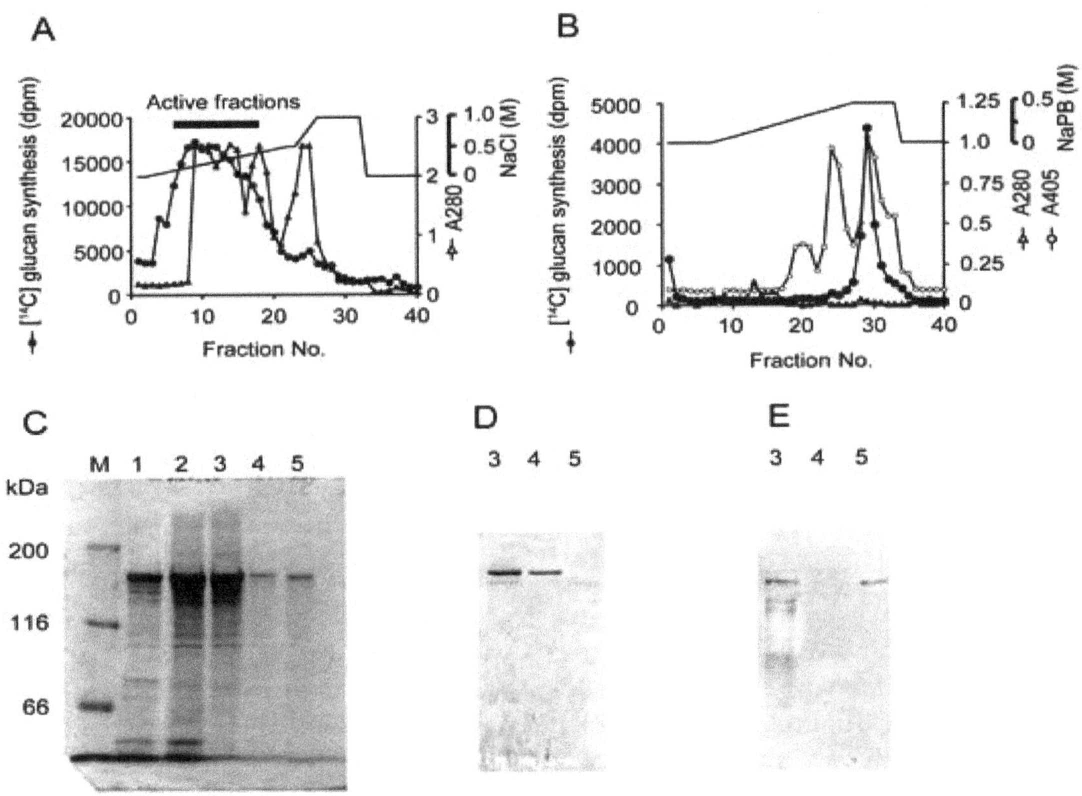

Figure 7. Purification of GTFB and GTFC from *S. mutans* MT8148, by sequential chromatography on. DEAE Sepharose FF column (collecting No. 6 to No. 17 fractions) (**A**) and Bio-Scale CHT10-I column (collecting No.29 and No.24 fraction as purified GTFB and GTFC, respectively) (**B**). The sample in each purification step was separated by SDS-PAGE (**C**) and assessed with Western blot analyses using anti-GTF-I (**D**), anti-GTF-SI (**E**) antiserum. Lane M, molecular weight marker; 1, 8 M-urea extraction; 2, precipitant of 1 by ammonium sulfate; 3, GTF-active fraction eluted with DEAE Sepharose column; 4, No. 29 fraction eluted with CHT10-I column; No. 24 fraction eluted with CHT10-I column. Cited from Reference [49] with permission.

Native WSG-synthesizing GTF, for example, GTFR was purified from *Streptococcus oralis* (*S. oralis*) ATCC 10557 [53], cultured in dialyzed TTY medium [50]. The culture supernatant was precipitated by 60% saturated ammonium sulfate and then applied to a Q Sepharose FF column and eluted with a linear gradient of 0 to 1.0 M NaCl [51]. Active fractions (indicated by bars) were pooled, applied to a Bio-Scale CHT10-I column and then eluted with a 10 to 500 mM KPB linear gradient [51]. To select the GTFR, the glucan synthesis assay and SDS-PAGE were carried out (Figure 8) [53].

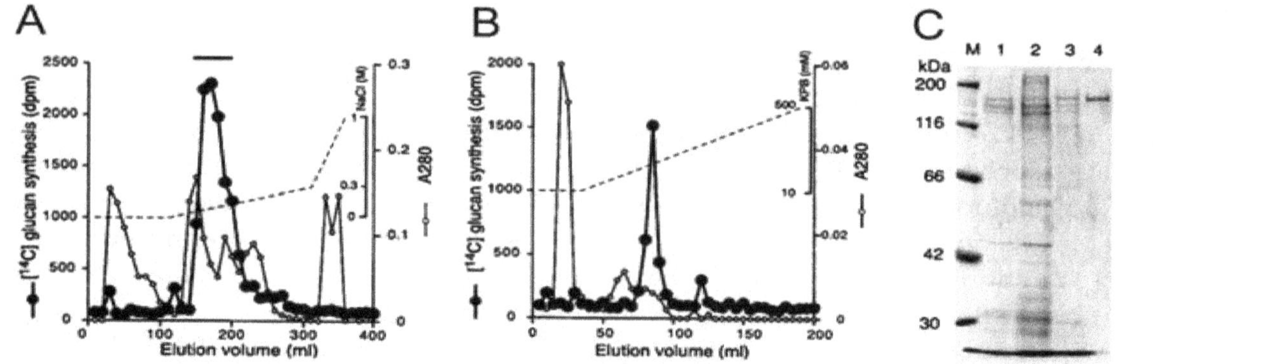

Figure 8. Purification of GTFR from *Streptococcus oralis* (*S. oralis*) ATCC 10557 by sequential chromatography on a Q Sepharose FF column (eluted with a linear gradient of 0 to 0.3 M NaCl) (**A**) and Bio-Scale CHT10-I column (**B**). Elution was done with a 10 to 500 mM KPB linear gradient. (**C**) SDS-PAGE of GTase preparations at different stages of purification. Lanes: 1, culture supernatant; 2, ammonium sulfate precipitate; 3, pooled active fractions from Q-ion-exchange chromatography; 4, pooled active fraction from CHT-10 hydroxylapatite chromatography; M, molecular mass markers. Cited from Reference [53] with permission.

In summary, purification of oral streptococcal GTFs would be commonly carried out by three steps method, ammonium sulfate precipitation, ion-exchange chromatography and hydroxyapatite chromatography [54–58]. Recombinant GTF (rGTF) would be produced as the other approach of GTF preparation using expression vector [59–63]. rGTF would be purified by ammonium sulfate precipitation, chromatography using His-tag and so on. These native and/or recombinant GTFs were used for the suppression analysis of glucan production by inhibitor and the recovery analysis of biofilm formation by addition of GTF. For these reasons, preparation of oral streptococcal GTFs would be important in the study of prevention of oral infectious diseases such as dental caries, periodontitis and so on.

3.3. Inhibitors of Oral Streptococcal GTFs

In GTFR from *S. oralis*, some inorganic salts suppressed the synthesis of water-soluble glucan. The synthesis of water-soluble glucan was reduced especially by divalent cation. Therefore, divalent cation could be inhibitors. However, in water-insoluble GTF from *Streptococcus sobrinus* 6715, high concentrations of monovalent (above 100 mM) and divalent (above 20 mM) cations stimulated the formation of insoluble glucan, whereas lower concentrations of monovalent (below 10 mM) and divalent (below 1 mM) cations reduced the formation of insoluble glucan to a negligible amount [64]. Thus, it would be difficult to adopt inorganic salts an inhibitor of oral streptococcal GTFs, considering their opposing actions between high and low concentrations.

It has been well known that natural products, for example, hydrolysable tannins (gallotannin, ellagitannin), condensed tannins (proanthocyanin, catechins), complex tannins, as from plant origin such as green tea, Oolong tea, cocoa, coffee and traditional Chinese medicine, inhibit glucan synthesis of oral streptococcal GTFs [65–71]. Especially, polyphenol mixtures from Oolong tea or cacao beans among them inhibited glucan-synthesis activity of GTFs from *S. mutans*. For example, OTF6, one of polyphenol fraction extracted from Oolong tea inhibited glucan-synthesis activity of rGTFB, rGTFC and rGTFD (Figure 9) [72]. With the increase of substrate of GTF, the production of glucan reached the plateau (near saturation) level. Even if the substrate concentration is enough, OTF6 effectively inhibited the production of glucan, suggesting its application to the dental plaque and caries. Since they can be inhibitors against other diseases, for example, stomatitis, periodontitis and aspiration pneumonia, they are expected to inhibit the formation of various glucan-biofilm, which contains some pathogenic organisms [73].

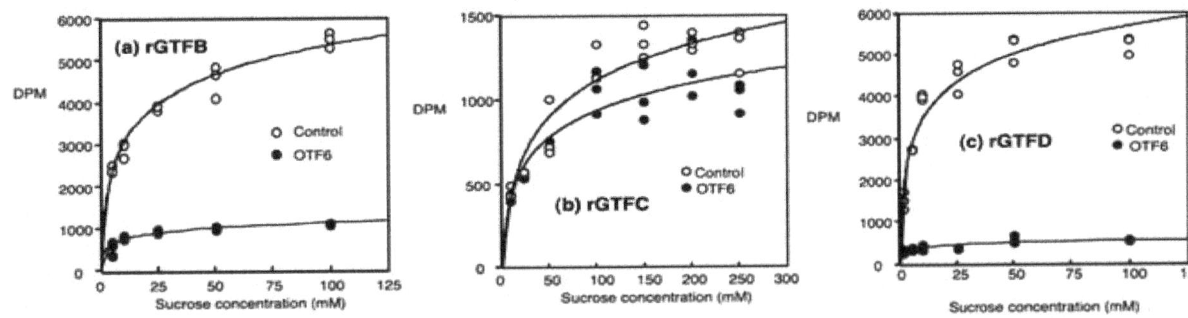

Figure 9. Changes in the quantity of glucan produced by recombinant GTFs. GTF activity was measured with [14C-glucose] sucrose. The OTF6 concentration in all displayed data was 1.0 mg/mL. Data are given in counts per minute. GTFs and sucrose were reacted without (○) and with (●) OTF6. Cited from Reference [72] with permission.

Nearly half of the commensal bacterial population of the human body is present in the oral cavity. An increase in the number of oral microorganisms may produce infective endocarditis, aspiration pneumonia and oral infections. When hydroxypropylcellulose strips containing green tea catechin were applied once a week for 8 weeks in pockets as a slow release local delivery system, the patient's periodontal status was significantly improved [74]. Gel-entrapped catechin (GEC) was manufactured by mixing catechins (epigallocatechin, epigallocatechin gallate, epicatechin, epicatechin gallate, gallocatechin, catechin and gallocatechin gallate) with polysaccharide, dextrin, citric acid, potassium chloride and stevia, to maintain the moistness in the oral cavity of elderly patients. GEC inhibited the growth of the Actinomyces, periodontopathic bacteria and Candida strains, possibly due to the produced hydrogen peroxide [75]. Local treatment of GEC seems to be important, since orally-administered catechin have been reported to increase the blood mitochondrial heme amounts and catalase activity, that may neutralize the antimicrobial activity of GEC [76].

4. Lignin-Carbohydrate Complex (LCC) as Anti-HIV Resources of the Natural Kingdom

We have previously reported anti-HV activity of three major polyphenols, tannins, flavonoids and lignin-carbohydrate complex (LCC), that were purified by our group. The potency of anti-HIV activity (SI) was calculated from the following equation: SI = CC_{50}/EC_{50}, where the CC_{50} is the concentration that reduced the viable cell number of the uninfected cells by 50% and the EC_{50} is the concentration that increased the viable cell number of the HIV-infected cells up to 50% that of the control (mock-infected, untreated) cells. Among them, LCC from pine cones of *Pinus parviflora* Sieb. et Zucc, pine cone of *Pinus elliottii var.* Elliottii, pine seed shell of *Pinus parviflora* Sieb. et Zucc, bark of *Erythroxylum catuaba* Arr. Cam, husk and mass of cacao beans of Theobroma, *Lentinus edodes* mycelia extract (L·E·M) and from precipitating fiber fraction of mulberry juice [77–84] showed the highest value (SI = 14, 28, 12, 43, 311, 46, 94 and 7), although much lower than that of popular anti-IIV agents (dextran sulfate, curdlan sulfate, azidothymidine, 2′,3′-dideoxycytidine) (SI = 2956 to 23261) (Table 3). Lignin but not carbohydrate moiety, seems to be essential to exert the anti-HIV activity, since synthetic lignin, manufactured by dehydrogenation polymerization of phenylpropenoids showed the comparable anti-HIV activity [85], whereas neutral and uronic acid-containing polysaccharides were inactive (SI = 1) [86]. We also found that monomer of phenylpropanoid monomers (*p*-coumaric acid, ferulic acid, caffeic acid) were inactive (SI < 1) [85], suggesting the importance of higher-ordered complicated structures for anti-HIV activity induction.

On the other hand, both hydrolysable and condensed tannins (see Figure 1A for classification) [87] (SI = 1.8 to 7.3 and 1.1) and flavonoids (Figure 1B) [88] (SI = 1.5) showed much lower anti-HIV activity. It is noted that anti-HIV activity of hydrolysable tannins increased with degree of polymerization: monomer (SI = 1.8) < dimer (SI = 2.3) < timer (SI = 3.4) < tetramer (SI = 7.3) [87].

Table 3. Anti-HIV activity of natural products.

Samples	Anti-HIV activity (SI)	Ref.
Lignin-carbohydrate complex		
Pine cone of *Pinus parviflora* Sieb. et Zucc	14	[77]
Pine cone of *Pinus elliottii* var. Elliottii	28	[78]
Pine seed shell of *Pinus parviflora* Sieb. et Zucc	12	[79]
Bark of *Erythroxylum catuaba* Arr. Cam.	43	[80]
Husk of cacao beans of Theobroma	311	[81]
Mass of cacao beans of Theobroma	46	[82]
Lentinus edodes mycelia extract (L·E·M)	94	[83]
Precipitating fiber fraction of mulberry juice	7	[84]
Dehydrogenation polymers of phenylpropenoids (n = 23)	105	[85]
Polysaccharides		
Neutral polysaccharides of pine cone of *P. parviflora* Sieb. et Zucc	1	[86]
Uronic acid-containing polysaccharides of pine cone	1	[86]
Lower molecular weight polyphenols		
Hydrolysable tannins (monomer) (MW: 484–1255) (n = 21)	1.8 ± 2.8	[87]
Hydrolysable tannins (dimer) (MW: 1571–2282) (n = 39)	2.3 ± 3.2	[87]
Hydrolysable tannins (trimer) (MW: 2354–2658) (n = 4)	3.4 ± 3.7	[87]
Hydrolysable tannins (tetramer) (MW: 3138–3745) (n = 3)	7.3 ± 6.5	[87]
Condensed tannins (MW: 290–1764) (n = 8)	1.1 ± 0.4	[87]
Flavonoids (MW: 84–648) (n = 92)	1.5 ± 1. 9	[88]
Herb extracts		
Green tea leaves — Hot water extraction		[89]
Alkaline extraction	3	
Oolong tea leaves — Hot water extraction	<0.033	[89]
Alkaline extraction	13	
Orange flower — Hot water extraction	<0.5	[89]
Alkaline extraction	>15	
Licorice root — Hot water extraction	4	[90]
Alkaline extraction	42	
Alkaline extract of leaves of *Sasa* sp.	86	[86]
Kampo medicines (n = 10)	1.0 ± 0.0	[91]
Constituent plant extracts of Kampo medicines (n = 25)	1.3 ± 0.8	[91]
Chromones		
(*E*)-3-(4-Hydroxystyryl)- 6-methoxy-4*H*-chromen-4-one	<1	[30]
(*E*)-3-(4-Chlorostyryl)-7-methoxy-2*H*-chromene	<1	[30]
Positive Controls		
Dextran sulfate (molecular mass, 5 kDa)	2956	
Curdlan sulfate (molecular mass, 79 kDa)	11718	
Azidothymidine	23261	
2′,3′-Dideoxycytidine (ddC)	2974	

Alkaline extraction of green tea leaves, oolong tea leaves, orange flower, licorice root was more efficient than hot water extraction to recover the anti-HIV substances: SI = 3 *vs* < 0.022; 13 *vs* < 0.033; > 15 *vs* < 0.5; 42 *vs* 4, respectively [89,90]. Likewise, alkaline extract of leaves of *Sasa* sp. showed much higher anti-HIV activity (SI = 86) than Japanese traditional medicines, Kampo (SI = 1.0) and constituent plant extracts (SI = 1.3) [91]. Chromone, such (*E*)-3-(4-hydroxystyryl)-6-methoxy-4*H*-chromen-4-one and (*E*)-3-(4-Chlorostyryl)-7-methoxy-2*H*-chromene were inactive [30] (Table 3).

5. Alkaline Extract of the Leaves of *Sasa* sp. (SE)

5.1. *Prominent Anti-HIV, Anti-UV, Anti-Inflammation and Neuroprotective Activities (in vitro)*

Although alkaline extracts of plants showed much higher anti-HIV activity than corresponding hot water extracts [86,89–91], only three papers from other groups have reported the anti-angiogenic and neuroprotective activity of alkaline extracts [92–94]. Also, only two papers have been published on the isolation and fractionation of lignin from bamboo, however, they reported no data of biological activity [95,96]. Based on these backgrounds, we reviewed mostly our research topics of SE.

Alkaline extract of the leaves of *Sasa* sp. (SE) is an over-the counter (OTC) drug in Japan, which is available in the drug store without the prescription of doctors. SE (dry weight: 58.8 mg/mL) contains Fe (II)-chlorophyllin, LCC and its degradation products and so forth. SE showed higher anti-HIV [86], anti-UV [97,98], anti-inflammatory [99] and neuroprotection activities [100], as compared with other lower molecular polyphenols (Table 4). SE has many good partners for exerting synergistic actions: anti-HIV activity with azidothymidine, 2′,3′-dideoxycytidine, dextran sulfate or curdlan sulfate [101]; anti-HSV activity with acyclovir [101], anti-bacterial activity with isopropyl methylphenol [102] and anti-UV activity [103] and radical scavenging activity with vitamin C [104]. SE also showed osteogenic activity [105].

Among three SE products, produc. A (100% pure SE that contains Fe(II)-chlorophyllin) showed 1~5-fold higher anti-HIV, anti-UV and hydroxyl radical scavenging activity and 3~7-fold lower CYP3A4 inhibitory activity than product B (contain Cu(II)-chlorophyllin and less LCC) and product C (product B further supplemented with ginseng and *Pinus densiflora* leaf extracts) [106]. Based on this finding, we used produc. A for the following studies and manufacturing the toothpaste.

Table 4. SE shows prominent anti-HIV, anti-UV, anti-inflammation and neuroprotective activities.

Samples *(Target cells)*	**Anti-HIV** (T-cell leukemia)	**Anti-UV** (HSC-2)	**Anti-Inflammation** (HPLF)	**Neuroprotection** (Differentiated PC12)
Evaluated by	CC_{50}/EC_{50} (+HIV)	CC_{50}/EC_{50}(+UV)	CC_{50}/EC_{50}(+IL-1β)	CC_{50}/EC_{50}(+A$\beta_{25\text{-}35}$)
SE	86	38.5	>96.8	56.8
Curcumin		<1.0	1.5	17.3
Gallic acid	<1.0	5.4	0.9	
Ferulic acid	<1.0		>2.9	
p-Coumaric acid	<1.0		>3.1	
EGCG	<1.0	7.7		10.7
Resveratrol		<1.0		<1.0
Rikkosan	<1.0	24.1	>4.3	
Hangesyashinto	<1.0	>4.9	285	
Glycyrrhiza	<1.0	4.3	59	
Ref.	[84]	[97,98]	[99]	[100]

5.2. Improvement of Lichenoid Dysplasia by SE

Oral *lichen planus* is a chronic mucocutaneous disease that affects tongue and oral mucosa, characterized by white lacy streaks on the mucosa or as smaller papules. The cause of lichen planus is not known. A biopsy was taken from a 43-year-old male patient and diagnosed as lichenoid dysplasia in 7 July 7 2003 (physician in charge: Dr. K. Mori). Treatment with vitamin B_1 improved the patient's symptoms but discontinuation of the treatment resulted in the disease recurrence. The patient was subjected to the SE treatment for 11 months (12 April 2011 until 12 March 2012), according to the guideline of Intramural Ethic Committee (no. A0901). The patient was orally administered 13.3 ml SE (diluted two-fold with water, thus containing 33 mg dried materials/mL) three times-a-day, 30 min before each meal. At each administration, the patient swallowed and retained SE in the oral cavity for 1 min before washing it down. The patient did not take any other medications during the treatment period. The patient's oral cavity was photographed with a digital camera and the total saliva was collected just before lunch and then every two weeks, after the start of SE administration.

When a patient had been treated for 12 months with SE, white areas of lacy streaks in the several areas of buccal mucosa progressively reduced (Figure 10A). Oral intake of SE also improved the patient's symptoms of pollen allergy and loose teeth, giving an impression that the oral mucosa became much tighter. Three weeks after treatment, uneven, rough and cut mucosa became much smoother. At four weeks, the rough mucosa was narrowed into a smaller area and the patient could eat without any pungent feeling on the oral mucosa. SE treatment reduced the salivary concentration of IL-6 from 0.052 $\pm$ 0.030 ng/mL (n = 5) to 0.01 ng/mL and that of IL-8 from 5.25 $\pm$ 1.06 ng/mL (n = 5) to 1.11 ng/mL [107].

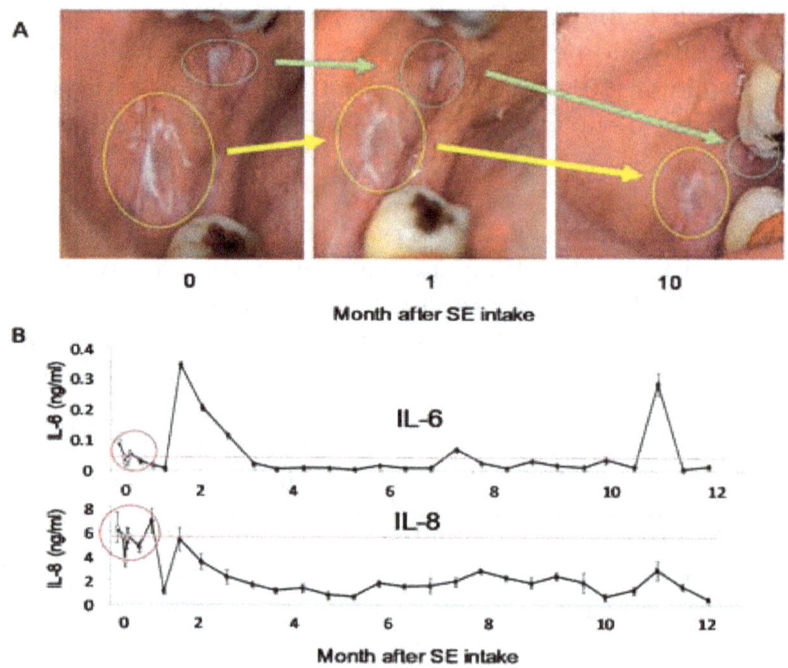

Figure 10. Effect of SE treatment on the oral lichenoid dysplasia. (**A**) Oral inspection with a digital camera, (**B**) salivary IL-6 and IL-8 concentrations. Cited from Reference [107] with permission.

5.3. Anti-Oxidative Stress Effect of SE in Chronic Dialysis Patients

With the cooperation of 10 maintenance dialysis patients in Masuko Memorial Hospital for 2 years from 2000, clinical data of SE were accumulated (Figure 11A–E).

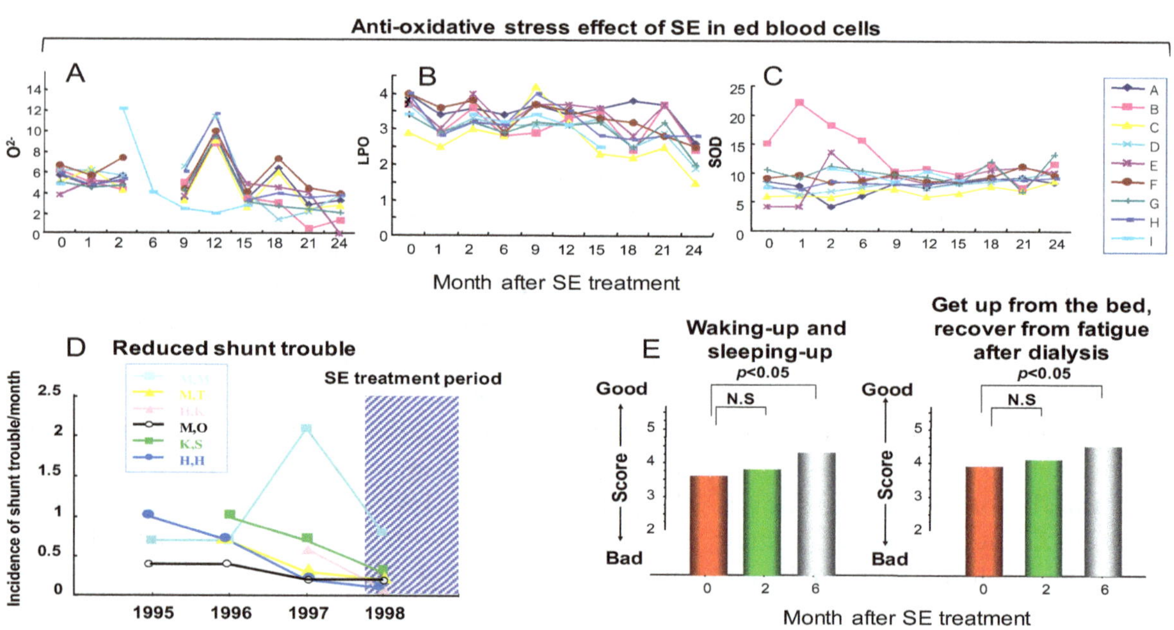

Figure 11. Anti-oxidative stress effects on chronic dialysis patients. (**A**) Superoxide (O^{2-}) (measured by luciferin chemiluminescence method), (**B**) LPO (measured by HPLC), (**C**) SOD activity (xanthine · xanthine oxidase reaction) of red blood cells. (**D**) Incidence of shunt problem from 1996–1998. Patients were treated with SE after 1 November 1997. (**E**) Questionnaire about the clinical effect of SE. Cited from Reference [108] with permission.

By treatment with SE, superoxide (O^{2-}) was gradually declined. Although the drift was seen in the middle of 12 months, possibly due to the measuring problem with instruments and after

24 months, cases exceeding the initial level were not observed (A). Likewise, LPO showed a decreasing tendency, possibly due to the elimination of O^{2-}, although no significant difference was observed (B). In support of this finding, the SOD activity gradually increased (C), suggesting the enhancement of the antioxidant action. Concentration of markers for the impairment of vascular endothelium (thrombomodulin and von Willebrand factor) did not show any significant fluctuation (measured by SRL Inc.), with large variation of the data due to small numbers of patients [108].

A shunt, which is a bypass connecting the artery and vein of the brachium to perform blood maintenance dialysis, is indispensable. However, the pressure due to the dialysis causes expansion, the bending and extension of blood vessel, the thickening of vein wall and the ectopic calcification due to the repeated puncture, leading to the blockage due to the decreased blood pressure, stagnation of blood flow and enhancement of coagulability. All patients frequently repeat the clotting in the part of shunt during dialysis. However, the incidences of such shunt troubles were apparently reduced by SE treatment (D) and questionnaire on the clinical effects of SE showed the good outcome (E) (Figure 11). Although this clinical trial has ended once in 2 years, one patient (84 years old) still receives the clinical trial, with little or no trouble of the shunt, possibly due to the preservation of blood fluidity and maintenance of blood vessel possibly by iron chlorophyllin and antioxidants in SE [108].

5.4. Anti-Halitosis Effect of Toothpaste Supplemented with SE

Considering the potent anti-HIV, anti-inflammatory effects of SE, we have manufactured SE containing toothpaste (SETP) for the first time. The SETP is composed of 26.2% SE, 0.1% isopropylmethylphenol, base materials, cleaning agents, humectants, flavoring substances, sweetening agent, stabilizers, binding agent and washing soap). We have selected the 26.2% SE, since treatment of periodontal ligament fibroblasts for 1 min with 50% of SE did not affect the cell viability and approximately 8 ml of saliva were produced and accumulated in the oral cavity by 5 min of tooth brushing. SETP can be obtained at the drug store. We investigated its anti-halitosis effect with the collaboration of a total of 12 volunteers, according to the guideline of Intramural Ethic Committee (no. A1219). They brushed their teeth immediately after meals three times each day with STEP or placebo toothpaste (omitting only SE). Halitosis in the breath and bacterial number on the tongue were measured by portable apparatuses at 11:00 AM in the morning. We found that SETP significantly reduced halitosis ($p = 0.046$) but not the number of bacterial on the tongue ($p = 0.60$) [109].

5.5. Other Unpublished Case Reports

The female subject (28 years old) was bothered by atopy since her infancy. When her living environment changed by getting a job three years ago, the symptoms worsened further especially in early spring, rainy season and dry winter. She unexpectedly found that pasting the *Sasa* sp. extract-immersed cotton on her skin improved the symptoms. In another when red eczema and skin roughness became apparent (A), she applied just a pearl-size amount of "Moisture Creamy Gel" (containing to 1.8% *Sasa* sp. extract), her skin of cheek and face line three times a day. The creamy gel produced no bleeding, in contrast to other commercially available lotions. After 1 week, area of red eczema began to diminish and rough skin became smooth, thus reducing the application time to twice a day. After 2 weeks, eczema has completely healed (B) (Figure 12).

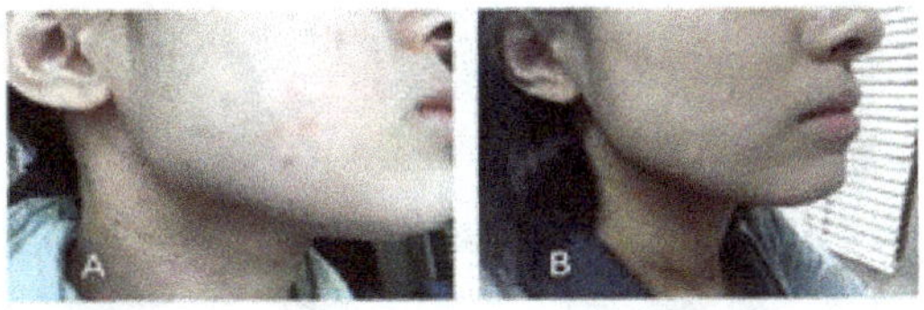

Figure 12. Facial photo before (**A**) and two weeks after application (**B**) of SE Moisture Creamy Gel.

Recently, diacetyl (2,3-butanedione), mostly produced by *Staphylococcus aureus* and *Staphylococcus epidermidis*, has been reported to be a key contributor to unpleasant odors emanating from the axillae, feet and head regions [110]. There was one case report that when male healthy volunteer (69 years old) take daily drink of SE (40 mL, 2.4 g dry weight) mixed with lemon and orange juice after lunch except for Sunday, he experienced the significant reduction in the fecal smell (after 1 week), tongue cloth (after 1 month) and body odor (after three months) and no stress-induced stomatitis for 7 months.

6. Kampo Medicines

Xerostomia is a disease in which a reduction in salivary secretion causes oral dryness and it may also be further complicated with odontonecrosis, periodontal disease, candidiasis, and taste disorders. The exacerbation of these diseases has a substantial effect on the QOL, so it is necessary in such cases to clarify the causes and select the most appropriate treatment. Herbal treatment alleviated thirst and oral dryness in most cases but many cases showed a slower increase in salivary production than the cases administered cevimeline hydrochloride [111] (Figure 13).

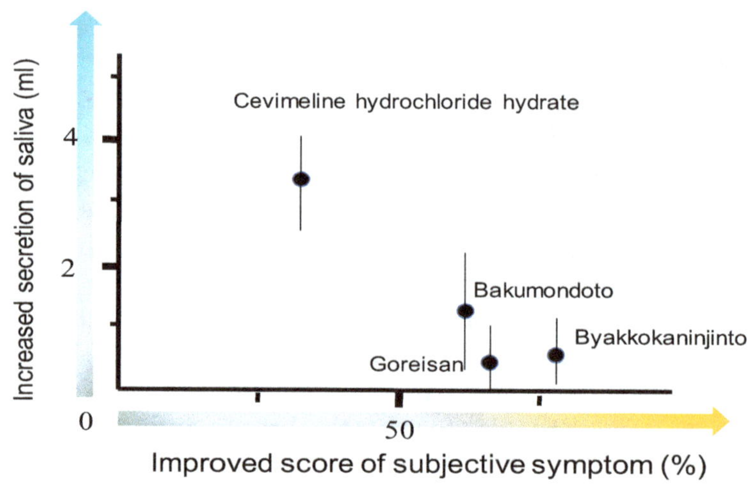

Figure 13. Regarding subjective symptoms, a questionnaire is issued about (i) mouth dryness, (ii) swallowing difficulty and (iii) oral pain, using the VAS method. When the average of these three items is 0, 1~20, 21~40, 41~60, 61~80, 81~100, the score is counted as 1, 2, 3, 4 and 5 points, respectively. The extent of subjective symptom improvement was calculated by dividing the subjective symptom score before the administration by that before starting administration and the multiplied by 100. Cited from Reference [111] with permission.

When the patient with xerostomia-induced glossitis was treated with Byakkokaninjinto (3 g three times a day) for two months, glossitis largely disappeared, and the subjective symptoms decreased (Figure 14).

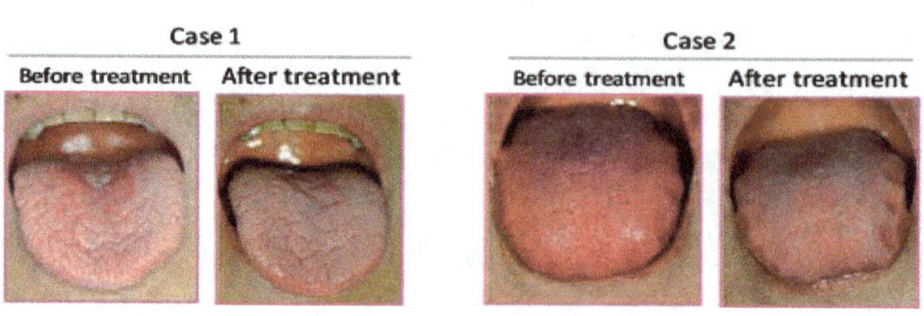

Figure 14. Effect of *Byakkokaninjinto* on glossitis. Cited from Reference [112] with permission.

7. Dental Application of Angiotensin II Receptor Blocker for Severe Periodontitis

7.1. Angiotensin II Receptor Blocker (ARB) in Marfan Syndrome

Marfan syndrome is an autosomal dominant connective tissue disease that affects about one in 5000 individuals [113]. The responsible gene of this syndrome is FBN1 which encodes the extracellular matrix protein fibrillin-1 [113]. FBN1 mutations lead to defects in multiple organs including skeletal, cardiovascular and ocular systems [114]. Among them, the most serious problems are seen in the cardiovascular system, such as, aortic regurgitation, aneurysm and dissection of the aortic root, mitral valve prolapse and mitral regurgitation, causing a short life expectancy in patients [115].

Fibrillin-1 regulates the function of endogenous transforming growth factor (TGF)-β by targeting the respective complexes to the extracellular cell matrix [116]. Studies of animal [117] and human [118] reported that TGF-β signaling drives aneurysm progression in the aorta [119]. Since Marfan syndrome patients have cardiovascular problems, the surgical replacement of aortic and mitral valve and aortic roots is often required [115]. It is known that effects of angiotensin II are mediated by two receptors, type 1 (AT1) and type 2 (AT2) receptor [120]. AT1-receptor signaling can increase the production of TGF-β ligands and receptors [121]. Angiotensin II-receptor blockers (ARBs) selectively block the binding of angiotensin II to its receptor within the renin–angiotensin system [122]. AT1-receptor blockade decreases TGF-β signaling and thus inhibit the phosphorylation of Smad2. Recently, losartan, one of ARBs, have been reported to suppress the progression of aortic root dilation by inhibiting TGF-β signaling [117,123]. Application of ARBs are now providing great benefit to Marfan syndrome patients by improving cardiovascular conditions.

7.2. Periodontal Disease Frequently Seen in Marfan Syndrome

Oral manifestations are not included as diagnostic criteria of Marfan syndrome but this disease is frequently affected with severe periodontitis [124–126]. Periodontitis affects periodontal tissues, including gingiva, periodontal ligament (PDL) and alveolar bone [127]. Approximately 15% of the adult population has an advanced form of periodontitis, making multiple negative impacts on quality of life [128,129]. Consequences of periodontitis include negative esthetics and functional problems in occlusion, chewing and speaking and finally result in tooth loss [130,131]. Periodontitis is initiated by chronic inflammation and immune reactions to bacterial pathogens [132]. Several bacteria play important roles in the pathogenesis of periodontitis but *Porphyromonas gingivalis* plays a central role in pathogenesis of periodontitis [133]. It is reported that 87.5% of Marfan syndrome patients had periodontitis with more than 4 mm of periodontal pocket depth, while only 35.7% of healthy volunteers showed such manifestation [134]. Interestingly, higher percentage of periodontitis with more than 4 mm of periodontal pocket depth was seen in patients with cardiovascular disease than those without cardiovascular disease [135]. Many Marfan syndrome patients have these cardiovascular problems, often necessitating the surgical replacement of aortic and mitral valve and aortic roots [115]. Because of this surgical replacement, it is essential to prevent dental infection, such as infectious endocarditis caused by the periodontitis.

The reason of higher incidence of severe periodontitis in Marfan in not known. However, the lower number of caries has been reported in adult Marfan syndrome patients than in healthy volunteers [124]. This implies that periodontal tissues but not teeth have structural problems making susceptible to severe periodontitis. The abnormal alignment of collagen fibers was observed in one of the model mice of Marfan syndrome (MgR mice). Homozygous MgR mice show the 72% of reduction in Fbn1 (encoding mouse fibrillin-1) expression because of transcriptional interference by insertion of the PGKneo-cassette [136] and resemble the phenotype of Marfan syndrome by showing 10% longer long bones than wild-type (WT) littermates. A comparable level of type I collagen, which is the most major collagen in periodontal ligaments, was expressed in PDL-cells of homozygous MgR mice as in WT mice [137]. However, multi-oriented collagen fiber bundles with a thinner appearance were noted in homozygous mice. These observations were never seen in WT mice showing well-organized definite collagen fiber bundles. This suggests that normal level of fibrillin-1 is essential for the normal architecture of periodontal ligament.

7.3. Progression of Periodontal Disease and Application of ARB

Telmisartan (4′-[[4-methyl-6-(1-methyl-1*H*-benzimidazol-2-yl)-2-propyl-1*H*-benzimidazol-1-yl] methyl]biphenyl-2-carboxylic acid) is a non-peptide ARBs used in the management of hypertension [138,139] and expected as an effective drug for the management of vascular condition in Marfan syndrome [140]. This drug has a binding affinity 3,000 times higher for AT1 than AT2 [141]. Heterozygous MgΔ mice, another mice model of Marfan syndrome, show half level of Fbn1 as WT mice [136]. Six-week-old male heterozygous MgΔ and WT mice were challenged with *P. gingivalis* with and without telmisartan application [142]. Infection of *P. gingivalis* induced alveolar bone resorption in both heterozygous MgΔ and wild-type mice. The amount of alveolar bone resorption was significantly larger in the former than the latter. Interleukin (IL)-17 and tumor necrosis factor (TNF)-α levels were significantly higher in infected MgΔ mice than infected WT mice. Telmisartan treatment significantly suppressed the alveolar bone resorption of infected Mg mice. Telmisartan also significantly reduced the levels of TGF-β, IL-17 and TNF-α in infected MgΔ mice to those seen in infected WT mice. These suggest that ARB can prevent the severe periodontitis frequently seen in Marfan syndrome. Combination with Chinese medicine and angiotensin-converting enzyme inhibitors (ACEI) or ARB showed kidney protection effect [143,144] and tannic acid inhibited AT1 gene expression and cellular response [145]. However, previous studies have not yet investigated whether traditional medicines and dietary polyphenols inhibit the periodontitis through blocking the AT1.

8. Future Direction

The present article demonstrated that chromone derivatives show high tumor-specificity, low keratinocyte toxicity, without or with induction of apoptosis, suggesting that apoptosis induction is not the absolute necessity for exploration of anticancer drugs. Chromone ring is a natural material, distributing into many flavonoids. By introducing an appropriate substituent thereto with the guidance of QSAR analysis, more active derivatives can be manufactured. Synthesis of ^{13}C-labled chromone derivatives is underway to investigate the cellular uptake and binding to the specific acceptor molecules in the cells. Since all data of chromone derivatives are produced in vitro, in vivo study with implanted tumors are necessary to confirm the selective action against tumor cells. Also, possibility of synergistic action with anticancer drugs and effects on CYP-3 enzymes that affect the stability of accompanying drugs should be monitored before the clinical application.

LCC and SE, both are extracted from plants by alkaline extraction showed extremely higher anti-HIV, anti-inflammatory and neuroprotective activity. Our recent study demonstrated that SE stimulated the growth of differentiated neuronal cells and human gingival epithelial progenitor (HGEP) at lower concentration. This hormetic action of SE may explain its ability to protect the cells from amyloid peptides. The pathogenesis of dementia is thought to be due to the collapse of cerebral nerve cells and the reduction of neurotransmitters by the senile plaques produced by the accumulation of amyloid beta (Aβ) and tau protein (Tau) in the brain. It remains to be investigated whether SE prevent the dementia, if so by what mechanism.

We have previously reported that LCC of SE, prepared by repeated acid-precipitation and alkaline solubilization, has greenish color (absorption peak = 655 nm), characteristic to chlorophyllin (absorption peak = 629 nm) and that 68.5% of SE eluted as a single peak at the retention time of 22.175 min in HPLC [146]. This suggests that LCC in SE may easily bind to or entangled with chlorophyllin and other components to make large molecule under physiological condition. Such arge molecule may non-specifically bind to many cell surface receptors including dectin-2, causing its unique biological activity.

This review suggests the efficacy of GTF inhibitors and ARBs to prevent the biofilm formation and periodontitis, respectively. It is crucial to search for these inhibitors and blockers from the natural kingdom and elucidate their action mechanism.

Author Contributions: H.S., T.O. and T.Y. organized the review; T.W. and T.H. wrote the section of GTFs: N.S. wrote section of ARBs; K.M. wrote the section of Kampo; N.Y. wrote the section of anti-oxidative stress effect; H.K. wrote the section of anti-eczema effect; T.G. wrote the section of body odor; J.N. and Y.U. performed the QSAR analysis; K.T. and Y.S. synthesized chromone derivatives.

Acknowledgments: The authors acknowledge Daiwa Biological Research Institute Co., Ltd for the supply of SE and Meikai University School of Dentistry for the support for the research.

Abbreviations

ARB	Angiotensin II receptor blocker
AT1	Angiotensin II type 1 receptor
AT2	Angiotensin II type 2 receptor
AZT	Azidothymidine
CC_{50}	50% cytotoxic concentration
CDP-choline	Cytidine diphosphate-choline
CPT	Camptothecin
DNR	Daunorubicin
DOC	Docetaxel
DXR	Doxorubicin
EGCG	Epigallocatechin-3-gallate
ELISA	EnzymelLinked immunoSorbent assay
ETP	Etoposide
FBN1	Gene that codes fibrillin-1 in humans
5-FU	5-Fluorouracil
GTF	Glucosyltransferase GTF
HIV	Human immuno-deficiency virus
HPLC	High-performance liquid chromatography HPLC
HSVV	Herpes simplex virus
IL	Interleukin
LCC	Lignin carbohydrate complex
LPO	Lipid peroxide
MEL	Melphalan
MgR mice	model mice of Marfan syndrome
MMC	Mitomycin C
O^{2-}	Superoxide
OSCC	Oral squamous cell carcinoma
PDL	Periodontal ligament
QASR	Quantitative structure-activity relationship
Sasa sp.	*Sasa* species
SA	Senescence-associated
SE	Alkaline extract of the leaves of *Sasa* sp.
SN-38	Active metabolite of irinotecan
SOD	Superoxide dismutase
TGF	Transforming growth factor
TNF	Tumor necrosis factor
TRL	Toll-like receptor

TS	Tumor-specificity
TS_E	Tumor-specificity determined with human normal oral epithelial cells *vs* OSCC cells
TS_M	Tumor-specificity determined with human normal oral mesenchymal cells *vs* OSCC cells
UV	Ultraviolet
WIG	water-insoluble glucan
WSG	water-soluble glucan WSG

References

1. Queiroz, S.I.M.L.; Silva, M.V.A.D.; Medeiros, A.M.; Oliveira, P.T.; Gurgel, B.C.V.; Silveira, É.J.D.D. Recurrent aphthous ulceration. An epidemiological study of etiological factors, treatment and differential diagnosis. *An. Bras. Dermatol.* **2018**, *93*, 341–346. [CrossRef]
2. Chiang, C.P.; Chang, J.; Wang, Y.P.; Wu, Y.H.; Wu, Y.C.; Sun, A. Recurrent aphthous stomatitis—Etiology, serum autoantibodies, anemia, hematinic deficiencies, and management. *J. Formos. Med. Assoc.* **2018**. [CrossRef] [PubMed]
3. Abdel Moneim, A.E.; Guerra-Librero, A.; Florido, J.; Shen, Y.Q.; Fernández-Gil, B.; Acuña-Castroviejo, D.; Escames, G. Oral Mucositis: Melatonin Gel an Effective New Treatment. *Int. J. Mol. Sci.* **2017**, *18*, 1003. [CrossRef] [PubMed]
4. Sakagami, H. Biological activities and possible dental application of three major groups of polyphenols. *J. Pharmacol. Sci.* **2014**, *126*, 92–106. [CrossRef] [PubMed]
5. Okuda, T.; Yoshida, T.; Hatano, T. Hydrolyzable tannins and related polyphenols. In *Fortschritte der Chemie Organischer Naturstoffe/Progressinthe Chemistry of Organic Natural Products*; Springer: Vienna, Austria, 1995; pp. 1–117.
6. Nomura, T.; Hano, Y.; Fukai, T. Chemistry and biosynthesis of isoprenylated flavonoids from Japanese mulberry tree. *Proc. Jpn. Acad. Ser. B Phys. Biol. Sci.* **2009**, *85*, 391–408. [CrossRef] [PubMed]
7. Cendrowski, A.; Ścibisz, I.; Mitek, M.; Kieliszek, M.; Kolniak-Ostek, J. Profile of the Phenolic Compounds of Rosa rugosa Petals. *J. Food Qual.* **2017**, *2017*. [CrossRef]
8. Cendrowski, A.; Ścibisz, I.; Kieliszek, M.; Kolniak-Ostek, J.; Mitek, M. UPLC-PDA-Q/TOF-MS profile of polyphenolic compounds of liqueurs from Rose petals (Rosa rugosa). *Molecules* **2017**, *22*, 1832. [CrossRef] [PubMed]
9. Sakagami, H.; Hashimoto, K.; Suzuki, F.; Ogiwara, T.; Satoh, K.; Ito, H.; Hatano, T.; Takashi, Y.; Fujisawa, S. Molecular requirements of lignin-carbohydrate complexes for expression of unique biological activities. *Phytochemistry* **2005**, *66*, 2108–2120. [CrossRef]
10. Olsen, I.; Singhrao, S.K. Can oral infection be a risk factor for Alzheimer's disease? *J. Oral. Microbiol.* **2015**, *7*, 29143. [CrossRef]
11. Furuta, M.; Yamashita, Y. Oral health and swallowing problems. *Curr. Phys. Med. Rehabil. Rep.* **2013**, *1*, 216–222. [CrossRef]
12. Olmsted, J.L.; Rublee, N.; Zurkawski, E.; Kleber, L. Public health dental hygiene. An option for improved quality of care and quality of life. *J. Dent. Hyg.* **2013**, *87*, 299–308.
13. Hägglund, P.; Olai, L.; Ståhlnacke, K.; Persenius, M.; Hägg, M.; Andersson, M.; Koistinen, S.; Carlsson, E. Study protocol for the SOFIA project: Swallowing function, Oral health, and Food Intake in old Age. A descriptive study with a cluster randomized trial. *BMC Geriatr.* **2017**, *78*. [CrossRef] [PubMed]
14. Bardellini, E.; Amadori, F.; Majorana, A. Oral hygiene grade and quality of life in children with chemotherapy-related oral mucositis. A randomized study on the impact of a fluoride toothpaste with salivary enzymes, essential oils, proteins and colostrum extract versus a fluoride toothpaste without menthol. *Int. J. Dent. Hyg.* **2016**, *14*, 314–319. [CrossRef] [PubMed]
15. Siddiqui, I.A.; Sanna, V. Impact of nanotechnology on the delivery of natural products for cancer prevention and therapy. *Mol. Nutr. Food Res.* **2016**, *60*, 1330–1341. [CrossRef] [PubMed]
16. Feller, L.; Khammissa, R.A.; Chandran, R.; Altini, M.; Lemmer, J. Oral candidosis in relation to oral immunity. *J. Oral. Pathol. Med.* **2014**, *43*, 563–569. [CrossRef]
17. Pang, Y.; Shen, Z.; Sun, J.; Wang, W. Does the use of targeted agents in advanced gastroesophageal cancer increase complete response. A meta-analysis of 18 randomized controlled trials. *Cancer Manag. Res.* **2018**, *10*, 5505–5514. [CrossRef] [PubMed]

18. Zhou, S.; Zuo, L.; He, X.; Pi, J.; Jin, J.; Shi, Y. Efficacy and safety of rh-endostatin (Endostar) combined with pemetrexed/cisplatin followed by rh-endostatin plus pemetrexed maintenance in non-small cell lung cancer. A retrospective comparison with standard chemotherapy. *Thorac. Cancer.* **2018**, *9*, 1354–1360. [CrossRef]
19. Harada, T.; Ijima, A. Pharmacological profile and clinical findings of palbociclib (IBRANCE®capsule 25 mg/125 mg). *Folia Pharmacol. Jpn.* **2018**, *152*, 206–318. (In Japanese) [CrossRef] [PubMed]
20. Lulli, D.; Carbone, M.L.; Pastore, S. Epidermal growth factor receptor inhibitors trigger a type I interferon response in human skin. *Oncotarget* **2016**, *7*, 47777–47793. [CrossRef] [PubMed]
21. Ferrari, D.; Codecà, C.; Bocci, B.; Crepaldi, F.; Violati, M.; Viale, G.; Careri, C.; Caldiera, S.; Bordin, V.; Luciani, A.; et al. Anti-epidermal growth factor receptor skin toxicity. A matter of topical hydration. *Anticancer Drugs* **2016**, *27*, 144–146. [CrossRef]
22. Benjakul, R.; Kongkaneramit, L.; Sarisuta, N.; Moongkarndi, P.; Müller-Goymann, C.C. Cytotoxic effect and mechanism inducing cell death of α-mangostin liposomes in various human carcinoma and normal cells. *Anticancer Drugs* **2015**, *26*, 824–834. [CrossRef] [PubMed]
23. Do, N.; Weindl, G.; Grohmann, L.; Salwiczek, M.; Koksch, B.; Korting, H.C.; Schäfer-Korting, M. Cationic membrane-active peptides–anticancer and antifungal activity as well as penetration into human skin. *Exp. Dermatol.* **2014**, *23*, 326–331. [CrossRef] [PubMed]
24. Moreno Garcia, V.; Thavasu, P.; Blanco Codesido, M.; Molife, L.R.; Vitfell Pedersen, J.; Puglisi, M.; Basu, B.; Shah, K.; Iqbal, J.; de Bono, J.S.; et al. Association of creatine kinase and skin toxicity in phase I trials of anticancer agents. *Br. J. Cancer* **2012**, *107*, 1797–1800. [CrossRef] [PubMed]
25. Benedict, A.L.; Knatko, E.V.; Dinkova-Kostova, A.T. The indirect antioxidant sulforaphane protects against thiopurine-mediated photo-oxidative stress. *Carcinogenesis* **2012**, *33*, 2457–2466. [CrossRef] [PubMed]
26. Fischel, J.L.; Formento, P.; Ciccolini, J.; Etienne-Grimaldi, M.C.; Milano, G. Lack of contribution of dihydrofluorouracil and Alpha-fluoro-beta-alanine to the cytotoxicity of 5′-deoxy-5-fluorouridine on human keratinocytes. *Anticancer Drugs* **2004**, *15*, 969–974. [CrossRef] [PubMed]
27. Sakagami, H.; Okudaira, N.; Masuda, Y.; Amano, O.; Yokose, S.; Kanda, Y.; Suguro, M.; Natori, T.; Oizumi, H.; Oizumi, T. Induction of apoptosis in human oral keratinocyte by doxorubicin. *Anticancer Res.* **2017**, *37*, 1023–1029.
28. Miyamoto, M.; Sakagami, H.; Minagawa, K.; Kikuchi, H.; Nishikawa, H.; Satoh, K.; Komatsu, N.; Fujimaki, M.; Nakashima, H.; Gupta, M.; et al. Tumor-specificity and radical scavenging activity of poly-herbal formula. *Anticancer Res.* **2002**, *22*, 1217–1224.
29. Gaspar, A.; Matos, M.J.; Garrido, J.; Uriarte, E.; Borges, F. Chromone. A valid scaffold in medicinal chemistry. *Chem Rev.* **2014**, *114*, 4960–4992. [CrossRef]
30. Shimada, C.; Uesawa, Y.; Ishii-Nozawa, R.; Ishihara, M.; Kagaya, H.; Kanamto, T.; Terakubo, S.; Nakashima, H.; Takao, K.; Sugita, Y.; et al. Quantitative structure–cytotoxicity relationship of 3-styrylchromones. *Anticancer Res.* **2014**, *34*, 5405–5412.
31. Sakagami, H.; Shimada, C.; Kanda, Y.; Amano, O.; Sugimoto, M.; Ota, S.; Soga, T.; Tomita, M.; Sato, A.; Tanuma, S.; et al. Effects of 3-styrylchromones on metabolic profiles and cell death in oral squamous cell carcinoma cells. *Toxocol. Rep.* **2015**, *2*, 1281–1290. [CrossRef]
32. Uesawa, Y.; Sakagami, H.; Kagaya, H.; Yamashita, M.; Takao, K.; Sugita, Y. Quantitative structure-cytotoxicity relationship of 3-benzylidenechromanones. *Anticancer Res.* **2016**, *36*, 5803–5812. [CrossRef] [PubMed]
33. Uesawa, Y.; Ishihara, M.; Kagaya, H.; Kanamoto, T.; Terakubo, S.; Nakashima, H.; Yahagi, H.; Takao, K.; Sugita, Y. Quantitative structure–cytotoxicity relationship of 3-styryl-2*H*-chromenes. *Anticancer Res.* **2015**, *35*, 5299–5308. [PubMed]
34. Sakagami, H.; Okudaira, N.; Uesawa, Y.; Takao, K.; Kagaya, H.; Sugita, Y. Quantitative structure-cytotoxicity relationship of 2-azolylchromones. *Anticancer Res.* **2018**, *38*, 763–770. [PubMed]
35. Shi, H.; Nagai, J.; Sakatsume, T.; Bandow, K.; Okudaira, N.; Sakagami, H.; Tomomura, M.; Tomomura, A.; Uesawa, Y.; Takao, K.; et al. Quantitative structure–cytotoxicity relationship of 2-(*N*-cyclicamino)chromone derivatives. *Anticancer Res.* **2018**, *38*, 3897–3906. [CrossRef] [PubMed]
36. Shi, H.; Nagai, J.; Sakatsume, T.; Bandow, K.; Okudaira, N.; Uesawa, Y.; Sakagami, H.; Tomomura, M.; Tomomura, A.; Takao, K.; et al. Quantitative structure–cytotoxicity relationship of 3-(*N*-cyclicamino)chromone derivatives. *Anticancer Res.* **2018**, *38*, 4459–4467. [CrossRef]
37. Uesawa, Y.; Sakagami, H.; Shi, H.; Hirose, M.; Takao, K.; Sugita, Y. Quantitative structure-cytotoxicity relationship of furo[2,3-*b*]chromones. *Anticancer Res.* **2018**, *38*, 3283–3290. [CrossRef]

38. Nagai, J.; Shi, H.; Kubota, Y.; Bandow, K.; Okudaira, N.; Uesawa, Y.; Sakagami, H.; Tomomura, M.; Tomomura, A.; Takao, K.; et al. Quantitative structure–cytotoxicity relationship of pyrano[4,3-*b*]chromones. *Anticancer Res.* **2018**, *38*, 4449–4457. [CrossRef]
39. Pleszczyńska, M.; Wiater, A.; Bachanek, T.; Szczodrak, J. Enzymes in therapy of biofilm-related oral diseases. *Biotechnol. Appl. Biochem.* **2017**, *64*, 337–346. [CrossRef]
40. Kalesinskas, P.; Kačergius, T.; Ambrozaitis, A.; Pečiulienė, V.; Ericson, D. Reducing dental plaque formation and caries development. A review of current methods and implications for novel pharmaceuticals. *Stomatologija* **2014**, *16*, 44–52.
41. Hehre, E. Enzymic synthesis of polysaccharides. A biological type of polymerization. *Adv. Enzymol. Relat. Subj. Biochem.* **1951**, *11*, 297–337.
42. Kuramitsu, H.K. Virulence factors of mutans streptococci: Role of molecular genetics. *Crit. Rev. Oral Biol. Med.* **1993**, *4*, 159–176. [CrossRef]
43. Caufield, P.W. Dental caries. An infectious and transmissible disease. *Compend. Contin. Educ. Dent.* **2005**, *26*, 10–16. [PubMed]
44. Miller, W.D. *The Microorganisms of the Human Mouth; Ko"nig KG*; Karger: Basel, Switzerland, 1973.
45. Touger-Decker, R.; van Loveren, C. Sugars and dental caries. *Am. J. Clin. Nutr.* **2003**, *78*, 881S–892S. [CrossRef] [PubMed]
46. Hoshino, T.; Fujiwara, T.; Kawabata, T. Evolution of Cariogenic Character in Streptococcus Mutans: Horizontal Transmission of Glycosyl Hydrase Family 70 Genes. *Sci. Rep.* **2012**, *2*, 518. [CrossRef] [PubMed]
47. Jeanmougin, F.; Thompson, J.D.; Gouy, M.; Higgins, D.G.; Gibson, T.J. Multiple sequence alignment with Clustal, X. *Trends. Biochem. Sci.* **1998**, *23*, 403–405. [CrossRef]
48. Tamura, K.; Dudley, J.; Nei, M.; Kumar, S. MEGA4: Molecular evolutionary genetics analysis (MEGA) software version 4.0. *Mol. Biol. Evol.* **2007**, *24*, 1596–1599. [CrossRef] [PubMed]
49. Hoshino, T.; Kondo, Y.; Saito, K.; Terao, Y.; Okahashi, N.; Kawabata, S.; Fujiwara, T. Novel epitopic region of glucosyltransferase B from Streptococcus mutans. *Clin. Vaccine Immunol.* **2011**, *18*, 1552–1561. [CrossRef] [PubMed]
50. Hamada, S.; Torii, M. Effect of sucrose in culture media on the location of glucosyltransferase of Streptococcus mutans and cell adherence to glass surfaces. *Infect. Immun.* **1978**, *20*, 592–599. [PubMed]
51. Hamada, S.; Horikoshi, T.; Minami, T.; Okahashi, N.; Koga, T. Purification and characterization of cell-associated glucosyltransferase synthesizing water-insoluble glucan from serotype c *Streptococcus mutans*. *J. Gen. Microbiol.* **1989**, *135*, 335–344. [CrossRef]
52. Tomita, Y.; Zhu, X.; Ochiai, K.; Namiki, Y.; Okada, T.; Ikemi, T.; Fukushima, K. Evaluation of three individual glucosyltransferases produced by Streptococcus mutans using monoclonal antibodies. *FEMS Microbiol. Lett.* **1996**, *145*, 427–432. [CrossRef]
53. Fujiwara, T.; Hoshino, T.; Ooshima, T.; Sobue, S.; Hamada, S. Purification, characterization, and molecular analysis of the gene encoding glucosyltransferase from *Streptococcus oralis*. *Infect. Immun.* **2000**, *68*, 2475–2483. [CrossRef] [PubMed]
54. Mukasa, H.; Tsumori, H.; Shimamura, A. Isolation and characterization of an extracellular glucosyltransferase synthesizing insoluble glucan from *Streptococcus mutans* serotype c. *Infect. Immun.* **1985**, *49*, 790–796. [PubMed]
55. Shimamura, A.; Tsumori, H.; Mukasa, H. Purification and properties of *Streptococcus mutans* extracellular glucosyltransferase. *Biochim. Biophys. Acta* **1982**, *702*, 72–80. [CrossRef]
56. Mukasa, H.; Shimamura, A.; Tsumori, H. Purification and characterization of basic glucosyltransferase from Streptococcus mutans serotype c. *Biochim. Biophys. Acta* **1982**, *719*, 81–89. [CrossRef]
57. Grahame, D.; Mayer, R. Purification, and comparison, of two forms of dextransucrase from *Streptococcus sanguis*. *Carbohydr. Res.* **1985**, *142*, 285–298. [CrossRef]
58. Kobs, S.; Husman, D.; Cawthern, K. Mayer R Affinity purification of dextransucrase from *Streptococcus sanguis* ATCC 10558. *Carbohydr. Res.* **1990**, *203*, 156–161. [CrossRef]
59. Aoki, H.; Shiroza, T.; Hayakawa, M.; Sato, S.; Kuramitsu, H. Cloning of a *Streptococcus mutans* glucosyltransferase gene coding for insoluble glucan synthesis. *Infect. Immun.* **1986**, *53*, 587–594. [PubMed]
60. Shiroza, T.; Ueda, S.; Kuramitsu, H. Sequence analysis of the gtfB gene from *Streptococcus mutans*. *J. Bacteriol.* **1987**, *169*, 4263–4270. [CrossRef] [PubMed]

61. Hanada, N.; Kuramitsu, H. Isolation and characterization of the *Streptococcus mutans* gtfC gene, coding for synthesis of both soluble and insoluble glucans. *Infect. Immun.* **1988**, *56*, 1999–2005. [PubMed]

62. Fukushima, K.; Ikeda, T.; Kuramitsu, H. Expression of *Streptococcus mutans* gtf genes in Streptococcus milleri. *Infect. Immun.* **1992**, *60*, 2815–2822. [PubMed]

63. Honda, O.; Kato, C.; Kuramitsu, H. Nucleotide sequence of the *Streptococcus mutans* gtfD gene encoding the glucosyltransferase-S enzyme. *J. Gen. Microbiol.* **1990**, *136*, 2099–2105. [CrossRef] [PubMed]

64. Mukasa, H.; Shimamura, A.; Tsumori, H. Effect of salts on water-insoluble glucan formation by glucosyltransferase of *Streptococcus mutans*. *Infect. Immun.* **1979**, *23*, 564–570. [PubMed]

65. Sakanaka, S.; Kim, M.; Taniguchi, M.; Yamamoto, T. Antibacterial substances in Japanese green tea extract against *Streptococcus mutans*, a cariogenic bacterium. *Agric. Biol. Chem.* **1989**, *53*, 2307–2311. [CrossRef]

66. Hattori, M.; Kusumoto, I.; Namba, T.; Ishigami, T.; Hara, Y. Effect of tea polyphenols on glucan synthesis by glucosyltransferase from *Streptococcus mutans*. *Chem. Pharm. Bull.* **1990**, *38*, 717–720. [CrossRef] [PubMed]

67. Nakahara, K.; Kawabata, S.; Ono, H.; Ogura, K.; Tanaka, T.; Ooshima, T.; Hamada, S. Inhibitory effect of oolong tea polyphenols on glycosyltransferases of *mutans Streptococci*. *Appl. Environ. Microbiol.* **1993**, *59*, 968–973. [PubMed]

68. Ooshima, T.; Minami, T.; Aono, W.; Izumitani, A.; Sobue, S.; Fujiwara, T.; Kawabata, S.; Hamada, S. Oolong tea polyphenols inhibit experimental dental caries in SPF rats infected with *mutans streptococci*. *Caries Res.* **1993**, *27*, 124–129. [CrossRef] [PubMed]

69. Otake, S.; Makimura, M.; Kuroki, T.; Nishihara, Y.; Hirasawa, M. Anticaries effects of polyphenolic compounds from Japanese green tea. *Caries Res.* **1991**, *25*, 438–443. [CrossRef] [PubMed]

70. Kakiuchi, N.; Hattori, M.; Nishizawa, M.; Yamagishi, T.; Okuda, T.; Namba, T. Studies on dental caries prevention by traditional medicines. VIII. Inhibitory effect of various tannins on glucan synthesis by glucosyltransferase from *Streptococcus mutans*. *Chem. Pharm. Bull.* **1986**, *34*, 720–725. [CrossRef] [PubMed]

71. Wu-Yuan, C.; Chen, C.; Wu, R. Gallotannins inhibit growth, water-insoluble glucan synthesis, and aggregation of *mutans streptococci*. *J. Dent. Res.* **1988**, *67*, 51–55. [CrossRef]

72. Matsumoto, M.; Hamada, S.; Ooshima, T. Molecular analysis of the inhibitory effects of oolong tea polyphenols on glucan-binding domain of recombinant glucosyltransferases from *Streptococcus mutans* MT8148. *FEMS Microbiol. Lett.* **2003**, *228*, 73–80. [CrossRef]

73. Karygianni, L.; Al-Ahmad, A.; Argyropoulou, A.; Hellwig, E.; Anderson, A.C.; Skaltsounis, A.L. Natural Antimicrobials and Oral Microorganisms. A Systematic Review on Herbal Interventions for the Eradication of Multispecies Oral Biofilms. *Front. Microbiol.* **2015**, *6*, 1529. [CrossRef] [PubMed]

74. Hirasawa, M.; Takada, K.; Makimura, M.; Otake, S. Improvement of periodontal status by green tea catechin using a local delivery system. A clinical pilot study. *J. Period. Res.* **2002**, *37*, 433–438. [CrossRef]

75. Tamura, M.; Saito, H.; Kikuchi, K.; Ishigami, T.; Toyama, Y.; Takami, M.; Ochiai, K. Antimicrobial activity of Gel-entrapped catechins toward oral microorganisms. *Biol. Pharm Bull.* **2011**, *34*, 638–643. [CrossRef] [PubMed]

76. Cueno, M.E.; Tamura, M.; Imai, K.; Ochiai, K. Orally supplemented catechin increases heme amounts and catalase activities in rat heart blood mitochondria. A comparison between middle-aged and young rats. *Exp Gerontol.* **2013**, *48*, 1319–1322. [CrossRef] [PubMed]

77. Lai, P.K.; Donovan, J.; Takayama, H.; Sakagami, H.; Tanaka, A.; Konno, K.; Nonoyama, M. Modification of human immunodeficiency viral replication by pine cone extracts. *AIDS Res. Hum. Retrovirus.* **1990**, *6*, 205–217. [CrossRef] [PubMed]

78. Satoh, K.; Kihara, T.; Ida, Y.; Sakagami, H.; Koyama, N.; Premanathan, M.; Arakaki, R.; Nakashima, H.; Komatsu, N.; Fujimaki, M.; et al. Radical modulation activity of pine cone extracts of *Pinus elliottii* var. Elliottii. *Anticancer Res.* **1999**, *19*, 357–364. [PubMed]

79. Sakagami, H.; Yoshihara, M.; Fujimaki, M.; Wada, C.; Komatsu, N.; Nakashima, H.; Murakami, T.; Yamamoto, N. Effect of pine seed shell extract on microbial and viral infection. *Lett. Appl. Microbiol.* **1992**, *6*, 13–16.

80. Manabe, H.; Sakagami, H.; Ishizone, H.; Kusano, H.; Fujimaki, M.; Wada, C.; Komatsu, N.; Nakashima, H.; Murakami, T.; Yamamoto, N. Effects of Catuaba extracts on microbial and HIV infection. *In Vivo* **1992**, *6*, 161–165. [PubMed]

81. Sakagami, H.; Satoh, K.; Fukamachi, H.; Ikarashi, T.; Shimizu, A.; Yano, K.; Kanamoto, T.; Terakubo, S.; Nakashima, H.; Hasegawa, H.; et al. Anti-HIV and vitamin C-synergized radical scavenging activity of cacao husk lignin fractions. *In Vivo* **2008**, *22*, 327–332. [PubMed]
82. Sakagami, H.; Kawano, M.; Thet, M.M.; Hashimoto, K.; Satoh, K.; Kanamoto, T.; Terakubo, S.; Nakashima, H.; Haishima, Y.; Maeda, Y.; Sakurai, K. Anti-HIV and immunomodulation activities of cacao mass lignin carbohydrate complex. *In Vivo* **2011**, *25*, 229–236. [PubMed]
83. Kawano, M.; Sakagami, H.; Satoh, K.; Shioda, S.; Kanamoto, T.; Terakubu, S.; Nakashima, H.; Makino, T. Lignin-like activity of *Lentinus edodes* mycelia extract (LEM). *In Vivo* **2010**, *24*, 543–551. [PubMed]
84. Sakagami, H.; Asano, K.; Satoh, K.; Takahashi, K.; Kobayashi, M.; Koga, N.; Takahashi, H.; Tachikawa, R.; Tashiro, T.; Hasegawa, A.; et al. Anti-stress, anti-HIV and vitamin C-synergized radical scavenging activity of mulberry juice fractions. *In Vivo* **2007**, *21*, 499–505. [PubMed]
85. Nakashima, H.; Murakami, T.; Yamamoto, N.; Naoe, T.; Kawazoe, Y.; Konno, K.; Sakagami, H. Lignified materials as medicinal resources. V. Anti-HIV (human immunodeficiency virus) activity of some synthetic lignins. *Chem. Pharm. Bull.* **1992**, *40*, 2102–2105. [CrossRef] [PubMed]
86. Sakagami, H.; Kushida, T.; Oizumi, T.; Nakashima, H.; Makino, T. Distribution of lignin carbohydrate complex in plant kingdom and its functionality as alternative medicine. *Pharmacol. Ther.* **2010**, *128*, 91–105. [CrossRef] [PubMed]
87. Nakashima, H.; Murakami, T.; Yamamoto, N.; Sakagami, H.; Tanuma, S.; Hatano, T.; Yoshida, T.; Okuda, T. Inhibition of human immunodeficiency viral replication by tannins and related compounds. *Antivir. Res.* **1992**, *18*, 91–103. [CrossRef]
88. Fukai, T.; Sakagami, H.; Toguchi, M.; Takayama, F.; Iwakura, I.; Atsumi, T.; Ueha, T.; Nakashima, H.; Nomura, T. Cytotoxic activity of low molecular weight polyphenols against human oral tumor cell lines. *Anticancer Res.* **2000**, *20*, 2525–2536. [PubMed]
89. Sakagami, H.; Ohkoshi, E.; Amano, S.; Satoh, K.; Kanamoto, T.; Terakubo, S.; Nakashima, H.; Sunaga, K.; Otsuki, T.; Ikeda, H.; et al. Efficient utilization of plant resources by alkaline extraction. *Altern. Integr. Med.* **2013**, *2*, 2013.
90. Ohno, H.; Miyoshi, S.; Araho, D.; Kanamoato, T.; Terakubo, S.; Nakashima, H.; Tsuda, T.; Sunaga, K.; Amano, S.; Ohkoshi, E.; et al. Efficient utilization of licorice root by alkaline extraction. *In Vivo* **2014**, *28*, 785–794. [PubMed]
91. Kato, T.; Horie, N.; Matsuta, T.; Umemura, N.; Shimoyama, T.; Kaneko, T.; Kanamoto, T.; Terakubo, S.; Nakashima, H.; Kusama, K.; et al. Anti-UV/HIV activity of Kampo medicines and constituent plant extracts. *In Vivo* **2012**, *26*, 1007–1013. [PubMed]
92. Huang, W.; Yu, X.; Liang, N.; Ge, W.; Kwok, H.F.; Lau, C.B.; Li, Y.; Chung, H.Y. Anti-angiogenic Activity and Mechanism of Sesquiterpene Lactones from Centipeda minima. *Nat. Prod. Commun.* **2016**, *11*, 435–438.
93. Huang, W.; Wang, J.; Liang, Y.; Ge, W.; Wang, G.; Li, Y.; Chung, H.Y. Potent anti-angiogenic component in Croton crassifolius and its mechanism of action. *J. Ethnopharmacol.* **2015**, *175*, 185–191. [CrossRef] [PubMed]
94. Ho, Y.S.; Yu, M.S.; Lai, C.S.; So, K.F.; Yuen, W.H.; Chang, R.C. Characterizing the neuroprotective effects of alkaline extract of Lycium barbarum on beta-amyloid peptide neurotoxicity. *Brain Res.* **2007**, *16*, 123–134. [CrossRef] [PubMed]
95. Yuan, Z.; Wen, Y.; Kapu, N.S.; Beatson, R.; Mark Martinez, D. A biorefinery scheme to fractionate bamboo into high-grade dissolving pulp and ethanol. *Biotechnol. Biofuels* **2017**, *10*, 38. [CrossRef] [PubMed]
96. Xie, J.; Hse, C.Y.; De Hoop, C.F.; Hu, T.; Qi, J.; Shupe, T.F. Isolation and characterization of cellulose nanofibers from bamboo using microwave liquefaction combined with chemical treatment and ultrasonication. *Carbohydr. Polym.* **2016**, *151*, 725–734. [CrossRef] [PubMed]
97. Sakagami, H.; Sheng, H.; Okudaira, N.; Yasui, T.; Wakabayashi, H.; Jia, J.; Natori, T.; Suguro-Kitajima, M.; Oizumi, H.; Oizumi, T. Prominent Anti-UV activity and possible cosmetic potential of lignin-carbohydrate complex. *In Vivo* **2016**, *30*, 331–339. [PubMed]
98. Nanbu, T.; Shimada, J.; Kobayashi, M.; Hirano, K.; Koh, T.; Machino, M.; Ohno, H.; Yamamoto, M.; Sakagami, H. Anti-UV activity of lignin-carbohydrate complex and related compounds. *In Vivo* **2013**, *27*, 133–140.
99. Kato, T.; Segami, N.; Sakagami, H. Anti-inflammatory activity of hangeshashinto in IL-1β -stimulated gingival and periodontal ligament fibroblasts. *In Vivo* **2016**, *30*, 257–264. [PubMed]

100. Sakagami, H.; Shi, H.; Bandow, K.; Tomomura, M.; Tomomura, A.; Horiuchi, M.; Fujisawa, T.; Oizumi, T. Search of neuroprotective polyphenols using the "overlay" isolated method. *Molecules* **2018**, *23*, 1840. [CrossRef]
101. Sakagami, H.; Fukuchi, K.; Kanamoto, T.; Terakubo, S.; Nakashima, H.; Natori, T.; Suguro-Kitajima, M.; Oizumi, H.; Yasui, T.; Oizumi, T. Synergism of alkaline extract of the leaves of *Sasa senanensis* Rehder and antiviral agents. *In Vivo* **2016**, *30*, 421–426.
102. Sakagami, H.; Amano, S.; Yasui, T.; Satoh, K.; Shioda, S.; Kanamoto, T.; Terakubo, S.; Nakashima, H.; Watanabe, K.; Sugiura, T.; et al. Biological interaction between *Sasa senanensis* Rehder leaf extract and toothpaste ingredients. *In Vivo* **2013**, *27*, 275–284.
103. Matsuta, T.; Sakagami, H.; Kitajima, M.; Oizumi, H.; Oizumi, T. Anti-UV activity of alkaline extracts of the leaves of *Sasa senanensis* Rehder. *In Vivo* **2011**, *25*, 751–755. [PubMed]
104. Sakagami, H.; Amano, S.; Kikuchi, H.; Nakamura, Y.; Kuroshita, R.; Watanabe, S.; Satoh, K.; Hasegawa, H.; Nomura, A.; Kanamoto, T.; et al. Antiviral, antibacterial and vitamin C-synergized radical scavenging activity of *Sasa senanensis* Rehder extract. *In Vivo* **2008**, *22*, 471–476. [PubMed]
105. Tomomura, M.; Tomomura, A.; Oizumi, T.; Yasui, T.; Sakagami, H. Extract of *Sasa senanensis* Rehder leaf promotes osteoblast differentiation in MC3T3-E1 cells. *J. Meikai Dent. Med.* **2017**, *46*, 111–116.
106. Sakagami, H.; Iwamoto, S.; Matsuta, T.; Satoh, K.; Shimada, C.; Kanamoto, T.; Terakubo, S.; Nakashima, H.; Morita, Y.; Ohkubo, A.; et al. Comparative study of biological activity of three commercial products of *Sasa senanensis* Rehder leaf extract. *In Vivo* **2012**, *26*, 259–264. [PubMed]
107. Matsuta, T.; Sakagami, H.; Tanaka, S.; Machino, M.; Tomomura, M.; Tomomura, A.; Yasui, T.; Itoh, K.; Sugiura, T.; Kitajima, M.; et al. Pilot clinical study of *Sasa senanensis* Rehder leaf extract treatment on lichenoid dysplasia. *In Vivo* **2012**, *26*, 957–962. [PubMed]
108. Yamauchi, N.; Nakagawa, R.; Namiki, K.; Hayashi, T.; Iguchi, A.; Kubota, I.; Oizumi, T.; Ito, A. *Effect of Fe Chlorophyllin on Shunt Clot*; Kidney and Free Radical Series 4; Tokyo Igakusha: Tokyo, Japan, 1998; pp. 66–70.
109. Sakagami, H.; Sheng, H.; Ono, K.; Komine, Y.; Miyadai, T.; Terada, Y.; Nakada, D.; Tanaka, S.; Matsumoto, M.; Yasui, T.; et al. Anti-halitosis effect of toothpaste supplemented with alkaline extract of the leaves of *Sasa senanensis* Rehder. *In Vivo* **2016**, *30*, 107–111. [PubMed]
110. Hara, T.; Matsui, H.; Shimizu, H. Suppression of microbial metabolic pathways inhibits the generation of the human body odor component diacetyl by *Staphylococcus* spp. *PLoS ONE* **2014**, *9*, e111833. [CrossRef] [PubMed]
111. Mori, K.; Shoda, H.; Tanura, N.; Takeshima, H.; Shimada, J. Comparisons between the effects of herb treatments and cases in which cevimeline hydrochloride (Saligren®) is administered for xerostomia. *Jpn. J. Oral Diagnos. Oral Med.* **2008**, *21*, 205–211. (In Japanese)
112. Mori, K.; Onuki, H.; Yoshida, A.; Tamura, N.; Maekawa, Y.; Konno, C.; Iida, S.; Shimada, J. Two cases of Xerostomia that showed an improvement after being treated with Chinese herbal medicine. *J. Meikai Dent. Med.* **2008**, *37*, 153–158. (In Japanese)
113. Dietz, H.C. Marfan syndrome caused by a recurrent de novo missense mutation in the fibrillin gene. *Nature* **1991**, *352*, 337–339. [CrossRef]
114. McKusick, V.A. The defect in Marfan syndrome. *Nature* **1991**, *352*, 279–281. [CrossRef] [PubMed]
115. Judge, D.P.; Dietz, H.C. Marfan's syndrome. *Lancet* **2005**, *366*, 1965–1976. [CrossRef]
116. Ramirez, F.; Dietz, H.C. Extracellular microfibrils in vertebrate development and disease processes. *J. Biol. Chem.* **2009**, *284*, 14677–14681. [CrossRef] [PubMed]
117. Habashi, J.P.; Judge, D.P.; Holm, T.M.; Cohn, R.D.; Loeys, B.L.; Cooper, T.K.; Myers, L.; Klein, E.C.; Liu, G.; Calvi, C.; et al. Losartan, an AT1 antagonist, prevents aortic aneurysm in a mouse model of Marfan syndrome. *Science* **2006**, *312*, 117–121. [CrossRef] [PubMed]
118. Brooke, B.S. Angiotensin II blockade and aortic-root dilation in Marfan's syndrome. *N. Engl. J. Med.* **2008**, *358*, 2787–2795. [CrossRef] [PubMed]
119. Neptune, E.R.; Frischmeyer, P.A.; Arking, D.E.; Myers, L.; Bunton, T.E.; Gayraud, B.; Ramirez, F.; Sakai, L.Y.; Dietz, H.C. Dysregulation of TGF-β activation contributes to pathogenesis in Marfan syndrome. *Nat. Genet.* **2003**, *33*, 407–411. [CrossRef]
120. Sumners, C.; Tang, W.; Zelezna, B.; Raizada, M.K. Angiotensin II receptor subtypes are coupled with distinct signal-transduction mechanisms in neurons and astrocytes from rat brain. *Proc. Natl. Acad. Sci. USA* **1991**, *88*, 7567–7571. [CrossRef]

121. Habashi, J.P.; Doyle, J.J.; Holm, T.M.; Aziz, H.; Schoenhoff, F.; Bedja, D.; Chen, Y.; Modiri, A.N.; Judge, D.P.; Dietz, H.C. Angiotensin II type 2 receptor signaling attenuates aortic aneurysm in mice through ERK antagonism. *Science* **2011**, *332*, 361–365. [CrossRef]
122. Holm, T.M.; Habashi, J.P.; Doyle, J.J.; Bedja, D.; Chen, Y.; van Erp, C.; Lindsay, M.E.; Kim, D.; Schoenhoff, F.; Cohn, R.D.; et al. Noncanonical TGFβ signaling contributes to aortic aneurysm progression in Marfan syndrome mice. *Science* **2011**, *332*, 358–361. [CrossRef]
123. Takagi, H.; Yamamoto, H.; Iwata, K.; Goto, S.N.; Umemoto, T.; ALICE (All-Literature Investigation of Cardiovascular Evidence) Group. An evidence-based hypothesis for beneficial effects of telmisartan on Marfan syndrome. *Int. J. Cardiol.* **2012**, *158*, 101–102. [CrossRef]
124. De Coster, P.J.; Martens, L.C.; De Paepe, A. Oral manifestations of patients with Marfan syndrome. A case-control study. *Oral Surg. Oral Med. Oral Pathol. Oral Radiol. Endod.* **2002**, *93*, 564–572. [CrossRef] [PubMed]
125. Shiga, M.; Saito, M.; Hattori, M.; Torii, C.; Kosaki, K.; Kiyono, T.; Suda, N. Characteristic phenotype of immortalized periodontal cells isolated from a Marfan syndrome type I patient. *Cell Tissue Res.* **2008**, *331*, 461–472. [CrossRef] [PubMed]
126. Suda, N.; Shiga, M.; Ganburged, G.; Moriyama, K. Marfan syndrome and its disorder in periodontal tissues. *J. Exp. Zool. B. Mol. Dev. Evol.* **2009**, *312B*, 503–509. [CrossRef] [PubMed]
127. Hujoel, P.; Zina, L.G.; Cunha-Cruz, J.; Lopez, R. Historical perspectives on theories of periodontal disease etiology. *Periodontology* **2012**, *58*, 153–160. [CrossRef] [PubMed]
128. Fox, C.H. New considerations in the prevalence of periodontal disease. *Curr. Opin. Dent.* **1992**, *2*, 5–11. [PubMed]
129. Fox, C.; Jette, A.M.; McGuire, S.M.; Feldman, H.A.; Douglass, C.W. Periodontal disease among New England elders. *J. Periodontol.* **1994**, *65*, 676–684. [CrossRef] [PubMed]
130. O'Dowd, L.K.; Durham, J.; McCracken, G.I.; Preshaw, P.M. Patients' experiences of the impact of periodontal disease. *J. Clin. Periodontol.* **2010**, *37*, 334–339. [CrossRef]
131. Pihlstrom, B.L. Periodontal risk assessment, diagnosis and treatment planning. *Periodontology* **2000**, *2001*, 37–58. [CrossRef]
132. Page, R.C.; Schroeder, H.E. *Periodontitis in Man and Other Animals. A Comparative Review*; Karger Medical and Scientific: Basel, Switzerland, 1982; pp. 5–41.
133. Christersson, L.A.; Zambon, J.J.; Genco, R.J. Dental bacterial plaques. Nature and role in periodontal disease. *J. Clin. Periodontol.* **1991**, *18*, 441–446. [CrossRef]
134. Suzuki, J.; Imai, Y.; Aoki, M.; Fujita, D.; Aoyama, N.; Tada, Y.; Akazawa, H.; Izumi, Y.; Isobe, M.; Komuro, I.; et al. High incidence and severity of periodontitis in patients with Marfan syndrome in Japan. *Heart Vessels* **2015**, *30*, 692–695. [CrossRef]
135. Suzuki, J.; Imai, Y.; Aoki, M.; Fujita, D.; Aoyama, N.; Tada, Y.; Wakayama, K.; Akazawa, H.; Izumi, Y.; Isobe, M.; et al. Periodontitis in cardiovascular disease patients with or without Marfan syndrome—A possible role of Prevotella intermedia. *PLoS ONE* **2014**, *9*, e95521. [CrossRef] [PubMed]
136. Pereira, L.; Lee, S.Y.; Gayraud, B.; Andrikopoulos, K.; Shapiro, S.D.; Bunton, T.; Biery, N.J.; Dietz, H.C.; Sakai, L.Y.; Ramirez, F. Pathogenetic sequence for aneurysm revealed in mice underexpressing fibrillin-1. *Proc. Natl. Acad. Sci. USA* **1999**, *96*, 3819–3823. [CrossRef] [PubMed]
137. Ganburged, G.; Suda, N.; Saito, M.; Yamazaki, Y.; Isokawa, K.; Moriyama, K. Dilated capillaries, disorganized collagen fibers and differential gene expression in periodontal ligaments of hypomorphic fibrillin-1 mice. *Cell Tissue Res.* **2010**, *341*, 381–395. [CrossRef] [PubMed]
138. Karlberg, B.E.; Lins, L.E.; Hermansson, K. Efficacy and safety of telmisartan, a selective AT1 receptor antagonist, compared with enalapril in elderly patients with primary hypertension. TEES Study Group. *J. Hypertens.* **1999**, *17*, 293–302. [CrossRef] [PubMed]
139. Benson, S.C.; Pershadsingh, H.A.; Ho, C.I.; Chittiboyina, A.; Desai, P.; Pravenec, M.; Qi, N.; Wang, J.; Avery, M.A.; Kurtz, T.W. Identification of telmisartan as a unique angiotensin II receptor antagonist with selective PPARgamma-modulating activity. *Hypertension* **2004**, *43*, 993–1002. [CrossRef]
140. Kaschina, E.; Schrader, F.; Sommerfeld, M.; Kemnitz, U.R.; Grzesiak, A.; Krikov, M.; Unger, T. Telmisartan prevents aneurysm progression in the rat by inhibiting proteolysis, apoptosis and inflammation. *J. Hypertens.* **2008**, *26*, 2361–2373. [CrossRef]

141. Ohno, K.; Amano, Y.; Kakuta, H.; Niimi, T.; Takakura, S.; Orita, M.; Miyata, K.; Sakashita, H.; Takeuchi, M.; Komuro, I.; et al. Unique "delta lock" structure of telmisartan is involved in its strongest binding affinity to angiotensin II type 1 receptor. *Biochem. Biophys. Res. Commun.* **2011**, *404*, 434–437. [CrossRef]
142. Suda, N.; Moriyama, K.; Ganburged, G. Effect of angiotensin II receptor blocker on experimental periodontitis in a mouse model of Marfan syndrome. *Infect. Immun.* **2013**, *81*, 182–188. [CrossRef]
143. Mao, W.; Zhang, L.; Zou, C.; Li, C.; Wu, Y.; Su, G.; Guo, X.; Wu, Y.; Lu, F.; Lin, Q.; et al. Rationale and design of the Helping Ease Renal failure with Bupi Yishen compared with the Angiotensin II Antagonist Losartan (HERBAAL) trial. A randomized controlled trial in non-diabetes stage 4 chronic kidney disease. *BMC Complement. Altern. Med.* **2015**, *15*, 316. [CrossRef]
144. Tu, X.; Ye, X.; Xie, C.; Chen, J.; Wang, F.; Zhong, S. Combination Therapy with Chinese Medicine and ACEI/ARB for the Management of Diabetic Nephropathy: The Promise in Research Fragments. *Curr. Vasc. Pharmacol.* **2015**, *13*, 526–539. [CrossRef]
145. Yesudas, R.; Gumaste, U.; Snyder, R.; Thekkumkara, T. Tannic acid down-regulates the angiotensin type 1 receptor through a MAPK-dependent mechanism. *Mol. Endocrinol.* **2012**, *26*, 458–470. [CrossRef] [PubMed]
146. Sakagami, H.; Zhou, L.; Kawano, M.; Thet, M.M.; Tanaka, S.; Machino, M.; Amano, S.; Kuroshita, R.; Watanabe, S.; Chu, Q.; et al. Multiple biological complex of alkaline extract of the leaves of *Sasa senanensis* Rehder. *In Vivo* **2010**, *24*, 735–743. [PubMed]

6

T and B Cells in Periodontal Disease: New Functions in A Complex Scenario

C.M. Figueredo [1,2,*], R. Lira-Junior [3] and R.M. Love [1]

[1] School of Dentistry and Oral Health, Griffith University, Queensland 4222, Australia
[2] Menzies Health Institute Queensland, Griffith University, Gold Coast, QLD 4222, Australia
[3] Division of Oral Diseases, Department of Dental Medicine, Karolinska Institutet, 141 04 Stockholm, Sweden
* Correspondence: c.dasilvafigueredo@griffith.edu.au

Abstract: Periodontal disease is characterised by a dense inflammatory infiltrate in the connective tissue. When the resolution is not achieved, the activation of T and B cells is crucial in controlling chronic inflammation through constitutive cytokine secretion and modulation of osteoclastogenesis. The present narrative review aims to overview the recent findings of the importance of T and B cell subsets, as well as their cytokine expression, in the pathogenesis of the periodontal disease. T regulatory (Treg), $CD8^+$ T, and tissue-resident $\gamma\delta$ T cells are important to the maintenance of gingival homeostasis. In inflamed gingiva, however, the secretion of IL-17 and secreted osteoclastogenic factor of activated T cells (SOFAT) by activated T cells is crucial to induce osteoclastogenesis via RANKL activation. Moreover, the capacity of mucosal-associated invariant T cells (MAIT cells) to produce cytokines, such as IFN-γ, TNF-α, and IL-17, might indicate a critical role of such cells in the disease pathogenesis. Regarding B cells, low levels of memory B cells in clinically healthy periodontium seem to be important to avoid bone loss due to the subclinical inflammation that occurs. On the other hand, they can exacerbate alveolar bone loss in a receptor activator of nuclear factor kappa-B ligand (RANKL)-dependent manner and affect the severity of periodontitis. In conclusion, several new functions have been discovered and added to the complex knowledge about T and B cells, such as possible new functions for Tregs, the role of SOFAT, and MAIT cells, as well as B cells activating RANKL. The activation of distinct T and B cell subtypes is decisive in defining whether the inflammatory lesion will stabilise as chronic gingivitis or will progress to a tissue destructive periodontitis.

Keywords: lymphocyte; T cells; B cells; cytokine; periodontal disease

---

1. Introduction

Periodontal disease is an inflammatory response to bacterial biofilm accumulation around teeth. This host inflammatory response is mediated mainly by neutrophils, monocytes/macrophages, and T and B lymphocytes (T and B cells). The development of the disease is characterised by a dense inflammatory infiltrate in the connective tissue, in which polymorphonuclear leukocytes and macrophages are abundant immune cells that firstly respond to the bacterial insult. When inflammation is not resolved, antigen-presenting cells (APCs) are activated by bacterial products and interact with naive T helper cells (Th0), driving their differentiation into several subsets, such as Th1, Th2, Th9, Th17, T-follicular helper (Tfh), and regulatory T cells (Treg) [1]).

Overexpression of the Th17/Treg axis is seen in disease initiation, followed by persistence of the Th17 response in periodontitis progression in a non-human primate model of periodontitis [2]. Tregs are required to keep periodontal health homeostasis, where their presence is essential to ensure a controlled response that minimises collateral tissue damage [3]. However, recent evidence suggested Th17 might not be the main source of interleukin (IL)-17A in periodontal tissues, suggesting Tregs may have a more prominent role in the pathogenesis of the periodontal disease [4]. These findings might change our understanding of the current literature. More recently, a new cell type named mucosal-associated invariant T (MAIT) cells has been associated with autoimmune and other inflammatory diseases in humans [5] and its role in the periodontal disease pathogenesis should be taken into consideration.

B cells, on the other hand, are part of the adaptive humoral immunity specialised in secreting antibodies and cytokines, as well as presenting antigens, and have been strongly associated with periodontal homeostasis and disease [5]. A minimal presence of B cells in healthy gingiva has been reported [6,7], which might be important to avoid bone loss due to the subclinical inflammation that occurs in the clinically healthy periodontium. B cells in periodontitis patients may contribute to chronic systemic inflammation through cytokine secretion [8]. Memory B cells can induce bone loss in rheumatoid arthritis [9], which led to the hypothesis that they express RANKL and regulate alveolar bone homeostasis during periodontitis [10]. The present narrative review aims to overview the recent findings of the importance of T and B cell subsets, as well as their cytokine expression, in the pathogenesis of the periodontal disease.

2. T and B Lymphocytes

2.1. T Lymphocytes

T lymphocytes (T cells) are immune cells involved in host defence and control of immune-mediated inflammatory disease development. They can be distinguished from other lymphocytes by the presence of a T-cell receptor (TCR) on the cell surface. Most T cells are composed of two glycoprotein chains named α (alpha) and β (beta) TCR chains. However, a smaller group of T cells, named $\gamma\delta$ T cells, presents a gamma/delta composition. They are an important subset of T cells as they can recognise a broad range of antigens without the presence of major histocompatibility complex (MHC) molecules [11]. T cells are subdivided into Th, Treg, T cytotoxic ($CD8^+$), natural killer, and memory cells. Also, T cell anergy has been defined as a mechanism of peripheral tolerance that determines the functional inactivation of T cells following antigen recognition under non-optimal conditions [12].

Naive $CD4^+$ T cells are activated after interaction with antigen-MHC complex and differentiate into specific subtypes depending on the cytokine microenvironment [13]. After such interactions, they become activated and differentiated into effector T cells, which are responsible for the production of effector molecules, such as pro-/anti-inflammatory cytokines and cytotoxic molecules. Most of the effector T cells undergo programmed cell death after the antigen clearance. The ones that survive differentiate into memory T cells. Th cells are classified as Th1, Th2, Th17, and Treg subpopulations based on their unique cytokine properties [14].

Besides the classical Th cell subpopulations, Tfh, Th9, and Th22 cells have recently been defined as new subpopulations that produce IL-21, IL-9, and IL-22, respectively [14,15]. Tfh is a specialised $CD4^+$ T-cell subset that provides survival, proliferation, and selection signals by engaging in cognate interactions with B cells [16]. Th9 cells have been shown to present both beneficial and detrimental functions. Among the beneficial functions is their ability to initiate antitumor immunity and immune response to helminth parasites [17]. Detrimental functions of Th9 cells include the promotion of allergic inflammation and the mediation of some types of autoimmunity [17]. Duhen et al. [18] showed that memory T cells with skin-homing properties from healthy donors are characterised by the production of IL-22 in the absence of IL-17 and IFN-γ. The authors found that several T cell clones isolated from psoriatic lesions were Th22. Their function is the specific production of IL-22, which has been linked to skin homeostasis and inflammation [14].

Cytotoxic T lymphocytes ($CD8^+$ T cells) are generated in the thymus and express a dimeric co-receptor, usually composed of one CD8α and one CD8β chain, and they recognise peptides presented by MHC class I molecules. $CD8^+$ T cells present three major mechanisms to kill infected or malignant cells: (a) secretion of cytokines, primarily TNF-α and IFN-γ, which have anti-tumor, anti-viral, and anti-microbial effects, (b) production and release of cytotoxic granules (also found in

NK cells), which contain two families of proteins, perforin and granzymes, and (c) destruction of infected cells via Fas/FasL interactions which can result in apoptosis of the target cell. Besides cytotoxic activities, CD8$^+$ T cells also have regulatory/suppressor functions (CD8$^+$ Treg), since they can control other leukocytes to avoid excessive immune activation and its pathological consequences [19].

Besides the T cells subgroups mentioned above, mucosal-associated invariant T (MAIT) cells represent a unique subset of innate-like T cells described in the late 1990s [20]. MAIT cells represent the most abundant innate-like T-cell population within human beings, comprising up to ~5% of the total T-cell population [21]. Characterisation of the MAIT cells in the buccal mucosa showed that the major subset displayed a tissue-resident and activated profile with high expression of CD69, CD103, HLA-DR, and PD-1. These tissue-resident MAIT cells produced higher IL-17 levels than tissue non-resident and circulating populations [22]. New research projects should be stimulated to better understanding the role of tissue-resident MAIT cells in the osteoclastogenesis activation in periodontal diseases.

2.2. *B Lymphocytes*

B lymphocytes (B cells) are part of the humoral component of the adaptive immune system and specialised in secreting antibodies. B cells can also present antigens and secrete cytokines. In mammals, B cells mature in the bone marrow, and B cell receptors (BCRs) mature on their cell membranes, which allow B cells to bind specific antigens initiating an antibody response. Such antigen recognition can happen through either low- or high-affinity binding modes [23]. After maturation, multiple subsets of B-cells co-expressing IgM and IgD emerge from the bone marrow and colonise compartments of secondary lymphoid organs [24].

B cell subpopulations can be distinguished in peripheral blood based on surface-marker expression, which mainly represents different developmental stages of the cell. Alterations in some of these populations have been associated with clinical phenotypes in immunodeficiency and autoimmune diseases. The second phase of B-cell development occurs after the antigen-dependent phase. Depending on various contacts and cytokine stimuli received by the activated cell, it will become either a memory cell to be activated once again in the future or it will become a plasma cell producing large amounts of antibodies [25].

Didactically, B cells can be subdivided as follows: plasmablasts (the immature precursor of plasmacytes), plasma cells (antibody-secreting cells arising from B cell differentiation), memory B cells (B2 cells and synonymous with classical B cells), marginal zone (MZ) B cells (specialized population of B cells that are located in the marginal zone of the spleen), B1 cells (subtype of B cells that are distinct from classical B cells with respect to their phenotype, distribution in the body, and function). Unlike classical B cells, B-1 cells are considered functionally to be part of the innate immune response [26]. Regulatory B cells (Breg) negatively regulate the immune response by producing regulatory cytokines and directly interacting with pathogenic T cells via cell-to-cell contact [27].

Abnormal B-cell recognition of self-antigens may lead to autoimmunity, which results in autoantibody production. Autoantibodies produced by B-cell-derived plasma cells provide diagnostic markers for autoimmunity, and also contribute significantly to disease pathogenesis [28]. Autoimmune diseases where B-cell functions are closely correlated with disease activity include systemic lupus erythematosus, rheumatoid arthritis, scleroderma, type 1 diabetes, and multiple sclerosis [28].

2.3. *T and B Lymphocytes in Periodontal Homeostasis*

2.3.1. T Lymphocytes

The characterisation of T lymphocytes in healthy gingiva has shown a dominance of CD4$^+$ helper T cells [6]. These cells play fundamental roles in the adaptive immune responses, and their cytokine production in response to specific immunological challenges led to the classical framework of distinct Th cell subsets [29]. CD8$^+$ T cells were the second most abundant T lymphocyte in healthy gingiva, followed by a small percentage of $\gamma\delta$T cells. Gingival CD8$^+$ T cells seem to have regulatory/suppressor properties important to the maintenance of gingival tissue integrity by downregulating inflammation under homeostatic conditions. These cells can produce IL-10 and TGF-β, which then suppress osteoclastogenesis [30]. Tissue-resident epithelial $\gamma\delta$ T cells have been reported to be the major T cell population in the epithelial tissues and are important in carrying out barrier surveillance and helping to keep tissue homeostasis, and to some extent, epithelial repair [31]. Gingival $\gamma\delta$ T cells accumulate after birth in response to barrier damage and are crucial for immune homeostasis. These cells produce amphiregulin, a wound healing-associated cytokine, which limits the development of periodontitis [32]. $\gamma\delta$ T cells are also the major source of IL-17 in homeostasis. Interestingly, ablation of $\gamma\delta$T cells resulted in increased gingival inflammation and alterations in the microbial diversity [33]. Within the CD4 compartment, about 15% are presumed to be Treg cells, which are crucial for periodontal homeostasis. Increased numbers of Tregs are associated with bone homeostasis, even in the presence of local inflammation [34] and may be related to the non-progression of gingivitis lesions in some patients, even after a long period of oral biofilm exposure. The new roles of $\gamma\delta$T cells and Tregs in periodontal tissue homeostasis are crucial to the understanding of periodontal disease initiation and progression.

Dutzan et al. [6] characterised memory and naive T-cell subsets in the gingiva, showing that approximately 80% of CD4$^+$ and 50% of CD8$^+$ T cells had a CD45RO$^+$ (activated T cell) memory phenotype. The CD4$^+$ cell compartment in gingiva had a minimal CD45RA$^+$ (naive T cell) population, but the CD8$^+$ T cell compartment had a substantial population of CD45RA$^+$/CCR7$^-$ cells (terminally differentiated effector T cells, T_{EMRA}) alongside a smaller population of naive CD45RA$^+$CCR7$^+$ cells [6,35]. CCR7 is a chemokine receptor that divides human memory T cells into two functionally distinct subsets. CCR7$^-$ memory cells express receptors for migration to inflamed tissues and display immediate effector function; CCR7$^+$ memory cells lack immediate effector function, but efficiently stimulate dendritic cells and differentiate into CCR7$^-$ effector cells upon secondary stimulation [36].

The combination of CD45RO and CCR7 (memory subset markers) with CD69 (a stimulatory receptor expressed at sites of chronic inflammation) was performed by Dutzan et al. [6] to analyse circulating and tissue-resident memory CD4$^+$ and CD8$^+$ T cell subsets. Their results showed that the majority of CD4 memory T cells in gingiva were CCR7$^-$CD69$^+$ (resident effector memory, rT_{EM} cells), followed almost equally by resident memory, effector memory (T_{EM}), and central memory (rT_{CM}; CCR7$^+$CD69$^+$) cells. Regarding CD8, memory CD45RO$^+$ cells were also rT_{EM} in their majority, followed by a large population of T_{EM} and a small population of central memory cells (T_{CM}). Increased proportions of resident memory T cells are common at barrier sites, where they have been reported to support early/immediate defence mechanisms, providing site-specific protection from pathogen challenges [37]. Resident memory T cells would then have special importance to protect the connective tissue form the bacterial products released in the periodontal sulcus.

Besides the T-cell characterisation, it is important to understand how these cells behave under physiological conditions. Having clinically healthy gingiva does not ensure that T cells are not being activated. Dutzan et al. [38], demonstrated in mouse gingiva that gingiva-resident Th17 cells developed via a commensal colonisation-independent mechanism. Th17 cells might accumulate at the gingiva in response to the physiological barrier damage that occurs, for instance, during mastication. The authors showed that physiological mechanical damage could induce the expression of IL-6 from epithelial cells, promoting an increase in gingival Th17 cell numbers.

2.3.2. B Lymphocytes

The characterisation of B cell subsets in gingival tissues was recently described by Mahanonda et al. [39]. The authors reported very few naïve B cells (<8%) in all stages of healthy and diseased tissues. Additionally, memory B cells (CD19$^+$CD27$^+$CD38$^-$) represented the majority of the B cell population in the clinically healthy gingiva and were detected in the connective tissue subjacent to the apical region of the junctional epithelium, which could be due to the local low-grade inflammatory response to a constant challenge of the biofilm. The authors highlighted the importance of detecting memory B cells in clinically healthy human gingiva since very little is known about memory B cells residing in human nonlymphoid tissues. The minimal presence of B cells in healthy gingiva was also reported by others [6,7,35,40]. Such low levels might be important to avoid bone loss around teeth due to the subclinical inflammation that occurs in the clinically healthy periodontium.

Another aspect of the B cell biology that is relevant for gingival homeostasis is the production of antibodies against periodontal pathogens, which can contribute to host protection [41,42]. Page et al. [43] demonstrated that immunisation using *P. gingivalis* as antigen could reduce the onset and progression of alveolar bone loss in non-human primates. Also, Shelburne et al. [41] suggested that anti-*P. gingivalis* HtpG antibodies predict health in patients susceptible to periodontal disease. The potential role of B cell humoral immunity in maintaining homeostasis needs further investigations. A description of the main functions of T and B cells' subsets in the periodontal tissues is presented in the Table 1.

2.4. Changes with Age

Furthermore, age is also a variable that needs to be considered when evaluating the lymphocyte function in healthy periodontium. The effects of aging on periodontal tissues are thought to intensify alveolar bone resorption in elderly individuals [44]. Witkowski et al. [45] reviewed the proteodynamics in aging human T cells and reported that the proteolytic elimination of altered proteins, as well as modulation of the activity of those remaining, leads to the dynamic change of proteome composition and function in aging lymphocytes. Ebersole et al. [44] reported that several B cell and plasmacyte genes are altered in aging healthy gingival tissues, which are mainly associated with antigen-dependent activation and B cell differentiation/maturation processes. Aging T and B cell dynamics requires further comprehensive analysis and may influence the pathophysiology of periodontal disease.

2.5. T and B Lymphocytes in Periodontal Inflammation

In 1983, Okada et al. [46] published a very elegant paper characterising the immunocompetent cells on histological sections from diseased human gingiva. According to the authors, human periodontitis contains numerous sets of infiltrating cells which are organized unusually, with a region rich in T lymphocytes and monocytes/macrophages just subjacent to the pocket or sulcular epithelium; and a region in the central lamina propria, located farther away from the microbial agent, which is rich in B cells and plasma cells and poor in T lymphocytes. Furthermore, the same group characterised the T lymphocyte subsets (T4+ and T8+) in the inflamed gingiva from human periodontitis and showed the ratio T4+/T8+ was lower in gingival tissue than in peripheral blood [47]. Dutzan et al. [6] evaluated the major cell subsets and revealed that the lymphocytic compartment, CD3+T cells remained the dominant population in both health and disease, yet in disease the total number of T cells is much greater, reflecting a 10 fold increase in total inflammatory cells [6].

The role of T cells in the immune dysregulation of periodontitis has been consistently revised by Campbell et al. [1]. Activated Th1, Th2, and Th17 cells can produce a variety of pro-inflammatory cytokines, such as IL-1β, IL-17E (IL-25) and IL-17, that activate other immune cells such as dendritic cells, neutrophils, and B cells. Activation of both T cells and subsequently, B cells can cause the production of the receptor activator of nuclear factor κ B -Ligand (RANKL), which leads to alveolar bone resorption by osteoclasts, resulting in tooth loss. Moreover, the activation of B cells by Tfh in either peripheral lymph nodes or tertiary lymph organs can result in clonal activation of B cells, which produce antibodies to recognise bacterial components; however, production of autoantibodies to collagen, fibronectin and laminin can contribute to local destruction of the gingival tissue. Finally, a lack of Treg cells or an inability of those present to reduce local inflammatory responses by other immune cells may play a role in the chronic inflammation associated with periodontitis [1].

Table 1. A summary of the main functions of mentioned T and B cells in periodontal health and disease.

Cell	Subtype	Function in the Periodontal Tissues
T cells	Treg	Periodontal homeostasis by producing IL-10 and TGF-β.
	MAIT	Largely unknown.
	Th	Specific immunological challenges lead to distinct cells' subsets; Th1, Th2, and Th17 cells can produce a variety of pro-inflammatory cytokines that activate other immune cells such as dendritic cells, neutrophils, and B cells. Th17 can also be produced in response to biological barrier damage in healthy tissue.
	Tissue-resident epithelial γδ	Barrier surveillance, tissue homeostasis, and epithelial repair; Major source of IL-17 in homeostasis.
	$CD8^+$	Downregulate inflammation and suppress osteoclastogenesis. IL-10 and TGF-β production.
	Tfh	Activation of B cells; IL-21 production.
	SOFAT	Induce osteoclastogenesis in a RANKL-independent manner.
B cells	Activated	Activation and expression of RANKL in the gingiva; promote osteoclastogenesis.
	Memory	To prevent bone loss due to subclinical inflammation in clinically healthy periodontium. Production of antibodies against periodontal pathogens.
	Immunoglobulin-bearing lymphocytes; plasma cells	Clinical progression of the periodontal lesion; Stimulate the expression of RANKL in the gingiva.
	B1	Associated with regulatory functions and the numbers might be decreased in periodontitis patients; produces antibodies against antigens and act as antigen-presenting cells.
	Breg/B10	Negatively regulates the inflammatory responses via IL-10.
	$CD138^+$ plasma cells	Association with the advancing front of the periodontal lesion.

Treg: regulatory T cells; MAIT cells: mucosal-associated invariant T cells; Th: helper T cells; CD: cluster of differentiation; SOFAT: secreted osteoclastogenic factor of activated T cells; Tfh: T-follicular helper; Breg: regulatory B cel.

T cells have a crucial role in the tissue secretion of IL-17, a cytokine strongly associated with bone loss around teeth. Chen et al. [48] reported that IL-17 and IFN-γ levels in biopsy specimens of gingival lesions from chronic periodontitis patients were higher than those in the healthy controls. Moreover, relative IFN-γ, IL-17A, and T-bet mRNA levels were also significantly higher in patients with chronic periodontitis compared to controls, suggesting that Th17 and Th1 cells might be involved in the pathogenesis of chronic periodontitis. Dutzan et al. [6,35] characterised IL-17-secreting cells within the hematopoietic compartment in healthy and periodontitis gingival samples and found a significant increase in IL-17$^+$ cells in diseased sites. The major source of IL-17 was CD4$^+$ T cells, with minimal contribution from CD8, $\gamma\delta$T, and non-T-cell sources.

Moreover, the percentage of CD4$^+$ T cells producing IL-17 significantly increased in periodontitis. CD4$^+$ T cells preferentially upregulated IL-17 and not IFN-γ in gingival tissue from periodontitis patients. The same group also reported that Th17 cells in periodontitis are dependent on the local dysbiotic microbiota, and both IL-6 and IL-23 are required for their accumulation. Also, pharmacologically targeting RORγt, a transcription factor relevant for Th17 differentiation, reduces alveolar bone loss in a murine model of periodontitis [49]. On the other hand, Parachuru et al. [4] presented an interesting paper that compared healthy/gingivitis tissues with chronic periodontitis tissues. Among other goals, they aimed to determine the identity of FoxP3 and IL-17A positive cells in periodontal tissues. The authors reported that Th17 cells either do not exist in periodontal disease or are present in small numbers and that, as with other chronic inflammatory lesions, the source of the relatively small amounts of IL-17 may be mast cells. Moreover, they also suggested that Tregs may have an important role in the pathogenesis of the chronic inflammatory periodontal disease. Such a statement needs to be better investigated since it might affect our present understanding of the Th17/Treg imbalance that leads to periodontal disease progression.

Besides the importance of IL-17 secreted by CD4$^+$ T cell or mast cells, a novel T cell-secreted cytokine, called secreted osteoclastogenic factor of activated T cells (SOFAT), that can induce osteoclastogenesis in a RANKL-independent manner, has been described in periodontal tissues [50]. The authors showed that the mRNA and protein levels of SOFAT were significantly higher in the gingival tissue of periodontitis patients compared to controls. More recently, Jarry et al. [51] demonstrated that B-lineage cells, including plasma cells, also exhibited strong staining for SOFAT in diseased periodontal tissue. Therefore, SOFAT might have an important role in periodontal disease by activating RANKL related osteoclastogenesis.

The characterisation and identification of interstitial T cells are relevant to understanding the immunopathogenesis of periodontitis. Bittner-Eddy et al. [52] have made an important contribution to this subject by describing a flow cytometry assay that distinguishes interstitial leukocytes in the oral mucosa of mice from those circulating within the vasculature or in post-dissection contaminating blood. They reported that, unlike circulating CD4 T cells, interstitial CD4 T cells were almost exclusively antigen-experienced cells (CD44^{hi}). The authors reported the presence of antigen-experienced *P. gingivalis*-specific CD4 T cells in nasal-associated lymphoid tissues following oral feeding of mice with *P. gingivalis*. Such differentiation might be critical for future understanding of the players driving alveolar bone destruction.

B cells infiltrate and dominate sites showing progressive chronic inflammatory periodontal disease in humans [53]. It has been shown that periodontitis lesions contain significant numbers of immunoglobulin-bearing lymphocytes and plasma cells, suggesting that the clinical progression of the periodontal lesion is followed by a shift in cellular infiltrates from predominantly immunoglobulin-negative lymphocytes to IgG and IgM-bearing lymphocytes and plasma cells [54]. Oliver-Bell et al. [55] demonstrated that B cells make a substantial contribution to alveolar bone loss in murine periodontitis, probably due to B-cell activation and expression of RANKL in the gingiva. Abe et al. [56] reported that ligature-induced periodontitis resulted in significantly less bone loss in B cell-deficient mice compared with wild-type controls, supporting the importance of B cells in periodontal bone loss. The authors also suggested that two cytokines of the TNF ligand superfamily, a proliferation-inducing ligand (APRIL) and B-lymphocyte stimulator (BLyS), might be potential therapeutic targets in periodontitis [56].

Mahanonda et al. [39] have characterised B cell subsets in gingivitis and periodontitis. The density of memory B cells in periodontitis lesions was significantly lower than in healthy and gingivitis tissues. On the other hand, Ab-secreting cells were the major cell type in the $CD19^+$ B cell population, with the mean percentage of Ab-secreting cells being significantly higher than that of memory B cells. Moreover, an abundance of $CD138^+$ plasma cells was observed in periodontitis tissues. The authors reported that plasma cells were arranged in clusters detected at the base of the periodontal pocket area and scattered throughout the gingival connective tissue, especially apically toward the advancing front of the lesion [39].

B cells in patients with periodontal disease may contribute to chronic systemic inflammation through constitutive secretion of IL-8 and IL-1β [8], but the in situ impact of such cytokine production should be elucidated. Kawai et al. [57] have demonstrated that B cells can be the cellular source of RANKL for bone resorption in homogenised gingival tissue from sites showing periodontal disease. Moreover, Malcolm et al. [58] have shown that the percentage of B cells expressing RANKL was elevated following *P. gingivalis* infection in gingival tissues. Oliver-Bell et al. [55] have also investigated the impact of *P. gingivalis* infection in the RANKL expression of B cells, showing that mice infected with *P. gingivalis* presented a significant increase in B-cell RANKL expression in the gingiva. Moreover, B-cell-deficient mice did not show *P. gingivalis*-induced alveolar bone loss. Recently, Kanzaki et al. [59] demonstrated that sRANKL and TNF-α cleaved from activated tumour necrosis factor-α-converting enzyme-bearing B cells might be important as an osteoclastogenic factor in periodontitis lesions.

Han et al. [10] suggested that B cells affect alveolar bone homeostasis in a murine model of periodontitis through antibody-independent and RANKL-dependent mechanisms. They reported that gingival memory B cells promote osteoclastogenesis and that this potential was increased by the development of periodontitis. Demoersman et al. [60] reported that a significantly higher percentage of $CD27^+$ memory B cells was observed in patients with severe periodontitis. At the same time, human B1 cells, which were previously associated with a regulatory function, decreased in such patients. The authors also reported that the RANKL expression increased in every B cell subset from severe periodontitis patients and was significantly greater in activated B cells than in the subjects without periodontitis. Moreover, an interesting literature review published by Zouali [54] supports that B cells are key participants in RANKL-mediated bone resorption. Activated RANKL-positive B cells can exacerbate alveolar bone loss in a RANKL-dependent manner in animal models. On the other hand, blocking RANKL, B-cell-activating factor (BAFF), and a proliferation-inducing ligand (APRIL) reduces alveolar bone loss in experimental models of periodontitis. Coat et al. [61] reported that periodontal parameters could be significantly improved after treatment with rituximab, concluding that anti-B lymphocyte therapy could be beneficial in improving de clinical conditions of patients with periodontitis.

Besides the fact that B cells positively activate immune responses, functioning as APCs and producing antibodies, regulatory B cells (Bregs) have been shown to exert a suppressive role in immune response [62]. B10 cells are a Breg cell subset that produces IL-10 and therefore, negatively regulates the inflammatory responses [63]. B10 cells are present in gingival tissues of patients with and without periodontal disease, but in significantly higher levels in periodontal disease lesions [5.89 ± 2.02) when compared to healthy tissues (0.1 ± 0.3, $p < 0.01$) [64]. Yu et al. [65] demonstrated that the local induction of IL-10 competency of B10 cells was associated with the inhibition of both inflammation and bone loss in ligature-induced experimental periodontitis. Wang et al. [66] also reported that the adoptive transfer of B10 cells significantly inhibited inflammation and bone loss in a mouse model of experimental periodontitis, suggesting a potential novel principle of treatment for periodontal diseases. It has been suggested that the in vitro treatment of B10 cells with a combination of IL-21, anti-Tim1, and CD40L might inhibit periodontal bone loss in ligature-induced experimental periodontitis [65]. A schematic of the lymphocyte subsets and their possible contribution to periodontal homeostasis and inflammation is presented in the Figure 1.

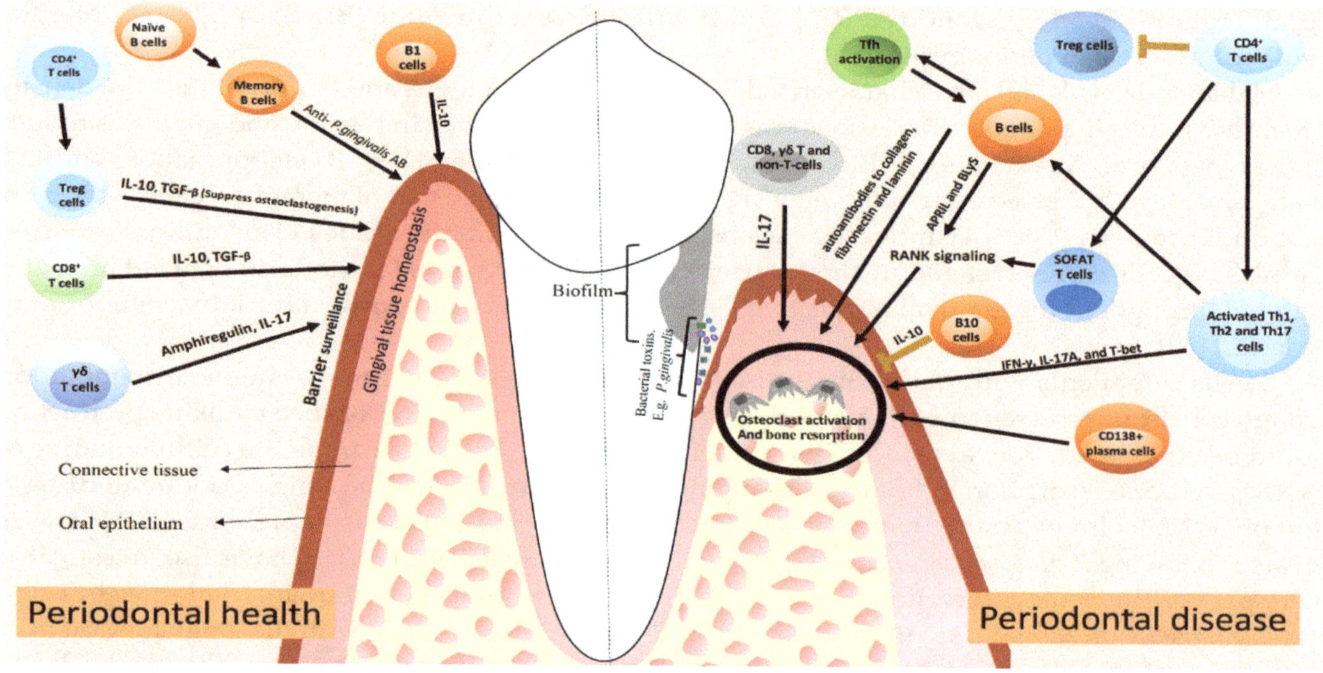

Figure 1. A summary of how mentioned T and B cells can contribute to periodontal health and disease. In periodontal health, Treg and CD8+ T cells contribute to periodontal homeostasis through the production of IL-10 and TGF-β. γδ T cells produce amphiregulin and IL-17 to promote periodontal homeostasis. B cells produce antibodies against periodontal pathogens, limiting the development of periodontal inflammation. In periodontal disease, activated Th1, Th2, and Th17 cells produce pro-inflammatory cytokines that contribute to tissue damage. Both T and B cells produce RANKL, which leads to osteoclast activation and alveolar bone resorption. Clonal activation of B cells by Tfh cells can lead to the production of autoantibodies to collagen, fibronectin and laminin, contributing to local tissue destruction. Lack of Treg cells or an impaired function probably impact on the development of periodontitis. IL-17 produced by other cells can also contribute to tissue damage via osteoclast activation. The figure was adapted from Lira-Junior & Figueredo [67].

The increased knowledge in T and B cells' biology, as well as their functions during gingival tissue homeostasis and inflammation might help in designing novel therapeutic strategies for bone disorders where these cells are a crucial part of the local tissue inflammation, such as periodontitis.

3. Conclusions

Several new roles have been discovered and added to the complex knowledge about T and B cells. These include different functions of Tregs, the role of γδ T cells in gingival homeostasis, the role of SOFAT in osteoclastogenesis, and the possible pathogenic role of MAIT cells. Also, the importance of B cells activating RANKL-mediated bone resorption adds to this complex scenario. During periodontal inflammation, the activation of distinct T and B-cell subtypes, as well as their cytokine production, are crucial in defining whether the inflammatory lesion will stabilise as chronic gingivitis or progress to tissue-destructive periodontitis.

References

1. Campbell, L.; Millhouse, E.; Malcolm, J.; Culshaw, S. T cells, teeth and tissue destruction—what do T cells do in periodontal disease? *Mol. Oral. Microbiol.* **2016**, *31*, 445–456. [CrossRef] [PubMed]

2. Ebersole, J.L.; Kirakodu, S.; Novak, M.J.; Stromberg, A.J.; Shen, S.; Orraca, L.; Orraca, L.; Gonzalez-Martinez, J.; Burgos, A.; Gonzalez, O.A. Cytokine gene expression profiles during initiation, progression and resolution of periodontitis. *J Clin Periodontol.* **2014**, *41*, 853–861. [CrossRef] [PubMed]
3. Alvarez, C.; Rojas, C.; Rojas, L.; Cafferata, E.A.; Monasterio, G.; Vernal, R. Regulatory T Lymphocytes in Periodontitis: A Translational View. *Mediators Inflamm.* **2018**, *2018*, 7806912. [CrossRef] [PubMed]
4. Parachuru, V.P.B.; Coates, D.E.; Milne, T.J.; Rich, A.M.; Seymour, G.J. FoxP3(+) regulatory T cells, interleukin 17 and mast cells in chronic inflammatory periodontal disease. *J. Periodontal Res.* **2018**, *53*, 622–635. [CrossRef] [PubMed]
5. Berglundh, T.; Liljenberg, B.; Tarkowski, A.; Lindhe, J. The presence of local and circulating autoreactive B cells in patients with advanced periodontitis. *J. Clin. Periodontol.* **2002**, *29*, 281–286. [CrossRef] [PubMed]
6. Dutzan, N.; Konkel, J.E.; Greenwell-Wild, T.; Moutsopoulos, N.M. Characterization of the human immune cell network at the gingival barrier. *Mucosal Immunol.* **2016**, *9*, 1163–1172. [CrossRef] [PubMed]
7. Artese, L.; Simon, M.J.; Piattelli, A.; Ferrari, D.S.; Cardoso, L.A.; Faveri, M.; Onuma, T.; Piccirilli, M.; Perrotti, V.; Shibli, J.A. Immunohistochemical analysis of inflammatory infiltrate in aggressive and chronic periodontitis: A comparative study. *Clin. Oral Investig.* **2011**, *15*, 233–240. [CrossRef] [PubMed]
8. Jagannathan, M.; Hasturk, H.; Liang, Y.; Shin, H.; Hetzel, J.T.; Kantarci, A.; Rubin, D.; McDonnell, M.E.; Van Dyke, T.E.; Ganley-Leal, L.M.; et al. TLR cross-talk specifically regulates cytokine production by B cells from chronic inflammatory disease patients. *J. Immunol.* **2009**, *183*, 7461–7470. [CrossRef]
9. Zundler, S.; Neurath, M.F. Interleukin-12: Functional activities and implications for disease. *Cytokine Growth Factor Rev.* **2015**, *26*, 559–568. [CrossRef]
10. Han, Y.K.; Jin, Y.; Miao, Y.B.; Shi, T.; Lin, X.P. Improved RANKL production by memory B cells: A way for B cells promote alveolar bone destruction during periodontitis. *Int. Immunopharmacol.* **2018**, *64*, 232–237. [CrossRef]
11. Bonneville, M.; O'Brien, R.L.; Born, W.K. Gammadelta T cell effector functions: A blend of innate programming and acquired plasticity. *Nat. Rev. Immunol.* **2010**, *10*, 467–478. [CrossRef] [PubMed]
12. Valdor, R.; Macian, F. Induction and stability of the anergic phenotype in T cells. *Semin Immunol.* **2013**, *25*, 313–320. [CrossRef] [PubMed]
13. Luckheeram, R.V.; Zhou, R.; Verma, A.D.; Xia, B. CD4(+)T cells: Differentiation and functions. *Clin. Dev. Immunol.* **2012**, *2012*, 925135. [CrossRef] [PubMed]
14. Jia, L.; Wu, C. The biology and functions of Th22 cells. *Adv. Exp. Med. Biol.* **2014**, *841*, 209–230. [PubMed]
15. Lee, N.; Kim, W.U. Microbiota in T cell homeostasis and inflammatory diseases. *Exp. Mol. Med.* **2017**, *49*, e340. [CrossRef] [PubMed]
16. Crotty, S. Follicular helper CD4 T cells (TFH). *Annu. Rev. Immunol.* **2011**, *29*, 621–663. [CrossRef] [PubMed]
17. Kaplan, M.H.; Hufford, M.M.; Olson, M.R. The development and in vivo function of T helper 9 cells. *Nat. Rev. Immunol.* **2015**, *15*, 295–307. [CrossRef] [PubMed]
18. Duhen, T.; Geiger, R.; Jarrossay, D.; Lanzavecchia, A.; Sallusto, F. Production of interleukin 22 but not interleukin 17 by a subset of human skin-homing memory T cells. *Nat. Immunol.* **2009**, *10*, 857–863. [CrossRef]
19. Xu, Z.; Ho, S.; Chang, C.C.; Zhang, Q.Y.; Vasilescu, E.R.; Vlad, G.; Suciu-Foca, N. Molecular and Cellular Characterization of Human CD8 T Suppressor Cells. *Front. Immunol.* **2016**, *7*, 549. [CrossRef]
20. Tilloy, F.; Treiner, E.; Park, S.H.; Garcia, C.; Lemonnier, F.; de la Salle, H.; Bendelac, A.; Bonneville, M.; Lantz, O. An invariant T cell receptor alpha chain defines a novel TAP-independent major histocompatibility complex class Ib-restricted alpha/beta T cell subpopulation in mammals. *J. Exp. Med.* **1999**, *189*, 1907–1921. [CrossRef]
21. Treiner, E.; Lantz, O. CD1d- and MR1-restricted invariant T cells: Of mice and men. *Curr. Opin. Immunol.* **2006**, *18*, 519–526. [CrossRef]
22. Sobkowiak, M.J.; Davanian, H.; Heymann, R.; Gibbs, A.; Emgard, J.; Dias, J.; Aleman, S.; Krüger-Weiner, C.; Moll, M.; Tjernlund, A.; et al. Tissue-resident MAIT cell populations in human oral mucosa exhibit an activated profile and produce IL-17. *Eur. J. Immunol.* **2018**. [CrossRef]
23. Cerutti, A.; Cols, M.; Puga, I. Activation of B cells by non-canonical helper signals. *EMBO Rep.* **2012**, *13*, 798–810. [CrossRef]
24. Cerutti, A.; Puga, I.; Cols, M. New helping friends for B cells. *Eur. J. Immunol.* **2012**, *42*, 1956–1968. [CrossRef]
25. Bonilla, F.A.; Oettgen, H.C. Adaptive immunity. *J. Allergy Clin. Immunol.* **2010**, *125*, S33–S40. [CrossRef]
26. Smith, F.L.; Baumgarth, N. B-1 cell responses to infections. *Curr. Opin. Immunol.* **2019**, *5*, 23–31. [CrossRef]

27. Yang, M.; Rui, K.; Wang, S.; Lu, L. Regulatory B cells in autoimmune diseases. *Cell Mol. Immunol.* **2013**, *10*, 122–132. [CrossRef]
28. Yanaba, K.; Bouaziz, J.D.; Matsushita, T.; Magro, C.M.; St Clair, E.W.; Tedder, T.F. B-lymphocyte contributions to human autoimmune disease. *Immunol. Rev.* **2008**, *223*, 284–299. [CrossRef]
29. Zhu, J.; Paul, W.E. CD4 T cells: Fates, functions, and faults. *Blood* **2008**, *112*, 1557–1569. [CrossRef]
30. Cardoso, E.M.; Arosa, F.A. CD8(+) T Cells in Chronic Periodontitis: Roles and Rules. *Front. Immunol.* **2017**, *8*, 145. [CrossRef]
31. Nielsen, M.M.; Witherden, D.A.; Havran, W.L. Gammadelta T cells in homeostasis and host defence of epithelial barrier tissues. *Nat. Rev. Immunol.* **2017**, *17*, 733–745. [CrossRef]
32. Krishnan, S.; Prise, I.E.; Wemyss, K.; Schenck, L.P.; Bridgeman, H.M.; McClure, F.A.; Zangerle-Murray, T.; O'Boyle, C.; Barbera, T.A.; Mahmood, F.; et al. Amphiregulin-producing gammadelta T cells are vital for safeguarding oral barrier immune homeostasis. *Proc. Natl. Acad. Sci. USA* **2018**, *115*, 10738–10743. [CrossRef]
33. Wilharm, A.; Tabib, Y.; Nassar, M.; Reinhardt, A.; Mizraji, G.; Sandrock, I.; Heyman, O.; Barros-Martins, J.; Aizenbud, Y.; Khalaileh, A.; et al. Mutual interplay between IL-17-producing gammadeltaT cells and microbiota orchestrates oral mucosal homeostasis. *Proc. Natl. Acad. Sci. USA* **2019**, *116*, 2652–2661. [CrossRef]
34. Arizon, M.; Nudel, I.; Segev, H.; Mizraji, G.; Elnekave, M.; Furmanov, K.; Eli-Berchoer, L.; Clausen, B.E.; Shapira, L.; Wilensky, A.; et al. Langerhans cells down-regulate inflammation-driven alveolar bone loss. *Proc. Natl. Acad. Sci. USA* **2012**, *109*, 7043–7048. [CrossRef]
35. Dutzan, N.; Abusleme, L.; Konkel, J.E.; Moutsopoulos, N.M. Isolation, Characterization and Functional Examination of the Gingival Immune Cell Network. *J. Vis. Exp.* **2016**, *108*, 53736. [CrossRef]
36. Sallusto, F.; Lenig, D.; Forster, R.; Lipp, M.; Lanzavecchia, A. Two subsets of memory T lymphocytes with distinct homing potentials and effector functions. *Nature* **1999**, *401*, 708–712. [CrossRef]
37. Sheridan, B.S.; Lefrancois, L. Regional and mucosal memory T cells. *Nat. Immunol.* **2011**, *12*, 485–491. [CrossRef]
38. Dutzan, N.; Abusleme, L.; Bridgeman, H.; Greenwell-Wild, T.; Zangerle-Murray, T.; Fife, M.E.; Bouladoux, N.; Linley, H.; Brenchley, L.; Wemyss, K.; et al. On-going Mechanical Damage from Mastication Drives Homeostatic Th17 Cell Responses at the Oral Barrier. *Immunity* **2017**, *46*, 133–147. [CrossRef]
39. Mahanonda, R.; Champaiboon, C.; Subbalekha, K.; Sa-Ard-Iam, N.; Rattanathammatada, W.; Thawanaphong, S.; Rerkyen, P.; Yoshimura, F.; Nagano, K.; Lang, N.P.; et al. Human Memory B Cells in Healthy Gingiva, Gingivitis, and Periodontitis. *J. Immunol.* **2016**, *197*, 715–725. [CrossRef]
40. Kim, Y.C.; Ko, Y.; Hong, S.D.; Kim, K.Y.; Lee, Y.H.; Chae, C.; Choi, Y. Presence of Porphyromonas gingivalis and plasma cell dominance in gingival tissues with periodontitis. *Oral Dis.* **2010**, *16*, 375–381. [CrossRef]
41. Shelburne, C.E.; Shelburne, P.S.; Dhople, V.M.; Sweier, D.G.; Giannobile, W.V.; Kinney, J.S.; Coulter, W.A.; Mullally, B.H.; Lopatin, D.E. Serum antibodies to Porphyromonas gingivalis chaperone HtpG predict health in periodontitis susceptible patients. *PLoS ONE* **2008**, *3*, e1984. [CrossRef]
42. Garlet, G.P. Destructive and protective roles of cytokines in periodontitis: A re-appraisal from host defense and tissue destruction viewpoints. *J. Dent. Res.* **2010**, *89*, 1349–1363. [CrossRef]
43. Page, R.C.; Lantz, M.S.; Darveau, R.; Jeffcoat, M.; Mancl, L.; Houston, L.; Braham, P.; Persson, G.R. Immunization of Macaca fascicularis against experimental periodontitis using a vaccine containing cysteine proteases purified from Porphyromonas gingivalis. *Oral Microbiol. Immunol.* **2007**, *22*, 162–168. [CrossRef]
44. Ebersole, J.L.; Kirakodu, S.S.; Novak, M.J.; Orraca, L.; Martinez, J.G.; Cunningham, L.L.; Thomas, M.V.; Stromberg, A.; Pandruvada, S.N.; Gonzalez, O.A. Transcriptome Analysis of B Cell Immune Functions in Periodontitis: Mucosal Tissue Responses to the Oral Microbiome in Aging. *Front. Immunol.* **2016**, *7*, 272. [CrossRef]
45. Witkowski, J.M.; Mikosik, A.; Bryl, E.; Fulop, T. Proteodynamics in aging human T cells—The need for its comprehensive study to understand the fine regulation of T lymphocyte functions. *Exp. Gerontol.* **2018**, *107*, 161–168. [CrossRef]
46. Okada, H.; Kida, T.; Yamagami, H. Identification and distribution of immunocompetent cells in inflamed gingiva of human chronic periodontitis. *Infect. Immun.* **1983**, *41*, 365–374.
47. Okada, H.; Kassai, Y.; Kida, T. T lymphocyte subsets in the inflamed gingiva of human adult periodontitis. *J. Periodontal Res.* **1984**, *19*, 595–598. [CrossRef]

48. Chen, M.L.; Sundrud, M.S. Cytokine Networks and T-Cell Subsets in Inflammatory Bowel Diseases. *Inflamm. Bowel Dis.* **2016**, *22*, 1157–1167. [CrossRef]
49. Dutzan, N.K.T.; Abusleme, L.; Greenwell-Wild, T.; Zuazo, C.E.; Ikeuchi, T.; Brenchley, L.; Abe, T.; Hurabielle, C.; Martin, D.; Morell, R.J.; et al. A dysbiotic microbiome triggers TH17 cells to mediate oral mucosal immunopathology in mice and humans. *Sci. Transl. Med.* **2018**, *10*, eaat0797. [CrossRef]
50. Jarry, C.R.; Duarte, P.M.; Freitas, F.F.; de Macedo, C.G.; Clemente-Napimoga, J.T.; Saba-Chujfi, E.; Passador-Santos, F.; de Araújo, V.C.; Napimoga, M.H. Secreted osteoclastogenic factor of activated T cells (SOFAT), a novel osteoclast activator, in chronic periodontitis. *Hum Immunol.* **2013**, *74*, 861–866. [CrossRef]
51. Jarry, C.R.; Martinez, E.F.; Peruzzo, D.C.; Carregaro, V.; Sacramento, L.A.; Araujo, V.C.; Weitzmann, M.N.; Napimoga, M.H. Expression of SOFAT by T- and B-lineage cells may contribute to bone loss. *Mol. Med. Rep.* **2016**, *13*, 4252–4258. [CrossRef]
52. Bittner-Eddy, P.D.; Fischer, L.A.; Tu, A.A.; Allman, D.A.; Costalonga, M. Discriminating between Interstitial and Circulating Leukocytes in Tissues of the Murine Oral Mucosa Avoiding Nasal-Associated Lymphoid Tissue Contamination. *Front. Immunol.* **2017**, *8*, 1398. [CrossRef]
53. Seymour, G.J.; Powell, R.N.; Davies, W.I. The immunopathogenesis of progressive chronic inflammatory periodontal disease. *J. Oral Pathol.* **1979**, *8*, 249–265. [CrossRef]
54. Zouali, M. The emerging roles of B cells as partners and targets in periodontitis. *Autoimmunity.* **2017**, *50*, 61–70. [CrossRef]
55. Oliver-Bell, J.; Butcher, J.P.; Malcolm, J.; MacLeod, M.K.; Adrados Planell, A.; Campbell, L.; Nibbs, R.J.; Garside, P.; McInnes, I.B.; Culshaw, S. Periodontitis in the absence of B cells and specific anti-bacterial antibody. *Mol. Oral Microbiol.* **2015**, *30*, 160–169. [CrossRef]
56. Abe, T.; AlSarhan, M.; Benakanakere, M.R.; Maekawa, T.; Kinane, D.F.; Cancro, M.P.; Korostoff, J.M.; Hajishengallis, G. The B Cell-Stimulatory Cytokines BLyS and APRIL Are Elevated in Human Periodontitis and Are Required for B Cell-Dependent Bone Loss in Experimental Murine Periodontitis. *J. Immunol.* **2015**, *195*, 1427–1435. [CrossRef]
57. Kawai, T.; Matsuyama, T.; Hosokawa, Y.; Makihira, S.; Seki, M.; Karimbux, N.Y.; Goncalves, R.B.; Valverde, P.; Dibart, S.; Li, Y.P.; et al. B and T lymphocytes are the primary sources of RANKL in the bone resorptive lesion of periodontal disease. *Am. J. Pathol.* **2006**, *169*, 987–998. [CrossRef]
58. Malcolm, J.; Awang, R.A.; Oliver-Bell, J.; Butcher, J.P.; Campbell, L.; Adrados Planell, A.; Lappin, D.F.; Fukada, S.Y.; Nile, C.J.; Liew, F.Y.; et al. IL-33 Exacerbates Periodontal Disease through Induction of RANKL. *J. Dent. Res.* **2015**, *94*, 968–975. [CrossRef]
59. Kanzaki, H.; Makihira, S.; Suzuki, M.; Ishii, T.; Movila, A.; Hirschfeld, J.; Mawardi, H.; Lin, X.; Han, X.; Taubman, M.A.; et al. Soluble RANKL Cleaved from Activated Lymphocytes by TNF-alpha-Converting Enzyme Contributes to Osteoclastogenesis in Periodontitis. *J. Immunol.* **2016**, *197*, 3871–3883. [CrossRef]
60. Demoersman, J.; Pochard, P.; Framery, C.; Simon, Q.; Boisrame, S.; Soueidan, A.; Pers, J.O. B cell subset distribution is altered in patients with severe periodontitis. *PLoS ONE.* **2018**, *13*, e0192986. [CrossRef]
61. Coat, J.; Demoersman, J.; Beuzit, S.; Cornec, D.; Devauchelle-Pensec, V.; Saraux, A.; Pers, J.O. Anti-B lymphocyte immunotherapy is associated with improvement of periodontal status in subjects with rheumatoid arthritis. *J. Clin. Periodontol.* **2015**, *42*, 817–823. [CrossRef]
62. Kalampokis, I.; Yoshizaki, A.; Tedder, T.F. IL-10-producing regulatory B cells (B10 cells) in autoimmune disease. *Arthritis Res. Ther.* **2013**, *15*, S1. [CrossRef]
63. Yanaba, K.; Yoshizaki, A.; Asano, Y.; Kadono, T.; Tedder, T.F.; Sato, S. IL-10-producing regulatory B10 cells inhibit intestinal injury in a mouse model. *Am. J. Pathol.* **2011**, *178*, 735–743. [CrossRef]
64. Dai, J.; Bi, L.; Lin, J.; Qi, F. Evaluation of interleukin-10 producing CD19(+) B cells in human gingival tissue. *Arch. Oral Biol.* **2017**, *84*, 112–117. [CrossRef]
65. Hu, Y.; Yu, P.; Yu, X.; Hu, X.; Kawai, T.; Han, X. IL-21/anti-Tim1/CD40 ligand promotes B10 activity in vitro and alleviates bone loss in experimental periodontitis in vivo. *Biochim. Biophys Acta Mol. Basis Dis.* **2017**, *1863*, 2149–2157. [CrossRef]
66. Wang, Y.; Yu, X.; Lin, J.; Hu, Y.; Zhao, Q.; Kawai, T.; Taubman, M.A.; Han, X. B10 Cells Alleviate Periodontal Bone Loss in Experimental Periodontitis. *Infect Immun.* **2017**, *85*, e00335-17. [CrossRef]
67. Lira-Junior, R.; Figueredo, C.M. Periodontal and inflammatory bowel diseases: Is there evidence of complex pathogenic interactions? *World J. Gastroenterol.* **2016**, 22, 7963. [CrossRef]

7

The Possible Causal Link of Periodontitis to Neuropsychiatric Disorders: More than Psychosocial Mechanisms

Sadayuki Hashioka [1,*], Ken Inoue [2], Tsuyoshi Miyaoka [1], Maiko Hayashida [1], Rei Wake, Arata Oh-Nishi [1] and Masatoshi Inagaki [1]

1 Department of Psychiatry, Shimane University, 89-1 Enya-cho, Izumo 693-8501, Japan
2 Health Service Center, Kochi University, 2-5-1 Akebono-cho, Kochi 780-8520, Japan
* Correspondence: hashioka@f2.dion.ne.jp

Abstract: Increasing evidence implies a possible causal link between periodontitis and neuropsychiatric disorders, such as Alzheimer's disease (AD) and major depression (MD). A possible mechanism underlying such a link can be explained by neuroinflammation induced by chronic systemic inflammation. This review article focuses on an overview of the biological and epidemiological evidence for a feasible causal link of periodontitis to neuropsychiatric disorders, including AD, MD, Parkinson's disease, and schizophrenia, as well as the neurological event, ischemic stroke. If there is such a link, a broad spectrum of neuropsychiatric disorders associated with neuroinflammation could be preventable and modifiable by simple daily dealings for oral hygiene. However, the notion that periodontitis is a risk factor for neuropsychiatric disorders remains to be effectively substantiated.

Keywords: periodontitis; neuropsychiatric disorders; Alzheimer's disease; Parkinson's disease; major depression; schizophrenia; neuroinflammation; microglia

---

1. Introduction

Periodontitis is a chronic, oral multi-bacterial infection affecting nearly 50% of the population worldwide and is the most prevalent inflammatory disease in adults [1,2]. Periodontitis is not only an oral localized inflammatory disease, but also elicits low-grade systemic inflammation via both the release of pro-inflammatory cytokines and the invasion of periodontitis bacteria (e.g., *Porphyromonas gingivalis* (*P. gingivalis*)) along with their components (e.g., lipopolysaccharide (LPS) and flagellin) into systemic circulation [3]. Periodontitis thus causes or hastens other chronic systemic inflammatory diseases, including atherosclerosis, cardiovascular diseases, diabetes, and rheumatoid arthritis [4]. In particular, the causal link between periodontitis and infective endocarditis has been known for many decades. Besides inducing systemic inflammation, increasing evidence implies that periodontitis provokes chronic inflammation associated with activation of microglia, the immune cells in the brain, which is referred to as neuroinflammation (reviewed in [5–7]).

The concept of neuroinflammation was originally proposed for neurodegenerative disorders in the 1980s, based on two historical discoveries. The first was the immunohistochemical identification of activated microglia in association with the lesions in Alzheimer's disease (AD) brains [8]. The second was the epidemiologic finding that rheumatoid arthritics, who regularly consume anti-inflammatory agents, were relatively spared from AD [9]. In the ensuing years, activated microglia have also been found in the lesions of Parkinson's disease (PD), multiple sclerosis, and amyotrophic lateral sclerosis [10]. Neuroinflammation has thus become considered as a common prominent feature among a variety of neurodegenerative disorders. Attention on the pathogenetic role of neuroinflammation has, over the past two decades, been expanded to psychiatric disorders. Immunohistochemistry and positron emission tomography studies have revealed microglial activation in the brain of patients with schizophrenia [11–13] and major depression (MD) [14,15], the representative endogenous psychoses. Neuroinflammation could thus be important in many pathological conditions of the brain, including both neurodegenerative disorders and psychiatric disorders (hereinafter referred to as neuropsychiatric disorders in this article).

Based on the aforementioned findings, chronic inflammation can be regarded as a common denominator of periodontitis and neuropsychiatric disorders. Specifically, neuroinflammation may causally link periodontitis to the clinical onset and development of neuropsychiatric disorders. Furthermore, through the biological mechanism of chronic inflammation, periodontitis could causally affect neuropsychiatric disorders, especially MD, because of its psychosocial effects, such as shame, loneliness, impaired quality of life (QOL), and impaired social status [16]. Nonetheless, this review article focuses on the biological and epidemiological evidence for possible causal links of periodontitis to the selected neuropsychiatric disorders, namely AD, MD, PD, and schizophrenia. This article also discusses an association between periodontitis and the neurological event of ischemic stroke.

2. How Does Periodontitis Cause Neuroinflammation?

Neuroinflammation is a key pathogenetic connector between periodontitis and neuropsychiatric disorders. The biological mechanisms by which periodontitis causes neuroinflammation can be presumed to consist of three possibilities, as follows (Figure 1).

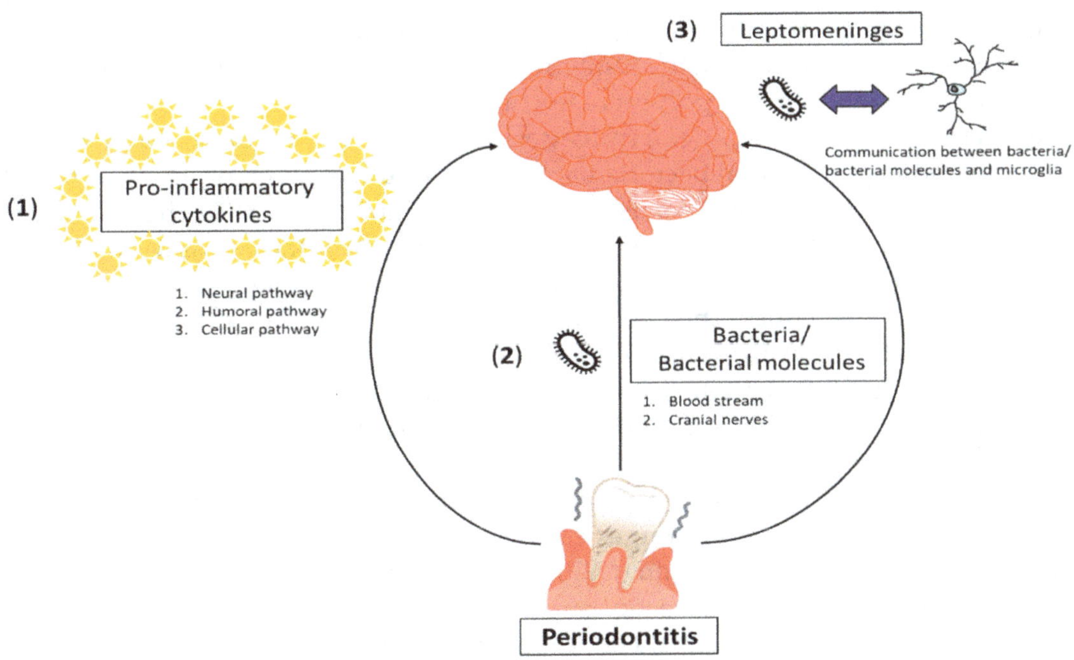

Figure 1. Scheme for presumed mechanisms by which periodontitis causes neuroinflammation. These consist of three possibilities as follows: **(1)** Peripheral pro-inflammatory cytokines associated with periodontitis communicate with the brain via the neural pathway, humoral pathway, and cellular pathway. **(2)** Periodontal bacteria/bacterial molecules can directly invade the brain either through the blood stream or via cranial nerves. **(3)** Communication between periodontal bacteria/bacterial molecules and brain-resident microglia could occur through the leptomeninges.

(1) Neuroinflammation can be caused by peripheral pro-inflammatory cytokines generated in systemic inflammation induced by periodontitis without the contact of periodontal bacteria/bacterial molecules with the brain tissue via three pathways, i.e., the neural pathway, the humoral pathway, and the cellular pathway. Through the neural pathway, systemic cytokines directly activate primary afferent nerves, such as the vagus nerve. The signal reaches the primary and secondary projection of the neural pathway, reaching first the nucleus tractus solitaries and subsequently, various hypothalamic brain nuclei [17]. It has been shown that subdiaphragmatic vagotomy blocks the LPS-induced sickness behavior in rats [18], while it does not affect the LPS-induced synthesis of pro-inflammatory cytokines at the periphery. The humoral pathway involves the choroid plexus and circumventricular organs, which lack an intact blood–brain barrier (BBB). These leaky regions may be access points for circulating pro-inflammatory cytokines to enter into the cerebral parenchyma by volume diffusion and elicit downstream signaling events, which are important in altering brain function [19]. The cellular pathway implicates systemic inflammation in association with both activation of endothelial cells (CECs) and an increase in circulating monocytes [19]. Systemic pro-inflammatory cytokines activate CECs, expressing receptors for TNF-α and IL-1β, which in turn, signal to the perivascular macrophages located immediately adjacent to CECs [20]. These perivascular macrophages subsequently communicate with microglia and thus lead to microglial activation. Activated microglia secrete not only pro-inflammatory cytokines but also proteases and chemokines, including monocyte chemoattractant protein (MCP)-1. MCP-1 is supposed to be responsible for the recruitment of monocytes into the motor cortex, hippocampus, and basal ganglia regions, areas of the brain known to be involved in the control of behavior [21].

(**2**) Periodontal bacteria/bacterial molecules can directly invade the brain either through the blood stream or via cranial nerves. In periodontitis, a periodontal pocket is filled with periodontal bacteria/bacterial molecules that form biofilms. Since periodontal bacteria are capable of invading an intact pocket epithelium, periodontal bacteria/bacterial molecules can gain access to the circulation [22]. It has been shown that LPS deteriorates the BBB and increases its permeability through abnormal activation of matrix metalloproteinase [23]. Circulating periodontal bacteria/bacterial molecules could then penetrate into the brain through the compromised BBB. In fact, *P. gingivalis* DNA has been identified by quantitative polymerase chain reaction (qPCR) in the brain of mice orally infected with *P. gingivalis* [24], and *P. gingivalis*-derived LPS has been detected in the brains of AD patients [25]. Circulating periodontal bacteria/bacterial molecules can also enter the brain through the circumventricular organs and choroid plexuses that lack the contiguous BBB. The cranial nerve may be another entry route for periodontal pathogens into the brain. The olfactory and trigeminal nerves are known to be used by periodontal bacteria to bypass the BBB [26]. The detection of oral *Treponemas* in the trigeminal ganglia supports the idea of neural pathways [27]. Via any of these pathways, infiltration of periodontal bacteria/bacterial molecules into the brain could result in inflammatory activation of microglia, since it has been demonstrated that either *P. gingivalis* infection or LPS of *P. gingivalis* activates microglia in vitro to produce pro-inflammatory cytokines, such as tumor necrosis factor (TNF)-α, interleukin (IL)-1β and IL-6 [28,29].

(**3**) The leptomeninges could be a site of communication between periodontal bacteria and brain-resident microglia. The leptomeninges covers the brain parenchyma surface and provides a physical boundary at the cerebrospinal fluid (CSF)-blood barrier. Leptomeningeal cells express Toll-like receptors (TLRs) 2 and 4 that are the receptors for *P. gingivalis* LPS. Leptomeningeal cells can be activated by circulating *P. gingivalis* LPS and subsequently produce pro-inflammatory cytokines for the brain [30,31]. The pro-inflammatory cytokines released from leptomeningeal cells activate microglia to evoke neuroinflammation. Accordingly, the leptomeninges could be harmful by transducing peripheral inflammation, including periodontitis, into neuroinflammation.

3. Alzheimer's Disease

AD is currently the best-known neuropsychiatric disease that is associated with periodontitis based on clinical and experimental evidence that is accumulating rapidly. Recent epidemiological studies have pointed out that periodontitis significantly elevates the risk for AD. A prospective pilot study using qPCR identified *P. gingivalis* DNA in the CSF in seven of the 10 clinically diagnosed AD patients who had mild to moderate cognitive impairment [24]. A cross-sectional study reported that plasma TNF-α and antibodies against periodontal bacteria were elevated in AD patients relative to normal controls and were independently associated with AD [32]. Another cross-sectional study demonstrated that the increased serum levels of TNF-α and IL-6 in patients with AD were significantly associated with periodontitis [33]. A case-control study established a significant association between AD and the increased number of deep periodontal pockets [34]. A retrospective matched cohort study on 9291 patients with periodontitis showed that chronic periodontitis exposure for 10 years was associated with a 1.707-fold increase in the risk of developing AD [35]. Another historical cohort study with the larger sample size of 262,349 participants who suffered from chronic periodontitis supports this finding [36]. Prospective cohort studies with relatively small sample sizes demonstrated that serum IgG antibody levels to periodontitis bacteria, such as *P. gingivalis*, *Tannerella forsythia* and *Treponema denticola* (the so-called "red complex"), were significantly increased in baseline serum drawn from subjects who were diagnosed with AD in later years compared to controls [37,38]. Even after the onset of AD, periodontitis may exacerbate cognitive impairment. A six-month observational cohort study tested cognitive function and serum pro-inflammatory markers in 52 patients with mild to moderate AD. The study showed that the presence of periodontitis at baseline was associated with a six-fold increase in the rate of cognitive decline in participants over the six-month follow-up period, and was also associated with a relative increase in the pro-inflammatory state over that period [39]. A meta-analysis based on one cross-sectional study [40] and two case-control studies [41,42], which have not been previously mentioned, and assessed as at a low risk of bias, came to the conclusion that periodontitis is significantly associated with AD (OR 1.69, 95% CI 1.21–2.35) [43]. Furthermore, severe forms of periodontitis show a more intense association with AD (OR 2.98, 95% CI 1.58–5.62) [43]. An interesting study comparing periodontal conditions between countries reported that periodontitis was more prevalent in Germany and that elderly German subjects had significantly more severe periodontal conditions and fewer remaining teeth compared to those in Japan, even after adjustment of the comprehensive risk factor [44]. Accordingly, it would be tempting to examine whether the AD prevalence in Germany is significantly higher than that of Japan by a direct comparison with the adjustment of confounding factors.

Growing evidence based on animal studies also strengthens a possible causal link of periodontitis to AD. Chronic intraperitoneal injection of *P. gingivalis* LPS (1 mg/kg/day, daily for 5 weeks) has been demonstrated to cause learning and memory deficits accompanied with intracellular amyloid β (Aβ) accumulation in neurons and microglial activation (i.e., increased expression of IL-1β and TLR2 restricted to microglia) in the hippocampus in middle-aged mice (12 months old), but not in young mice (2 months old) or in middle-aged cathepsin-B knockout mice [29]. Therefore, cathepsin B, known as an amyloid precursor protein (APP) secretase, may play a critical role in the periodontitis-exacerbated AD and could be a therapeutic target. Even a single intraperitoneal injection of *P. gingivalis* LPS (5 mg/kg) into 8-week old mice has been shown to impair spatial learning and memory with neuroinflammation (i.e., microglial activation, astrocytic activation, and increased expression of TNF-α, IL-1β, and IL-6 in the cortex and/or hippocampus) and activation of the TLR4/nuclear factor-kappa B (NF-κB) signaling pathway (i.e., up-regulation of TLR4, CD14, IL-1 receptor-associated kinase 1, and phospho-p65 in the cortex) [45]. These behavioral and immuno-biochemical findings were considerably abolished by the TLR4 inhibitor TAK242, suggesting that the *P. gingivalis* LPS-induced cognitive dysfunction and neuroinflammation are mediated by the TLR4/NF-κB signaling pathway [45]. Interestingly, this study also tested *E. coli* LPS and reported that either *P. gingivalis* LPS or *E. coli* LPS caused both cognitive impairment and neuroinflammation and there was no significant difference between the effects of the two LPS species [45]. Experimental chronic periodontitis, caused when live *P. gingivalis* (ATCC33277) was given by oral gavage every 48 h over 6 weeks, has been shown to impair learning and memory and elicit neuroinflammation (i.e., increased expression of TNF-α, IL-1β and IL-6 in the brain) in middle-aged mice (12 months old), although not in young individuals (4 weeks old) [46]. Experimental chronic periodontitis, induced by repeated oral application of another live *P. gingivalis* W83 every 48 h over 22 weeks, has been demonstrated to increase extracellular Aβ42 amyloid plaques, ser396 residue of tau protein phosphorylation, neurofibrillary tangle formation, and neuroinflammation (i.e., microglial activation, astrocytic activation, and increased expression of TNF-α, IL-1β and IL-6) in the hippocampus of 6-week old mice [47]. Currently, there is only one study that employed APP-transgenic (Tg) mice and the study implies that periodontitis exacerbates the hallmark pathology and symptoms of AD [48]. Specifically, APP-Tg mice with periodontitis induced by oral infection with *P. gingivalis* ATCC33277, showed greater deposition of Aβ40 and Aβ42 amyloid plaques in both the hippocampus and cortex and increased brain expression of TNF-α and IL-1β, compared with sham-infected APP-Tg mice. Furthermore, cognitive function was significantly impaired in the periodontitis-induced APP-Tg mice relative to sham-infected APP-Tg mice [48].

Postmortem studies have indicated the potentially causal presence of periodontopathic virulence products in AD brains. LPS from *P. gingivalis* was detected in the brain of four out of 10 AD cases by immunofluorescence and Western blot (WB) analyses, whereas *P. gingivalis* LPS was not detected in 10 age-matched non-AD controls. Dominiy et al. (2019) have performed a seminal study, identifying *P. gingivalis* DNA and gingipains, toxic proteases secreted from *P. gingivalis* in AD brains. Immunohistochemical analyses using tissue microarrays showed that gingipain immunoreactivity in AD brains was significantly greater than that in sex- and age-matched non-AD brains, and that gingipain immunoreactivity significantly correlates with tau and ubiquitin loads and AD diagnosis [24]. Using qPCR, the authors identified *P. gingivalis* DNA in the AD brains which were lysine gingipain-positive in WB and immunoprecipitated analyses [24]. In addition to postmortem brain studies, they carried out in vivo studies using wild-type mice and gingipain-knockout mice that were orally infected with *P. gingivalis* W83 every other day for 42 days. Colonization of *P. gingivalis* and Aβ42 levels were increased in the brains of the infected wild-type mice, while the colonization and Aβ42 levels were decreased in the brains of either the infected wild-type mice treated with the gingipain inhibitor COR119 or of the gingipain-knockout mice [24]. Because these findings suggest that gingipain inhibition reduces the *P. gingivali* load and Aβ42 production in the brain, gingipain inhibitors could have therapeutic potential for patients with both AD and periodontitis.

4. Major Depression

MD has also attracted attention and is currently the second elucidated neuropsychiatric disease with respect to its reciprocal association with periodontitis. A recent cross-sectional study on 108 subjects reported that patients with periodontitis showed a significantly higher comorbidity rate of depression (62.5%) compared to periodontally healthy subjects (38.86%), excluding smokers, pregnant women, subjects with systemic pathologies, and subjects taking antidepressants [49]. MD is susceptible to psychosocial factors and periodontitis could increase the risk for developing MD through the psychosocial effects that stem from periodontitis-causing oral troubles, such as halitosis, poor oral hygiene, and edentulousness [16]. Patients with malodorous wounds and poor oral hygiene often experience social isolation, depression, shame, and poor appetite, all of which have a negative impact on their QOL [50]. Also, tooth loss negatively affects the patients' QOL since it worsens not only chewing function, but also body image, self-esteem, and social status [16,51]. Because of all this, many early studies in this field were performed from a psychosocial viewpoint [52,53].

Although several studies have recently focused on the biological relationship between periodontitis and MD, most of them investigated periodontitis as an outcome influenced by MD [54,55]. The effects of antidepressants, which are known to possess anti-inflammatory and immunomodulatory properties [56,57], on chronic periodontitis have been studied in both MD animal models (systematically reviewed in [58]) and in MD patients [59,60]. The majority has established the therapeutic effects of antidepressants on chronic periodontitis. A recent cross-sectional study made by Gomes et al. (2018), who hypothesized that increased root canal LPS accompanying chronic apical periodontitis causes MD, showed that patients with periodontitis and MD had highly increased root canal endotoxin levels relative to patients with periodontitis without MD or normal controls. This study demonstrated a strong positive association between periodontitis or root canal endotoxin levels and the severity of MD, suggesting that the association between periodontitis and MD is attributable, at least in part, to root canal endotoxin levels [61]. In the study, periodontitis-related MD was accompanied with elevated levels of oxidative and nitrosative stress index, including nitric oxide metabolites and hydroperoxides, which are supposed to play a role in the pathogenesis of MD [62]. A recent cohort study composed of a high methodological quality with more than 60,000 participants and a 10-year follow-up period also supports the feasible causal link of periodontitis to MD. The study showed a higher incidence of subsequent depression in the periodontitis group (n = 12,708) than in the non-periodontitis group (n = 50,832) (HR 1.73, 95% CI 1.58–1.89), after adjustment of sex, age and comorbidities [63]. This result suggests that periodontitis is an independent risk factor for subsequent MD regardless of sex, age, and the comorbidities except for diabetes, alcohol abuse, and cancer. On the other hand, in a meta-analysis on four cross-sectional studies [64–67] that were assessed as moderate-high quality of the evidence and considered periodontitis as the outcome and MD as the exposure, the pooled estimate does not show association between periodontitis and MD (OR 0.96, 95% CI 0.84–1.10) [68]. Therefore, more prospective cohort studies that test periodontitis as the independent variable and MD as the outcome, or interventional studies, such as studies that determine the effects of periodontal treatment on MD, are clearly warranted to elucidate the causal relationship between periodontitis and MD.

5. Parkinson's Disease

Compared with AD and MD, any correlation between PD and periodontitis has, traditionally, been less effectively understood. Nevertheless, a few studies have noted an increased prevalence of periodontal disease among individuals with PD relative to age-matched controls [69,70]. PD causes motor disturbance (due to tremor, rigidity, akinesia, and involuntary movement), apathy, and cognitive impairment, all of which appear to make it difficult for patients to maintain daily oral hygiene. Therefore, periodontitis can be considered as a consequence of the poor oral hygiene related to clinical symptoms of PD. Recent epidemiological studies have investigated whether periodontitis increases the risk for developing PD. Chen et al. (2017) conducted a population-based retrospective matched-cohort study and reported that individuals with newly diagnosed periodontitis (n = 5396) had an increased risk of subsequent PD compared to individuals without periodontitis (n = 10,792), regardless of sex, age, comorbidities, and urbanization levels (HR 1.431, 95% CI 1.141–1.794) [71]. The authors also examined the effect of periodontal treatment on developing PD. Their population-based nested case-control study demonstrated that among individuals without periodontitis aged 40–69 (n = 5552), dental scaling over five consecutive years showed a protective effect against PD development, relative to individuals who did not undergo dental scaling (OR 0.204, 95% CI 0.047–0.886) [72]. Moreover, among individuals with periodontitis aged ≥70 (n = 3377), the discontinued scaling (i.e., not five consecutive years) or no treatment were significant risk factors for developing PD [35]. These findings suggest that early and consecutive dental scaling could prevent the development of PD. Although these seminal epidemiological studies imply a feasible causal link of periodontitis to PD and a preventive effect of periodontal treatment on PD development, experimental studies for verifying these concepts are lacking at the present time. Therefore, additional epidemiological studies and experimental studies along this line are required.

6. Schizophrenia

Evidence for a significant relationship between periodontitis and schizophrenia has not yet been accumulated. Only one cross-sectional study with a small sample size has concluded that patients with schizophrenia have a high risk of periodontitis and there is an even higher risk in those who are taking antipsychotics that reduce salivary secretion and cause xerostomia [73]. Intriguingly, human genome/gene analysis on insertion/deletion (D) polymorphism in the angiotensin-converting enzyme (ACE) gene has indicated that the D allele is a protective factor against schizophrenia [74] and chronic periodontitis [75]. Accordingly, the ACE D allele may be a clue to reveal any biological and reciprocal connection between these two diseases.

7. Ischemic Stroke

Epidemiological studies also suggest an association between periodontitis and ischemic stroke. Stroke is the second most common cause of mortality worldwide and approximately 80% of strokes are caused by focal cerebral ischemia [76]. A recent meta-analysis [76] has shown a significant association between periodontitis and ischemic stroke based on three cohort studies [77–79] (pooled RR 2.52, 95% CI 1.77–3.58) and five case-control studies (pooled RR 3.04, 95% CI 1.10–8.43) [80–84]. Chi et al. (2019) examined mice with both experimental periodontitis induced by periodontal injection of LPS and photothrombotic ischemia. The study has demonstrated that chronic periodontitis exacerbates ischemic stroke through increasing the activation of microglia/astrocytes and the expression of nod-like receptor protein 3 inflammasome and IL-1β [85], suggesting that chronic periodontitis is a driving force for neuroinflammation associated with ischemia.

8. Conclusions

The relationship between periodontitis and neuropsychiatric disorders, in particular AD, has recently attracted researchers' attention, and the evidence for their considerable reciprocal association has been accumulated. Specifically, various clinical and experimental studies imply the potentially causal link of periodontitis to neuropsychiatric disorders, and neuroinflammation seems to be a key pathological connector between them. After establishment of such a link, a broad spectrum of neuropsychiatric disorders associated with neuroinflammation may be preventable and modifiable by simple daily dealings for oral hygiene, even though the notion that periodontitis is a risk factor for neuropsychiatric disorders remains to be effectively substantiated.

Author Contributions: S.H. wrote the manuscript. All authors discussed and edited the manuscript. All authors read and approved the final manuscript.

Acknowledgments: Sincere appreciation is extended to Edith G. McGeer for her invaluable support.

References

1. Eke, P.I.; Dye, B.A.; Wei, L.; Thornton-Evans, G.O.; Genco, R.J. CDC Periodontal Disease Surveillance Workgroup. Prevalence of periodontitis in adults in the United States: 2009 and 2010. *J. Dent. Res.* **2012**, *91*, 914–920. [CrossRef] [PubMed]
2. Roman-Malo, L.; Bullon, P. Influence of the Periodontal Disease, the Most Prevalent Inflammatory Event, in Peroxisome Proliferator-Activated Receptors Linking Nutrition and Energy Metabolism. *Int. J. Mol. Sci.* **2017**, *18*, 1438. [CrossRef] [PubMed]
3. Gurav, A.N. Alzheimer's disease and periodontitis—An elusive link. *Rev. Assoc. Med. Bras.* **2014**, *60*, 173–180. [CrossRef] [PubMed]
4. Holmstrup, P.; Damgaard, C.; Olsen, I.; Klinge, B.; Flyvbjerg, A.; Nielsen, C.H.; Hansen, P.R. Comorbidity of periodontal disease: Two sides of the same coin? An introduction for the clinician. *J. Oral Microbiol.* **2017**, *9*, 1332710. [CrossRef] [PubMed]
5. Hashioka, S.; Inoue, K.; Hayashida, M.; Wake, R.; Oh-Nishi, A.; Miyaoka, T. Implications of Systemic Inflammation and Periodontitis for Major Depression. *Front. Neurosci.* **2018**, *12*, 483. [CrossRef] [PubMed]
6. Singhrao, S.K.; Olsen, I. Assessing the role of Porphyromonas gingivalis in periodontitis to determine a causative relationship with Alzheimer's disease. *J. Oral Microbiol.* **2019**, *11*, 1563405. [CrossRef] [PubMed]
7. Sochocka, M.; Zwolinska, K.; Leszek, J. The Infectious Etiology of Alzheimer's Disease. *Curr. Neuropharmacol.* **2017**, *15*, 996–1009. [CrossRef] [PubMed]

8. McGeer, P.L.; Itagaki, S.; Tago, H.; McGeer, E.G. Reactive microglia in patients with senile dementia of the Alzheimer type are positive for the histocompatibility glycoprotein HLA-DR. *Neurosci. Lett.* **1987**, *79*, 195–200. [CrossRef]
9. McGeer, P.L.; McGeer, E.; Rogers, J.; Sibley, J. Anti-inflammatory drugs and Alzheimer disease. *Lancet* **1990**, *335*, 1037. [CrossRef]
10. McGeer, P.L.; McGeer, E.G. History of innate immunity in neurodegenerative disorders. *Front. Pharmacol.* **2011**, *2*, 77. [CrossRef]
11. Doorduin, J.; de Vries, E.F.; Willemsen, A.T.; de Groot, J.C.; Dierckx, R.A.; Klein, H.C. Neuroinflammation in schizophrenia-related psychosis: A PET study. *J. Nucl. Med.* **2009**, *50*, 1801–1807. [CrossRef] [PubMed]
12. Fillman, S.G.; Cloonan, N.; Catts, V.S.; Miller, L.C.; Wong, J.; McCrossin, T.; Cairns, M.; Weickert, C.S. Increased inflammatory markers identified in the dorsolateral prefrontal cortex of individuals with schizophrenia. *Mol. Psychiatry* **2013**, *18*, 206–214. [CrossRef] [PubMed]
13. Van Berckel, B.N.; Bossong, M.G.; Boellaard, R.; Kloet, R.; Schuitemaker, A.; Caspers, E.; Luurtsema, G.; Windhorst, A.D.; Cahn, W.; Lammertsma, A.A.; et al. Microglia activation in recent-onset schizophrenia: A quantitative (R)-[11C]PK11195 positron emission tomography study. *Biol. Psychiatry* **2008**, *64*, 820–822. [CrossRef] [PubMed]
14. Su, L.; Faluyi, Y.O.; Hong, Y.T.; Fryer, T.D.; Mak, E.; Gabel, S.; Hayes, L.; Soteriades, S.; Williams, G.B.; Arnold, R.; et al. Neuroinflammatory and morphological changes in late-life depression: The NIMROD study. *Br. J. Psychiatry J. Ment. Sci.* **2016**, *209*, 525–526. [CrossRef] [PubMed]
15. Torres-Platas, S.G.; Cruceanu, C.; Chen, G.G.; Turecki, G.; Mechawar, N. Evidence for increased microglial priming and macrophage recruitment in the dorsal anterior cingulate white matter of depressed suicides. *Brain Behav. Immun.* **2014**, *42*, 50–59. [CrossRef] [PubMed]
16. Dumitrescu, A.L. Depression and Inflammatory Periodontal Disease Considerations-An Interdisciplinary Approach. *Front. Psychol.* **2016**, *7*, 347. [CrossRef] [PubMed]
17. Capuron, L.; Miller, A.H. Immune system to brain signaling: Neuropsychopharmacological implications. *Pharmacol. Ther.* **2011**, *130*, 226–238. [CrossRef]
18. Bluthé, R.M.; Walter, V.; Parnet, P.; Layé, S.; Lestage, J.; Verrier, D.; Poole, S.; Stenning, B.E.; Kelley, K.W.; Dantzer, R. Lipopolysaccharide induces sickness behaviour in rats by a vagal mediated mechanism. *C. R. L'Académie Sci. Ser. III Sci. Vie* **1994**, *317*, 499.
19. D'Mello, C.; Swain, M.G. Immune-to-Brain Communication Pathways in Inflammation-Associated Sickness and Depression. *Curr. Top. Behav. Neurosci.* **2017**, *31*, 73–94. [CrossRef]
20. Perry, V.H. The influence of systemic inflammation on inflammation in the brain: Implications for chronic neurodegenerative disease. *Brain Behav. Immun.* **2004**, *18*, 407–413. [CrossRef]
21. D'Mello, C.; Le, T.; Swain, M.G. Cerebral microglia recruit monocytes into the brain in response to tumor necrosis factoralpha signaling during peripheral organ inflammation. *J. Neurosci.* **2009**, *29*, 2089–2102. [CrossRef] [PubMed]
22. Kamer, A.R.; Craig, R.G.; Dasanayake, A.P.; Brys, M.; Glodzik-Sobanska, L.; de Leon, M.J. Inflammation and Alzheimer's disease: Possible role of periodontal diseases. *Alzheimers Dement.* **2008**, *4*, 242–250. [CrossRef] [PubMed]
23. Frister, A.; Schmidt, C.; Schneble, N.; Brodhun, M.; Gonnert, F.A.; Bauer, M.; Hirsch, E.; Muller, J.P.; Wetzker, R.; Bauer, R. Phosphoinositide 3-kinase gamma affects LPS-induced disturbance of blood-brain barrier via lipid kinase-independent control of cAMP in microglial cells. *Neuromol. Med.* **2014**, *16*, 704–713. [CrossRef] [PubMed]
24. Dominy, S.S.; Lynch, C.; Ermini, F.; Benedyk, M.; Marczyk, A.; Konradi, A.; Nguyen, M.; Haditsch, U.; Raha, D.; Griffin, C.; et al. Porphyromonas gingivalis in Alzheimer's disease brains: Evidence for disease causation and treatment with small-molecule inhibitors. *Sci. Adv.* **2019**, *5*, eaau3333. [CrossRef] [PubMed]
25. Poole, S.; Singhrao, S.K.; Kesavalu, L.; Curtis, M.A.; Crean, S. Determining the presence of periodontopathic virulence factors in short-term postmortem Alzheimer's disease brain tissue. *J. Alzheimers Dis.* **2013**, *36*, 665–677. [CrossRef]
26. Olsen, I.; Singhrao, S.K. Can oral infection be a risk factor for Alzheimer's disease? *J. Oral Microbiol.* **2015**, *7*, 29143. [CrossRef]

27. Riviere, G.R.; Riviere, K.H.; Smith, K.S. Molecular and immunological evidence of oral Treponema in the human brain and their association with Alzheimer's disease. *Oral Microbiol. Immunol.* **2002**, *17*, 113–118. [CrossRef]

28. Liu, Y.; Wu, Z.; Nakanishi, Y.; Ni, J.; Hayashi, Y.; Takayama, F.; Zhou, Y.; Kadowaki, T.; Nakanishi, H. Infection of microglia with Porphyromonas gingivalis promotes cell migration and an inflammatory response through the gingipain-mediated activation of protease-activated receptor-2 in mice. *Sci. Rep.* **2017**, *7*, 11759. [CrossRef]

29. Wu, Z.; Ni, J.; Liu, Y.; Teeling, J.L.; Takayama, F.; Collcutt, A.; Ibbett, P.; Nakanishi, H. Cathepsin B plays a critical role in inducing Alzheimer's disease-like phenotypes following chronic systemic exposure to lipopolysaccharide from Porphyromonas gingivalis in mice. *Brain Behav. Immun.* **2017**, *65*, 350–361. [CrossRef]

30. Liu, Y.; Wu, Z.; Zhang, X.; Ni, J.; Yu, W.; Zhou, Y.; Nakanishi, H. Leptomeningeal cells transduce peripheral macrophages inflammatory signal to microglia in reponse to Porphyromonas gingivalis LPS. *Mediat. Inflamm.* **2013**, *2013*, 407562. [CrossRef]

31. Wu, Z.; Zhang, J.; Nakanishi, H. Leptomeningeal cells activate microglia and astrocytes to induce IL-10 production by releasing pro-inflammatory cytokines during systemic inflammation. *J. Neuroimmunol.* **2005**, *167*, 90–98. [CrossRef] [PubMed]

32. Kamer, A.R.; Craig, R.G.; Pirraglia, E.; Dasanayake, A.P.; Norman, R.G.; Boylan, R.J.; Nehorayoff, A.; Glodzik, L.; Brys, M.; de Leon, M.J. TNF-alpha and antibodies to periodontal bacteria discriminate between Alzheimer's disease patients and normal subjects. *J. Neuroimmunol.* **2009**, *216*, 92–97. [CrossRef] [PubMed]

33. Cestari, J.A.; Fabri, G.M.; Kalil, J.; Nitrini, R.; Jacob-Filho, W.; de Siqueira, J.T.; Siqueira, S.R. Oral Infections and Cytokine Levels in Patients with Alzheimer's Disease and Mild Cognitive Impairment Compared with Controls. *J. Alzheimers Dis.* **2016**, *52*, 1479–1485. [CrossRef] [PubMed]

34. Holmer, J.; Eriksdotter, M.; Schultzberg, M.; Pussinen, P.J.; Buhlin, K. Association between periodontitis and risk of Alzheimer's disease, mild cognitive impairment and subjective cognitive decline: A case-control study. *J. Clin. Periodontol.* **2018**, *45*, 1287–1298. [CrossRef] [PubMed]

35. Chen, C.K.; Wu, Y.T.; Chang, Y.C. Association between chronic periodontitis and the risk of Alzheimer's disease: A retrospective, population-based, matched-cohort study. *Alzheimers Res. Ther.* **2017**, *9*, 56. [CrossRef] [PubMed]

36. Choi, S.; Kim, K.; Chang, J.; Kim, S.M.; Kim, S.J.; Cho, H.J.; Park, S.M. Association of Chronic Periodontitis on Alzheimer's Disease or Vascular Dementia. *J. Am. Geriatr. Soc.* **2019**. [CrossRef] [PubMed]

37. Noble, J.M.; Scarmeas, N.; Celenti, R.S.; Elkind, M.S.; Wright, C.B.; Schupf, N.; Papapanou, P.N. Serum IgG antibody levels to periodontal microbiota are associated with incident Alzheimer disease. *PLoS ONE* **2014**, *9*, e114959. [CrossRef]

38. Sparks Stein, P.; Steffen, M.J.; Smith, C.; Jicha, G.; Ebersole, J.L.; Abner, E.; Dawson, D., 3rd. Serum antibodies to periodontal pathogens are a risk factor for Alzheimer's disease. *Alzheimers Dement. J. Alzheimers Assoc.* **2012**, *8*, 196–203. [CrossRef]

39. Ide, M.; Harris, M.; Stevens, A.; Sussams, R.; Hopkins, V.; Culliford, D.; Fuller, J.; Ibbett, P.; Raybould, R.; Thomas, R.; et al. Periodontitis and Cognitive Decline in Alzheimer's Disease. *PLoS ONE* **2016**, *11*, e0151081. [CrossRef]

40. Syrjala, A.M.; Ylostalo, P.; Ruoppi, P.; Komulainen, K.; Hartikainen, S.; Sulkava, R.; Knuuttila, M. Dementia and oral health among subjects aged 75 years or older. *Gerodontology* **2012**, *29*, 36–42. [CrossRef]

41. De Souza Rolim, T.; Fabri, G.M.; Nitrini, R.; Anghinah, R.; Teixeira, M.J.; de Siqueira, J.T.; Cestari, J.A.; de Siqueira, S.R. Oral infections and orofacial pain in Alzheimer's disease: A case-control study. *J. Alzheimers Dis.* **2014**, *38*, 823–829. [CrossRef] [PubMed]

42. Gil-Montoya, J.A.; Sanchez-Lara, I.; Carnero-Pardo, C.; Fornieles, F.; Montes, J.; Vilchez, R.; Burgos, J.S.; Gonzalez-Moles, M.A.; Barrios, R.; Bravo, M. Is periodontitis a risk factor for cognitive impairment and dementia? A case-control study. *J. Periodontol.* **2015**, *86*, 244–253. [CrossRef] [PubMed]

43. Leira, Y.; Dominguez, C.; Seoane, J.; Seoane-Romero, J.; Pias-Peleteiro, J.M.; Takkouche, B.; Blanco, J.; Aldrey, J.M. Is Periodontal Disease Associated with Alzheimer's Disease? A Systematic Review with Meta-Analysis. *Neuroepidemiology* **2017**, *48*, 21–31. [CrossRef] [PubMed]

44. Hirotomi, T.; Kocher, T.; Yoshihara, A.; Biffar, R.; Micheelis, W.; Hoffmann, T.; Miyazaki, H.; Holtfreter, B. Comparison of periodontal conditions among three elderly populations in Japan and Germany. *J. Clin. Periodontol.* **2014**, *41*, 633–642. [CrossRef] [PubMed]
45. Zhang, J.; Yu, C.; Zhang, X.; Chen, H.; Dong, J.; Lu, W.; Song, Z.; Zhou, W. Porphyromonas gingivalis lipopolysaccharide induces cognitive dysfunction, mediated by neuronal inflammation via activation of the TLR4 signaling pathway in C57BL/6 mice. *J. Neuroinflamm.* **2018**, *15*, 37. [CrossRef] [PubMed]
46. Ding, Y.; Ren, J.; Yu, H.; Yu, W.; Zhou, Y. Porphyromonas gingivalis, a periodontitis causing bacterium, induces memory impairment and age-dependent neuroinflammation in mice. *Immun. Ageing* **2018**, *15*, 6. [CrossRef] [PubMed]
47. Ilievski, V.; Zuchowska, P.K.; Green, S.J.; Toth, P.T.; Ragozzino, M.E.; Le, K.; Aljewari, H.W.; O'Brien-Simpson, N.M.; Reynolds, E.C.; Watanabe, K. Chronic oral application of a periodontal pathogen results in brain inflammation, neurodegeneration and amyloid beta production in wild type mice. *PLoS ONE* **2018**, *13*, e0204941. [CrossRef] [PubMed]
48. Ishida, N.; Ishihara, Y.; Ishida, K.; Tada, H.; Funaki-Kato, Y.; Hagiwara, M.; Ferdous, T.; Abdullah, M.; Mitani, A.; Michikawa, M.; et al. Periodontitis induced by bacterial infection exacerbates features of Alzheimer's disease in transgenic mice. *NPJ Aging Mech. Dis.* **2017**, *3*, 15. [CrossRef] [PubMed]
49. Laforgia, A.; Corsalini, M.; Stefanachi, G.; Pettini, F.; Di Venere, D. Assessment of Psychopatologic Traits in a Group of Patients with Adult Chronic Periodontitis: Study on 108 Cases and Analysis of Compliance during and after Periodontal Treatment. *Int. J. Med. Sci.* **2015**, *12*, 832–839. [CrossRef]
50. Bale, S.; Tebbie, N.; Price, P. A topical metronidazole gel used to treat malodorous wounds. *Br. J. Nurs.* **2004**, *13*, S4–S11. [CrossRef]
51. Saintrain, M.V.; de Souza, E.H. Impact of tooth loss on the quality of life. *Gerodontology* **2012**, *29*, e632–e636. [CrossRef] [PubMed]
52. Monteiro da Silva, A.M.; Oakley, D.A.; Newman, H.N.; Nohl, F.S.; Lloyd, H.M. Psychosocial factors and adult onset rapidly progressive periodontitis. *J. Clin. Periodontol.* **1996**, *23*, 789–794. [CrossRef] [PubMed]
53. Moss, M.E.; Beck, J.D.; Kaplan, B.H.; Offenbacher, S.; Weintraub, J.A.; Koch, G.G.; Genco, R.J.; Machtei, E.E.; Tedesco, L.A. Exploratory case-control analysis of psychosocial factors and adult periodontitis. *J. Periodontol.* **1996**, *67*, 1060–1069. [CrossRef] [PubMed]
54. Breivik, T.; Gundersen, Y.; Murison, R.; Turner, J.D.; Muller, C.P.; Gjermo, P.; Opstad, K. Maternal Deprivation of Lewis Rat Pups Increases the Severity of Experi-mental Periodontitis in Adulthood. *Open Dent. J.* **2015**, *9*, 65–78. [CrossRef] [PubMed]
55. Solis, A.C.O.; Marques, A.H.; Dominguez, W.V.; Prado, E.B.A.; Pannuti, C.M.; Lotufo, R.F.M.; Lotufo-Neto, F. Evaluation of periodontitis in hospital outpatients with major depressive disorder. A focus on gingival and circulating cytokines. *Brain Behav. Immun.* **2016**, *53*, 49–53. [CrossRef]
56. Hashioka, S.; McGeer, P.L.; Monji, A.; Kanba, S. Anti-inflammatory effects of antidepressants: Possibilities for preventives against Alzheimer's disease. *Cent. Nerv. Syst. Agents Med. Chem.* **2009**, *9*, 12–19. [CrossRef]
57. Hashioka, S. Antidepressants and neuroinflammation: Can antidepressants calm glial rage down? *Mini Rev. Med. Chem.* **2011**, *11*, 555–564. [CrossRef]
58. Muniz, F.; Melo, I.M.; Rosing, C.K.; de Andrade, G.M.; Martins, R.S.; Moreira, M.; Carvalho, R.S. Use of antidepressive agents as a possibility in the management of periodontal diseases: A systematic review of experimental studies. *J. Investig. Clin. Dent.* **2018**, *9*. [CrossRef]
59. Bhatia, A.; Sharma, R.K.; Tewari, S.; Khurana, H.; Narula, S.C. Effect of Fluoxetine on Periodontal Status in Patients With Depression: A Cross-Sectional Observational Study. *J. Periodontol.* **2015**, *86*, 927–935. [CrossRef]
60. Bhatia, A.; Sharma, R.K.; Tewari, S.; Narula, S.C.; Khurana, H. Periodontal status in chronic periodontitis depressed patients on desvenlafaxine: An observational study. *J. Indian Soc. Periodontol.* **2018**, *22*, 442–446. [CrossRef]
61. Gomes, C.; Martinho, F.C.; Barbosa, D.S.; Antunes, L.S.; Povoa, H.C.C.; Baltus, T.H.L.; Morelli, N.R.; Vargas, H.O.; Nunes, S.O.V.; Anderson, G.; et al. Increased Root Canal Endotoxin Levels are Associated with Chronic Apical Periodontitis, Increased Oxidative and Nitrosative Stress, Major Depression, Severity of Depression, and a Lowered Quality of Life. *Mol. Neurobiol.* **2018**, *55*, 2814–2827. [CrossRef] [PubMed]
62. Maes, M.; Galecki, P.; Chang, Y.S.; Berk, M. A review on the oxidative and nitrosative stress (O&NS) pathways in major depression and their possible contribution to the (neuro)degenerative processes in that illness. *Prog. Neuro-Psychopharmacol. Biol. Psychiatry* **2011**, *35*, 676–692. [CrossRef]

63. Hsu, C.C.; Hsu, Y.C.; Chen, H.J.; Lin, C.C.; Chang, K.H.; Lee, C.Y.; Chong, L.W.; Kao, C.H. Association of Periodontitis and Subsequent Depression: A Nationwide Population-Based Study. *Medicine* **2015**, *94*, e2347. [CrossRef]
64. Delgado-Angulo, E.K.; Sabbah, W.; Suominen, A.L.; Vehkalahti, M.M.; Knuuttila, M.; Partonen, T.; Nordblad, A.; Sheiham, A.; Watt, R.G.; Tsakos, G. The association of depression and anxiety with dental caries and periodontal disease among Finnish adults. *Community Dent. Oral Epidemiol.* **2015**, *43*, 540–549. [CrossRef] [PubMed]
65. Khambaty, T.; Stewart, J.C. Associations of depressive and anxiety disorders with periodontal disease prevalence in young adults: Analysis of 1999–2004 National Health and Nutrition Examination Survey (NHANES) data. *Ann. Behav. Med.* **2013**, *45*, 393–397. [CrossRef] [PubMed]
66. Park, S.J.; Ko, K.D.; Shin, S.I.; Ha, Y.J.; Kim, G.Y.; Kim, H.A. Association of oral health behaviors and status with depression: Results from the Korean National Health and Nutrition Examination Survey, 2010. *J. Public Health Dent.* **2014**, *74*, 127–138. [CrossRef] [PubMed]
67. Persson, G.R.; Persson, R.E.; MacEntee, C.I.; Wyatt, C.C.; Hollender, L.G.; Kiyak, H.A. Periodontitis and perceived risk for periodontitis in elders with evidence of depression. *J. Clin. Periodontol.* **2003**, *30*, 691–696. [CrossRef]
68. Cademartori, M.G.; Gastal, M.T.; Nascimento, G.G.; Demarco, F.F.; Correa, M.B. Is depression associated with oral health outcomes in adults and elders? A systematic review and meta-analysis. *Clin. Oral Investig.* **2018**, *22*, 2685–2702. [CrossRef]
69. Einarsdóttir, E.R.; Gunnsteinsdóttir, H.; Hallsdóttir, M.H.; Sveinsson, S.; Jónsdóttir, S.R.; Olafsson, V.G.; Bragason, T.H.; Saemundsson, S.R.; Holbrook, W.P. Dental health of patients with Parkinson's disease in Iceland. *Spec. Care Dent.* **2009**, *29*, 123–127. [CrossRef]
70. Schwarz, J.; Heimhilger, E.; Storch, A. Increased periodontal pathology in Parkinson's disease. *J. Neurol.* **2006**, *253*, 608–611. [CrossRef]
71. Chen, C.K.; Huang, J.Y.; Wu, Y.T.; Chang, Y.C. Dental Scaling Decreases the Risk of Parkinson's Disease: A Nationwide Population-Based Nested Case-Control Study. *Int. J. Environ. Res. Public Health* **2018**, *15*, 1587. [CrossRef] [PubMed]
72. Chen, C.K.; Wu, Y.T.; Chang, Y.C. Periodontal inflammatory disease is associated with the risk of Parkinson's disease: A population-based retrospective matched-cohort study. *PeerJ* **2017**, *5*, e3647. [CrossRef] [PubMed]
73. Eltas, A.; Kartalci, S.; Eltas, S.D.; Dundar, S.; Uslu, M.O. An assessment of periodontal health in patients with schizophrenia and taking antipsychotic medication. *Int. J. Dent. Hyg.* **2013**, *11*, 78–83. [CrossRef] [PubMed]
74. Crescenti, A.; Gasso, P.; Mas, S.; Abellana, R.; Deulofeu, R.; Parellada, E.; Bernardo, M.; Lafuente, A. Insertion/deletion polymorphism of the angiotensin-converting enzyme gene is associated with schizophrenia in a Spanish population. *Psychiatry Res.* **2009**, *165*, 175–180. [CrossRef] [PubMed]
75. Gurkan, A.; Emingil, G.; Saygan, B.H.; Atilla, G.; Kose, T.; Baylas, H.; Berdeli, A. Renin-angiotensin gene polymorphisms in relation to severe chronic periodontitis. *J. Clin. Periodontol.* **2009**, *36*, 204–211. [CrossRef] [PubMed]
76. Leira, Y.; Seoane, J.; Blanco, M.; Rodriguez-Yanez, M.; Takkouche, B.; Blanco, J.; Castillo, J. Association between periodontitis and ischemic stroke: A systematic review and meta-analysis. *Eur. J. Epidemiol.* **2017**, *32*, 43–53. [CrossRef] [PubMed]
77. Beck, J.; Garcia, R.; Heiss, G.; Vokonas, P.S.; Offenbacher, S. Periodontal Disease and Cardiovascular Disease. *J. Periodontol.* **1996**, *67*, 1123–1137. [CrossRef] [PubMed]
78. Wu, T.; Trevisan, M.; Genco, R.J.; Dorn, J.P.; Falkner, K.L.; Sempos, C.T. Periodontal disease and risk of cerebrovascular disease: The first national health and nutrition examination survey and its follow-up study. *Arch. Intern. Med.* **2000**, *160*, 2749–2755. [CrossRef]
79. Jimenez, M.; Krall, E.A.; Garcia, R.I.; Vokonas, P.S.; Dietrich, T. Periodontitis and incidence of cerebrovascular disease in men. *Ann. Neurol.* **2009**, *66*, 505–512. [CrossRef]
80. Grau, A.J.; Becher, H.; Ziegler, C.M.; Lichy, C.; Buggle, F.; Kaiser, C.; Lutz, R.; Bultmann, S.; Preusch, M.; Dorfer, C.E. Periodontal disease as a risk factor for ischemic stroke. *Stroke* **2004**, *35*, 496–501. [CrossRef]
81. Dorfer, C.E.; Becher, H.; Ziegler, C.M.; Kaiser, C.; Lutz, R.; Jorss, D.; Lichy, C.; Buggle, F.; Bultmann, S.; Preusch, M.; et al. The association of gingivitis and periodontitis with ischemic stroke. *J. Clin. Periodontol.* **2004**, *31*, 396–401. [CrossRef] [PubMed]

82. Pradeep, A.R.; Hadge, P.; Arjun Raju, P.; Shetty, S.R.; Shareef, K.; Guruprasad, C.N. Periodontitis as a risk factor for cerebrovascular accident: A case-control study in the Indian population. *J. Periodontal. Res.* **2010**, *45*, 223–228. [CrossRef] [PubMed]

83. Sim, S.J.; Kim, H.D.; Moon, J.Y.; Zavras, A.I.; Zdanowicz, J.; Jang, S.J.; Jin, B.H.; Bae, K.H.; Paik, D.I.; Douglass, C.W. Periodontitis and the risk for non-fatal stroke in Korean adults. *J. Periodontol.* **2008**, *79*, 1652–1658. [CrossRef] [PubMed]

84. Lafon, A.; Tala, S.; Ahossi, V.; Perrin, D.; Giroud, M.; Bejot, Y. Association between periodontal disease and non-fatal ischemic stroke: A case-control study. *Acta Odontol. Scand.* **2014**, *72*, 687–693. [CrossRef] [PubMed]

85. Chi, L.; Cheng, X.; He, X.; Sun, J.; Liang, F.; Pei, Z.; Teng, W. Increased cortical infarction and neuroinflammation in ischemic stroke mice with experimental periodontitis. *Neuroreport* **2019**, *30*, 428–433. [CrossRef] [PubMed]

8

Periodontal Therapy for Improving Lipid Profiles in Patients with Type 2 Diabetes Mellitus

Siddharth Garde [1], Rahena Akhter [1], Mai Anh Nguyen [1], Clara K. Chow [2] and Joerg Eberhard [1,*]

[1] The University of Sydney School of Dentistry, Faculty of Medicine and Health, The University of Sydney, Camperdown 2006, Australia
[2] Westmead Applied Research Centre, Sydney Medical School, Westmead 2145, Australia
* Correspondence: joerg.eberhard@sydney.edu.au

Abstract: Periodontitis is a chronic inflammatory disorder often seen in patients with diabetes mellitus (DM). Individuals with diabetes are at a greater risk of developing cardiovascular complications and this may be related, in part, to lipid abnormalities observed in these individuals. The objective of this systematic review is to compile the current scientific evidence of the effects of periodontal treatment on lipid profiles in patients with type 2 diabetes mellitus. Through a systematic search using MEDLINE, EMBASE, PubMed, and Web of Science, 313 articles were identified. Of these, seven clinical trials which met all inclusion criteria were chosen for analysis. Between baseline and 3-month follow-up, there was a statistically significant reduction in the levels of total cholesterol (mean differences (MD) −0.47 mmol/L (95% confidence interval (CI), −0.75, −0.18, $p = 0.001$)), triglycerides (MD −0.20 mmol/L (95% CI −0.24, −0.16, $p < 0.00001$)) favouring the intervention arm, and a statistically significant reduction in levels of high density lipoprotein (HDL) (MD 0.06 mmol/L (95% CI 0.03, 0.08, $p < 0.00001$)) favouring the control arm. No significant differences were observed between baseline and 6-month follow-up levels for any lipid analysed. The heterogeneity between studies was high. This review foreshadows a potential benefit of periodontal therapy for lipid profiles in patients suffering from type 2 DM, however, well designed clinical trials using lipid profiles as primary outcome measures are warranted.

Keywords: periodontal therapy; type 2 diabetes mellitus; lipid profiles; inflammation

---

1. Introduction

Periodontal diseases are a group of inflammatory conditions affecting the connective tissues surrounding teeth. Periodontitis, a specific type of periodontal disease, is a major cause of tooth loss and the prevalence of its moderate to severe forms in adult Western populations is approximately 50% [1,2]. Periodontitis is caused by gram-negative bacteria which induce a host inflammatory response, resulting in the destruction of tissues that supports the teeth and also has adverse systemic effects [3].

Type 2 diabetes mellitus (type 2 DM) is a metabolic disorder ranging from insulin resistance to insulin deficiency, with poor glycaemic control presenting as a predominant feature [3]. Diabetes is also a major risk factor for periodontitis, and the risk of developing periodontitis is increased approximately three times in patients with diabetes compared with non-diabetic individuals [4]. There is an increasing prevalence of type 2 DM worldwide, and this is expected to contribute to an increase in diabetes-related complications [5].

Cardiovascular disease (CVD) is also one of the major complications associated with diabetes, and there is a high prevalence of cardiovascular risk factors and markers of cardiovascular organ injury in patients with type 2 DM. Ninety-seven percent of patients with diabetes are dyslipidaemic, with a characteristic pattern of increased plasma triglycerides and decreased high density lipoprotein (HDL) cholesterol. In a large clinical study with an average follow-up period of 3.9 years, low density lipoprotein (LDL) cholesterol, non-HDL cholesterol, apolipoprotein B, triglyceride, and homocysteine levels all increased over time, with most participants also having low HDL levels [6]. The downregulation of the enzyme lipoprotein lipase due to low insulin levels may be the cause of the dyslipidaemic profiles noted in diabetic individuals [7]. Other mechanisms involved linking diabetes to higher CVD risk involve chronic oxidative stress in diabetics, purportedly related to the metabolism of excess substrates (glucose and fatty acids [8]) and a state of chronic, low-level inflammation [9] in diabetes.

Recent intervention trials have demonstrated that anti-inflammatory periodontitis therapy may reduce serum levels of glycated haemoglobin (HbA1c) and high sensitivity C-reactive protein (hsCRP) [10–16], demonstrating the capacity to modulate glucose control and cardiovascular risk. However, little attention has been paid to the potential effects of periodontitis therapy in patients with diabetes to improve lipid profiles. This systematic review aims to evaluate the scientific evidence of the impact of periodontal therapy on lipid profiles in patients with type 2 DM.

2. Results

2.1. Selection of Studies

Six hundred and eighty-two studies were retrieved from the electronic databases PubMed, MEDLINE via Ovid, EMBASE via Ovid, and Web of Science. Three hundred and sixty-nine duplicates were removed, and the remaining abstracts were screened for eligibility, resulting in sixty-eight studies being further excluded. Two hundred and forty-five studies were then selected for full-text analysis. After reading of the full texts, seven studies [10–16] were included in the systematic review (Figure 1). Full text studies were excluded if they did not report lipid levels as an outcome or studies did not have appropriate intervention and control arms.

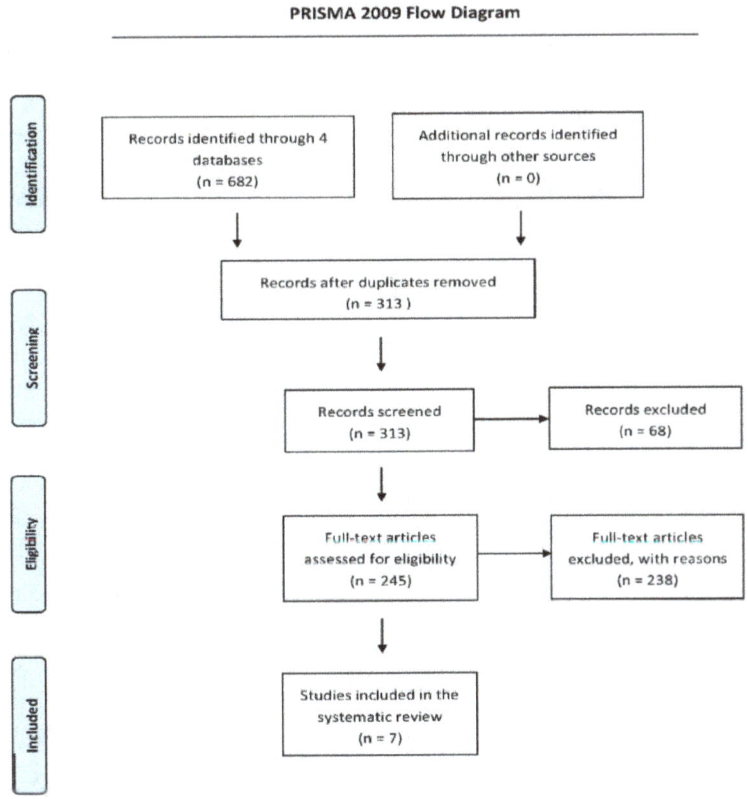

Figure 1. Study selection flow diagram.

2.2. *Characteristics of Studies*

The characteristics of the included studies are described in Table 1. In total, there were 411 individuals who underwent periodontal treatment (intervention arm) and 341 individuals who did not or received post-trial intervention (control arm). The total number of participants in each study ranged from 40 to 264. The follow-up times for the studies ranged from 3 to 12 months, however, for this review only the 3- and 6-month follow-up data has been analysed. Among seven studies, five studies reported 3-month follow-up [10,12,13,15,16] and three studies reported 6-month follow-up data [10,11,14].

The mean age of individuals in the studies ranged from 45.5 to 63.2 years old. Three out of seven studies [11,12,16] excluded patients with cardiovascular disease. Three studies [10,14,15] excluded patients with uncontrolled systemic diseases, however, did not specify whether cardiovascular disease was amongst this exclusion criteria. One study [13] did not specify whether participants with any uncontrolled systemic diseases were excluded or not. Two studies [11,14] specified that participants taking anti-hypertensive/cholesterol medications were included whereas five studies [10,12,13,15,16] did not specify whether patients taking anti-hypertensive/cholesterol medications were included or not. Six out of the seven studies [10–12,14–16] presented periodontal inclusion criteria and, among them, four different criteria were identified. All studies [10–16] reported diabetes inclusion criteria, and seven different criteria were identified (Table 1).

Table 1. Characteristics of included studies.

Author	Country	Intervention/ Control	Participants at Baseline (*n*)	Follow Up TIME (months)	Diabetes Inclusion Criteria	Periodontal Inclusion Criteria
D'Aiuto et al. 2018 [11]	United Kingdom	SPT + NSPT	133	12	Type 2 DM for >6 months (WHO diagnostic criteria)	>20 periodontal pockets with PD > 4mm and alveolar bone loss > 30%
		Supragingival SRP	131			
Masi et al. 2018 [14]	United Kingdom	NSPT	27	6	Diagnosed type 2 DM (WHO criteria)	>15 remaining teeth and >20 sites with PD >5mm
		Supragingival SRP	24			
Kapellas et al. 2017 [12]	Australia	NSPT	35	3	HbA1c > 6.5% or >47.5 mmol/mol	Joint Centers for Disease Control and Prevention and American Academy of Periodontology case definition
		No treatment	27			
Chen et al. 2012 [10]	China	NSPT	45	6	Type 2 DM for >12 months	American Academy of Periodontology criteria
		No treatment	44			
Moeintaghavi et al. 2012 [15]	Iran	NSPT	22	3	HbA1c > 7%	Mild-moderate periodontitis-American Academy of Periodontology criteria
		No treatment	18			
Sun et al. 2011 [16]	China	NSPT	82	3	Diagnosed type 2 DM for >12 months and HbA1c 7.5–9.5%	>20 remaining teeth, PD > 5 mm, more than 30% teeth CAL over 4 mm, or over 60% teeth with PD > 4 mm and CAL > 3 mm
		No treatment	75			
Kiran et al. 2005 [13]	Turkey	NSPT	22	3	HbA1c 6–8%	Not specified
		No treatment	22			

SPT: surgical periodontal treatment; NSPT: non-surgical periodontal treatment; SRP: scaling and root planing; DM: diabetes mellitus; HbA1c: glycated haemoglobin; WHO: World Health Organization; PD: pocket depth; CAL: clinical attachment loss.

2.3. *Risk of Bias within Studies*

The Cochrane Collaboration's tool for assessing risk of bias [17] was used to assess the risk of bias within the included studies which have been summarized in Figure 2. Of the seven clinical trials included [10–16], five studies described the methods of randomisation [10–12,14,15]. Three studies [11,12,14] used a computer-generated table for allocation concealment, two studies [10,15] assigned an independent individual to allocate participants, and two studies [13,16] did not specify allocation concealment. Blinding of patients and personnel was not possible due to the nature of the periodontal treatment. Blinding of investigators was conducted in four studies [10–12,14], two did not specify whether investigators were blinded [13,15], and one study was non-blinded [16]. Four studies had minimal/no participant drop out or the data for the participants who dropped out was excluded [13–16], two studies had a moderate number of participants drop out [10,11] and one study [12] had a high participant dropout rate indicating attrition bias. There was no evidence of selective reporting or any other form of bias in any of the studies.

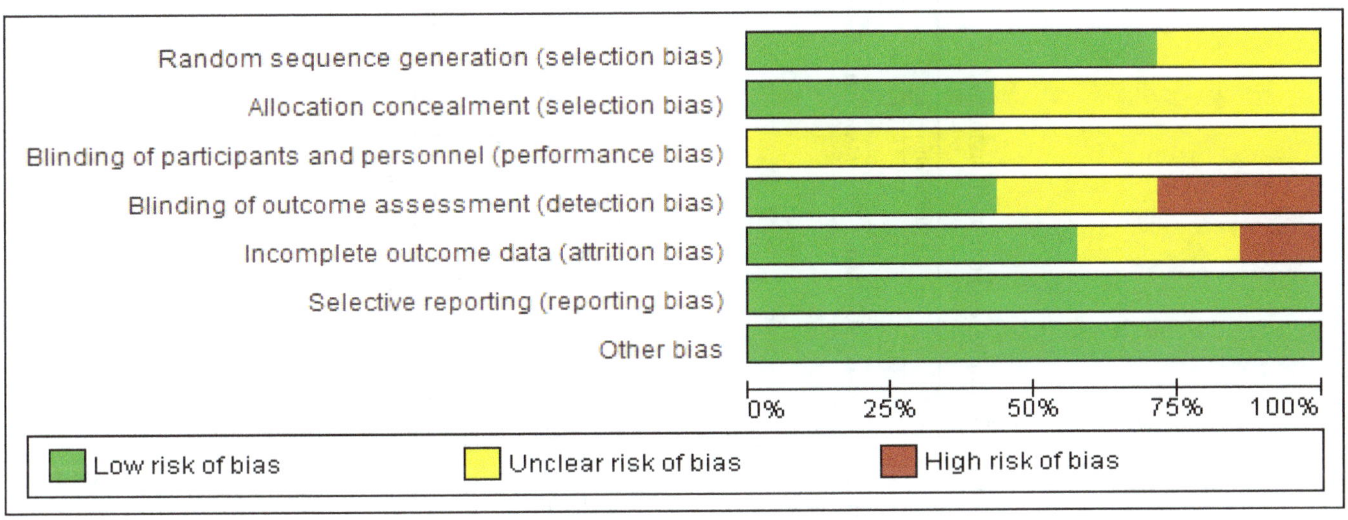

Figure 2. Risk of bias analysis of individual studies.

2.4. *Lipid Profiles*

Changes in lipid profiles between baseline and the 3- and 6-month follow-ups have been depicted in Table 2.

Table 2. Lipid profiles at baseline, 3 months, and 6 months in mmol/L.

Author	Groups		Baseline								3 Month Follow Up								6 Month Follow Up							
			TC		TG		LDL		HDL		TC		TG		LDL		HDL		TC		TG		LDL		HDL	
			Mean	SD	Mean	SD	Mean	SD	Mean	SD	Mean	SD	Mean	SD	Mean	SD	Mean	SD	Mean	SD	Mean	SD	Mean	SD	Mean	SD
D'Aiuto et al. 2018 [11]	Intervention	SPT+NSPT	4.2	1 *	1.6	1.2 *	2.2	0.9 *	1.2	0.4 *									4.3	0.1 *	1.7	0.1 *	2.3	0.1 *	1.3	0.0 *
	Control	SG SRP	4.3	1.1 *	1.6	1.1 *	2.4	0.9 *	1.3	0.4 *									4.2	0.1 *	1.5	0.1 *	2.3	0.1 *	1.2	0.0 *
Masi et al. 2018 [14]	Intervention	NSPT	4.3	1.1	1.48	1.13	2.3	0.9	1.3	0.4									4.2	0.9	1.4	0.9	2.2	0.7	1.4	0.4
	Control	SG SRP	4.3	1	2.3	2.6	2	0.9	1.3	0.4									4.1	1.1	2.2	1.9	2	0.8	1.2	0.5
Kapellas et al. 2017 [12]	Intervention	NSPT	4.8	1.1					1	0.3	4.5	1					1	0.3								
	Control	No tx	4.6	0.8					1.1	0.2	4.4	0.9					0.9	0.2								
Chen et al. 2012 [10]	Intervention	NSPT	2.63	1.32	6.02	1.57	3.5	1.3	1.31	0.46	2.2	1.33	5.61	1.41	3.37	1.3	1.23	0.39	2.15	1.93	5.26	1.41	3.04	1.23	1.14	0.39
	Control	No tx	2.35	1.78	6.37	1.87	3.79	1.48	1.44	0.53	2.3	2.16	5.94	1.22	3.5	1.17	1.36	0.49	2.25	1.98	5.81	1.61	1.26	0.5	3.25	1.27
Moeintaghavi et al. 2012 [15]	Intervention	NSPT	10.66	1.5	7.66	4.54	6.6	1.38	2.55	0.51	10.31	1.72	7.22	3.22	6.26	1.76	2.45	0.37								
	Control	No tx	10.69	1.5	8.4	1.51	6.51	1.9	2.57	0.69	10.95	1.51	8.19	1.62	6.36	2.12	2.44	0.54								
Sun et al. 2011 [16]	Intervention	NSPT			2.07	0.69	3.32	0.71	1.17	0.29			1.85	0.64	3.21	0.76	1.23	0.33								
	Control	No tx			2.1	0.68	3.37	0.74	1.15	0.28			2.08	0.66	3.31	0.75	1.16	0.3								
Kiran et al. 2005 [13]	Intervention	NSPT	10.4	2.13	7.6	5.5	6.31	1.35	2.87	0.77	10.17	1.73	6.82	3.1	6.15	1.73	2.94	0.85								
	Control	No tx	9.95	1.95	7.26	3.8	5.96	1.81	2.54	0.73	10.57	2.07	9.17	5.95	5.94	2.16	2.85	0.79								

TC: total cholesterol; TG: triglyceride; LDL: low-density lipoprotein; HDL: high-density lipoprotein; SD: standard deviation; *: standard error; NSPT: non-surgical periodontal treatment; SG SRP: supragingival scaling and root planning; tx: treatment.

2.4.1. Baseline vs. 3-Month Follow-Up

After a 3 month observation period data from five studies [10,12,13,15,16] were included in the meta-analysis (Figure 3). A total of 235 participants in four studies [10,12,13,15] were analysed for changes in their total cholesterol levels and there was a statistically significant differences in favour of the intervention group ($p = 0.001$, mean difference −0.47 mmol/L (95% CI, −0.75 mmol/L to −0.18 mmol/L)) with evidence of high heterogeneity ($Chi^2 = 35.22$, 3 df, $p < 0.00001$, $I^2 = 91\%$). A total of 330 patients in four studies [10,13,15,16] were analysed for changes in triglycerides, and there was a statistically significant difference in favour of the intervention treatment ($p < 0.00001$, mean difference −0.20 mmol/L (95% CI −0.24 mmol/L to −0.16 mmol/L, $Chi^2 = 179.34$, 3 df, $p < 0.00001$, $I^2 = 98\%$)), with evidence of high heterogeneity. A total of 330 patients in four studies [10,13,15,16] compared changes in LDL levels, and there was no significant difference between the intervention and the control treatment ($p = 0.21$, mean difference −0.02 mmol/L (95% CI −0.06 mmol/L to 0.01 mmol/L, $Chi^2 = 16.64$, 3 df, $p = 0.0008$, $I^2 = 82\%$)). A total of 392 patients in five studies [10,12,13,15,16] compared changes in HDL levels, and there was a statistically significant difference in favour of the control treatment ($p < 0.00001$, mean difference 0.06 mmol/L (95% CI 0.03 mmol/L to 0.08 mmol/L, $Chi^2 = 37.06$, 4 df, $p < 0.00001$, $I^2 = 89\%$)), with evidence of high heterogeneity.

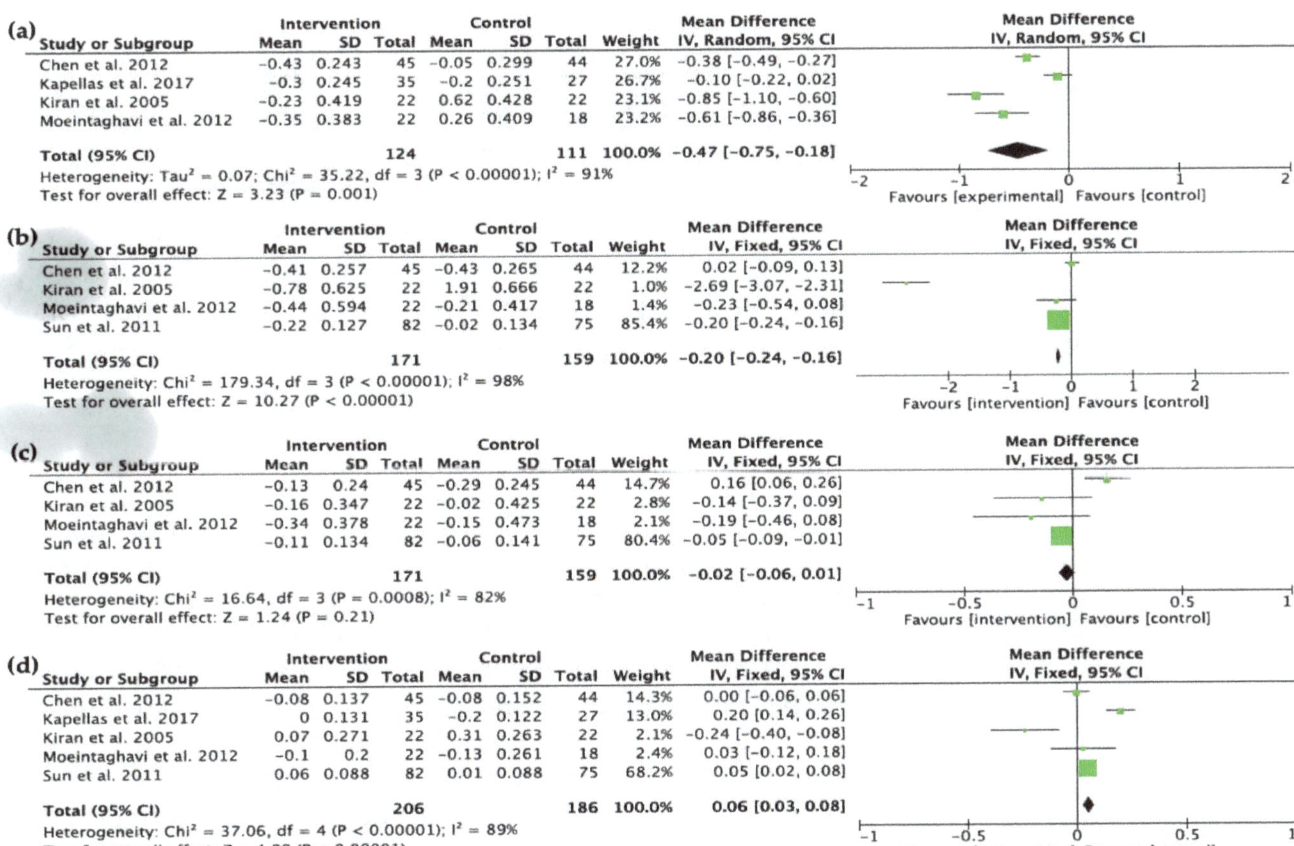

Figure 3. Forest plots depicting the changes of (**a**) total cholesterol, (**b**) triglycerides, (**c**) LDL, and (**d**) HDL (all in mmol/L) between the intervention and control groups at baseline and the 3-month follow-up.

2.4.2. Baseline vs. 6-Month Follow-Up

After 6 months, three studies [10,11,14] were included in a meta-analysis of total cholesterol, triglycerides, LDL and HDL. There were no statistically significant differences found for any lipid levels (Figure 4).

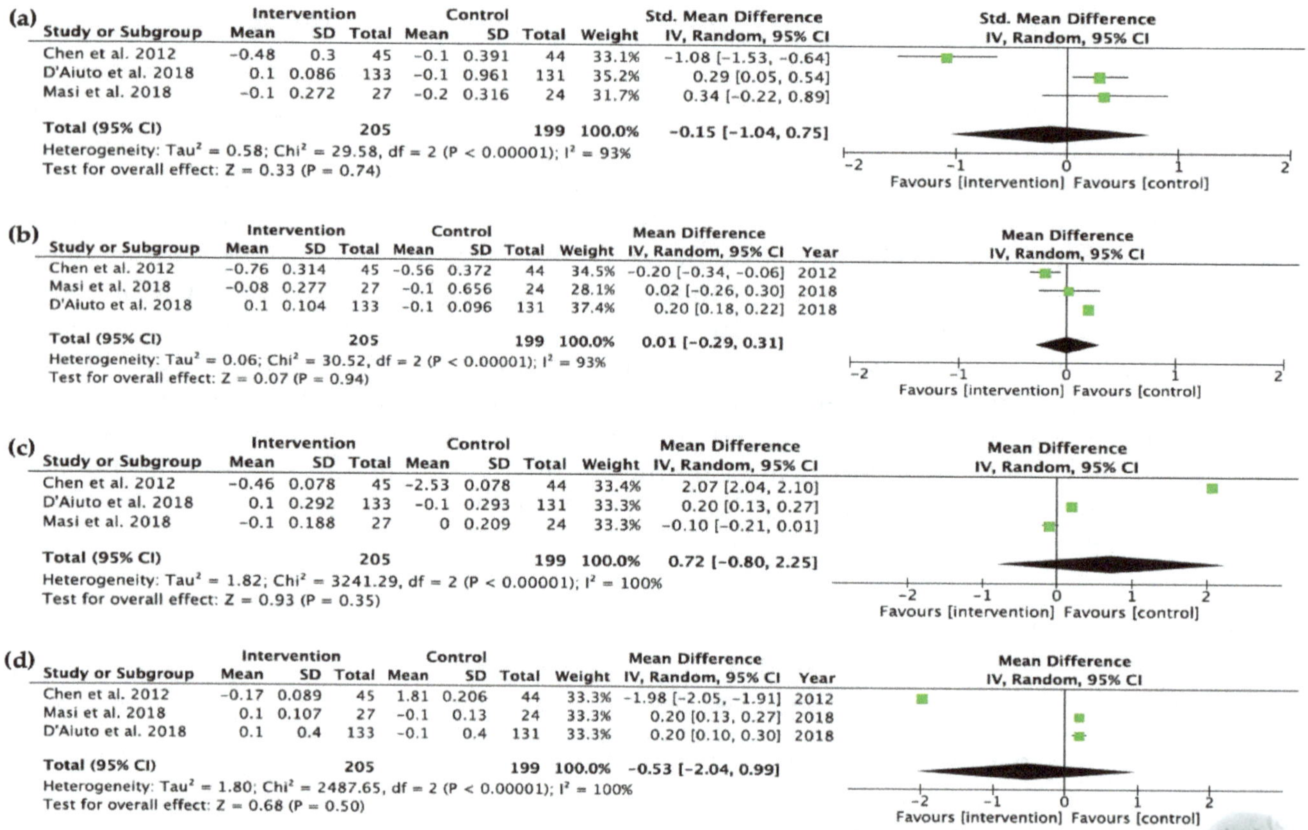

Figure 4. Forest plots depicting the changes of (**a**) total cholesterol, (**b**) triglycerides, (**c**) LDL, and (**d**) HDL (all in mmol/L) between the intervention and control groups at baseline and the 6-month follow-up.

2.5. Periodontal Outcomes

The periodontal parameters at baseline, 3 months, and 6 months are outlined in Table 3. At baseline, four studies [10,13,15,16] reported a mean periodontal probing depth of 2.93 mm for the intervention groups, compared to 2.82 mm in the control groups. Three months after therapy a mean PD of 2.30 mm was reported in the intervention groups (PD reduction of 0.63 mm), compared to 2.81 mm in the control groups (PD reduction of 0.1 mm). For the comparison between baseline vs. 6 months, three studies [10,11,14] reported a mean baseline PD of 3.46 mm in the intervention group and of 3.99 mm in the control group. After 6 months, a mean PD of 2.63 mm in the intervention group (PD reduction 0.83 mm) and a mean PD of 3.14 mm in the control groups (PD reduction 0.18 mm) was reported.

Two studies [10,13] reported changes in bleeding on probing (BOP) between baseline and 3-month follow-up. For the intervention group a mean BOP of 43.4% was calculated at baseline and of 18.0% at 3-month follow-up. For the control group the mean BOP at baseline was 42.2%, compared to 40.2% at 3-month follow-up. Three studies [10,11,14] reported BOP values for baseline and 6-month follow-up. For the intervention group a mean BOP of 56.5% was calculated at baseline and of 27.0% at the 6-month follow-up assessment. For the control group, the mean BOP at baseline was 56.3%, compared to 47.8% at 6-month follow-up.

Table 3. Periodontal parameters at baseline, and 3 and 6 months.

Author	Groups		Baseline				3-month Follow Up				6-month Follow Up			
			PD		BOP		PD		BOP		PD		BOP	
			Mean	SD	Mean	SD	Mean	SD	Mean	SD	Mean	SD	Mean	SD
D'Aiuto et al. 2018 [11]	Intervention	SPT + NSPT	3.9	0.1 *	65	2.0 *					2.9	0.1 *	33.0	2.0 *
	Control	SG SRP	3.9	0.1 *	63	2.0 *					3.7	0.1 *	57.0	2.0 *
Masi et al. 2018 [14]	Intervention	NSPT	3.9	0.8	70.0	20.0								
	Control	SG SRP	3.6	0.7	72.0	15.0								
Kapellas et al. 2017 [12]	Intervention	NSPT												
	Control	No treatment												
Chen et al. 2012 [10]	Intervention	NSPT	2.57	0.66	32.42	16.63	2.2	0.39	12.13	8.24	2.1	0.39	12.02	8.99
	Control	No treatment	2.47	0.57	34.01	18.91	2.38	0.47	28.53	14.42	2.42	0.5	28.37	13.5
Moeintaghavi et al. 2012 [15]	Intervention	NSPT	2.31	0.65			2.21	0.6						
	Control	No treatment	2.06	0.24			2.33	0.3						
Sun et al. 2011 [16]	Intervention	NSPT	4.53	0.83			2.97	0.78						
	Control	No treatment	4.49	0.85			4.28	0.81						
Kiran et al. 2005 [13]	Intervention	NSPT	2.29	0.49	54.38	18.75	1.8	0.25	23.9	12.73				
	Control	No treatment	2.24	0.7	50.48	26.1	2.26	0.63	51.91	27.38				
Total	**Intervention**		**3.3**	**0.6**	**55.5**	**16.1**	**2.3**	**0.5**	**18.0**	**10.7**	**2.6**	**0.5**	**27.0**	**13.1**
	Control		**3.1**	**0.6**	**54.9**	**17.8**	**2.8**	**0.3**	**40.2**	**21.9**	**3.1**	**0.5**	**47.8**	**13.0**

SPT: surgical periodontal treatment; NSPT: non-surgical periodontal treatment; SG SRP: supragingival scaling and root planing; PD: pocket depth (mm); SD: standard deviation; *: standard error; BOP: bleeding on probing (%).

3. Discussion

This is the first meta-analysis aimed to evaluate the effect of anti-inflammatory periodontal therapy on changes of lipid levels in patients with type 2 DM. Periodontal therapy involves the mechanical removal of dental plaque associated with periodontitis. The majority of the studies used non-surgical periodontal treatment as the intervention, however one study [11] used surgical periodontal treatment for select individuals in the intervention arm as well. The analyses demonstrated that total cholesterol and triglycerides were significantly reduced in the intervention arm 3 months after therapy to lower levels, while HDL levels were reduced in the control group. However, no significant differences were observed after 6 months. The studies included in this review showed considerable heterogeneity, which has to be recognized before any conclusion can be drawn. However, this systematic review highlighted the potential benefits of periodontitis therapy to reduce total cholesterol and triglycerides levels. These positive effects may reduce the risk for cardiovascular complications in patients with type 2 DM.

The studies included were selected using stringent selection criteria described in the methods section, however, none of the studies included were designed to analyse lipid profiles as primary outcome measures. This may contribute to the high heterogeneity of the outcomes, as well as factors affecting lipid levels in general, including how long the individuals have had type 2 DM, lifestyle factors, and diet, which have not been assessed or reported in the included studies. All studies demonstrated a substantial reduction of clinical parameters of periodontal disease, including PD and BOP in the intervention groups 3 and 6 months after therapy, indicative of a successful treatment of the inflammatory reaction involved in periodontal disease. By contrast, the control groups did not show obvious changes in assessed oral health parameters. The mean levels of investigated total cholesterol and triglycerides decreased 3 months after periodontitis therapy, however, no differences were observed after 6 months. A possible explanation for this fading effect on lipid profiles after prolonged observation periods is recolonization by the subgingival microbiota and subsequent inflammation [18] if supportive periodontal treatment is not provided. Even though the periodontal parameters were significantly improved at the 6-month follow-up relative to baseline, five out of the seven included studies [10,12,13,15,16] did not provide supportive periodontal therapy to participants in the intervention arm after the initial treatment. In these participants, it is very likely that the recolonization of the microflora re-induced the inflammatory reaction which may have adversely affected lipid parameters. It should also be noted that average periodontal probing depths and bleeding on probing percentages are lower at the 3-month follow-up compared to the 6-month follow-up. This observation indicates the necessity of a regular periodontal maintenance program aimed to minimise the recolonization of tooth surfaces with periodontal pathogens and the concordant inflammation of the adjacent tissues.

Three out of the seven studies included in the current review [14–16] showed a significant reduction in levels of glycated haemoglobin and four studies [10–13] did not show significant changes between baseline and follow-up. In those studies reporting a significant reduction of glycated haemoglobin after periodontal treatment, one study [15] showed improved levels of total cholesterol, one study [16] showed an improvement in levels of HDL, whereas in both studies, other lipid parameters showed no significant changes. The third study [16] did not find any difference in lipid parameters between baseline and follow-up despite the reduction in levels of glycated haemoglobin. Within the limitations of this comparison, a reduction in glycated haemoglobin may not necessarily be accompanied by changes in lipid levels.

Individuals with periodontitis have been noted to have an increased risk of hyperlipidaemia and hypercholesterolaemia [19]. As mentioned previously, periodontitis is a chronic infection of the tooth supporting structures [1], and local chronic infections have been shown to alter concentrations of cytokines and hormones which can result in changes in lipid metabolism [20]. Specifically, systemic exposure to infectious challenges such as bacterial lipopolysaccharide can result in the release of inflammatory cytokines including interleukin-1 (IL-1) and tumour necrosis factor alpha (TNF-α) that alter fat metabolism and promote hyperlipidaemia. Both TNF-α and IL-1 inhibit the production of lipoprotein lipase, which causes disturbances of lipid metabolism, including increased amounts of serum cholesterol and LDL [21]. A second mechanism by which bacterial lipopolysaccharides contribute to the development of atherosclerosis is by oxidative modification of increased LDL caused by macrophage activation. Oxidized LDL is taken up by macrophage scavengers, which leads to transformation of macrophages into foam cells, the hallmark of the atherosclerotic process. Oxidized LDL is also cytotoxic to endothelial cells and a potent chemoattractant for circulating human monocytes [22]. Conversely, it has also been demonstrated that a short-term high-fat diet results in prolonged impairment in the antibacterial function of polymorphonuclear leukocytes, which may cause damage of periodontal tissues [23]. Thus, a chronic hyperlipidaemic state may impair the host resistance to bacterial infection.

Cardiovascular disease is a major complication of type 2 DM and lipid abnormalities seen in diabetics are a serious contributor to this complication [6]. Glycaemic control via maintaining adequate levels of HbA1c is considered as an essential way to lower patients' risk of having diabetic complications and each 1% drop in HbA1c levels is associated with a risk reduction of 21% for diabetes-related deaths, 14% for myocardial infarction, and 37% for microvascular complications [24]. Several studies have indicated that periodontal infection caused by gram-negative bacteria had adverse effects on diabetic patients' glycaemic control [25,26]. By contrast, improved periodontal conditions following periodontal treatment can significantly improve HbA1c levels [11,27]. A lipid-lowering management in type 2 DM patients is also aimed at reducing the incidence of cardiovascular complications, and statins can be very effective in improving the lipid profile and are therefore the first line class of drugs [28]. In general, different statins have varying abilities to improve lipid profiles in patients, e.g., HDL cholesterol levels increase between 5% and 10% with statin therapy, LDL levels reduce, ranging from 27% to 60%, and triglycerides levels reduce between 11% and 40% [29]. The current analysis demonstrated a mean reduction of triglyceride levels by approximately 8% achieved by periodontitis treatment. Within the limitations of the available study data and the heterogeneity of studies, this will not be sufficient to annotate periodontitis treatment as an adjunct to a lipid-lowering management in patients suffering from type 2 DM. However, it may stimulate the interest in further exploring the benefits of good oral health for the prevention of diabetes complications and especially to setup well designed clinical trials with lipid profiles as the primary outcome.

4. Materials and Methods

4.1. Types of Studies

Randomized control trials of 3- or 6-month follow-ups were considered for this review.

4.2. Types of Participants

The participants of the included studies had a diagnosis of type 2 DM and periodontitis. Patients with type I diabetes were excluded.

4.3. Types of Intervention

All periodontal treatments using mechanical debridement (surgical and non-surgical, with and without adjunctive treatment) were included.

4.4. Types of Outcome Measures

Primary outcome measures were total cholesterol, triglycerides, LDL cholesterol, and HDL cholesterol between baseline and 3- or 6-month follow-ups. Secondary outcome measures were periodontal probing depths, clinical attachment loss, and bleeding on probing.

4.5. Search Methods

The search attempted to identify all relevant trials in English. The electronic databases searched were (date of most recent search 19 May 2019) PubMed, MEDLINE via Ovid, EMBASE via Ovid and Web of Science. A sensitive search strategy was developed following the PICO process for the question: Does periodontal treatment improve lipid profiles in individuals with type 2 DM?

- Patients = individuals with type 2 DM
- Intervention = anti-inflammatory surgical or non-surgical periodontal treatment
- Comparison = no periodontal treatment or only supragingival scaling and polishing
- Outcome = lipid profiles

The search strategy for PubMed is given as an example: ("periodontal treatment" OR "periodontitis treatment" OR "periodontal therapy" OR "periodontitis therapy" AND "diabet*"). Incomplete information and ambiguous data were researched further by contacting the author and/or researcher responsible for the study directly. If the corresponding author failed to reply, the studies were excluded. Cross-sectional studies, retrospective studies, literature reviews, systematic reviews, editors'/authors'/reviewers' comments, articles not in English, studies where the intervention was not periodontal treatment, studies which did not have an appropriate control arm, studies where lipids were not analysed both pre and post-trial, and trials involving individuals with diabetes other than type 2 DM were excluded.

4.6. Selection of Studies

Titles and abstracts were managed by downloading to Endnote X8 software. The selection of papers, the decision about eligibility, and data extraction were carried out independently, in duplicate, by three reviewers (S.G., J.E. and M.A.N.). Any disagreement was resolved by discussion. The full text of the included studies was evaluated by two authors (S.G. and M.A.N.). Data entry to a computer and data extraction was carried out by one reviewer (S.G.).

4.7. Data Extraction

The following data was extracted:

- General study characteristics: authors, year of study, country of origin, intervention/control, number of participants at baseline, follow-up period, diabetes and periodontal inclusion criteria
- Primary outcomes: lipid profiles (total cholesterol, triglycerides, LDL, HDL)
- Secondary outcomes: probing depth and bleeding on probing at baseline and 3- or 6-month follow-ups.

4.8. Quality Assessment

Quality assessment was done according to the guidelines of the Cochrane Handbook for Systematic Reviews of Interventions [17].

4.9. Data Synthesis

For continuous outcomes, mean differences (MD) and 95% CI were used to summarize the data for each group. All statistical analyses were conducted with Review Manager 5.3. Heterogeneity was assessed with Cochran's test for heterogeneity undertaken prior to each meta-analysis, and I^2 statistics.

Author Contributions: Conceptualization, S.G., C.K.C. and J.E.; methodology, S.G.; software, J.E.; validation, S.G. and M.A.N.; formal analysis, J.E.; investigation, S.G. and J.E.; resources, J.E.; data curation, S.G.; writing—original draft preparation, S.G., J.E. and R.A.; writing—review and editing, J.E., C.K.C. and R.A.; visualization, M.A.N.; supervision, J.E. and R.A.; project administration, J.E.

References

1. Ericsson, J.S.; Abrahamsson, K.H.; Ostberg, A.L.; Hellström, M.K.; Jönsson, K.; Wennström, J.L. Periodontal health status in Swedish adolescents: An epidemiological, cross-sectional study. *Swed. Dent. J.* **2009**, *33*, 131–139. [PubMed]
2. Li, Y.; Lee, S.; Hujoel, P.; Su, M.; Zhang, W.; Kim, J.; Zhang, Y.P.; De Vizio, W. Prevalence and severity of gingivitis in American adults. *Am. J. Dent.* **2010**, *23*, 9. [PubMed]
3. Negrato, C.A.; Tarzia, O.; Jovanovič, L.; Chinellato, L.E.M. Periodontal disease and diabetes mellitus. *J. Appl. Oral Sci.* **2013**, *21*, 1. [CrossRef] [PubMed]
4. Preshaw, P.; Alba, A.; Herrera, D.; Jepsen, S.; Konstantinidis, A.; Makrilakis, K.; Taylor, R. Periodontitis and diabetes: A two-way relationship. *Diabetologia* **2012**, *55*, 21–31. [CrossRef] [PubMed]
5. Capewell, S.; Buchan, I. Why have sustained increases in obesity and type 2 diabetes not offset declines in cardiovascular mortality over recent decades in Western countries? *Nutr. Metab. Cardiovasc. Dis. NMCD* **2012**, *22*, 307–311. [CrossRef] [PubMed]
6. Fagot-campagna, A.; Rolka, D.B.; Beckles, G.L.; Gregg, E.W.; Narayan, K. Prevalence of lipid abnormalities, awareness, and treatment in US adults with diabetes. *Diabetes* **2000**, *49*, A78.
7. Shen, G.X. Lipid disorders in diabetes mellitus and current management. *Curr. Pharm. Anal.* **2007**, *3*, 17–24. [CrossRef]
8. Nourooz-Zadeh, J.; Rahimi, A.; Tajaddini-Sarmadi, J.; Tritschler, H.; Rosen, P.; Halliwell, B.; Betteridge, D. Relationships between plasma measures of oxidative stress and metabolic control in NIDDM. *Diabetologia* **1997**, *40*, 647–653. [CrossRef]
9. Pickup, J.; Mattock, M.; Chusney, G.; Burt, D. NIDDM as a disease of the innate immune system: association of acute-phase reactants and interleukin-6 with metabolic syndrome X. *Diabetologia* **1997**, *40*, 1286. [CrossRef]
10. Chen, L.; Luo, G.; Xuan, D.; Wei, B.; Liu, F.; Li, J.; Zhang, J. Effects of non-surgical periodontal treatment on clinical response, serum inflammatory parameters, and metabolic control in patients with type 2 diabetes: A randomized study. *J. Periodontol.* **2012**, *83*, 435–443. [CrossRef]
11. D'Aiuto, F.; Gkranias, N.; Bhowruth, D.; Khan, T.; Orlandi, M.; Suvan, J.; Masi, S.; Tsakos, G.; Hurel, S.; Hingorani, A.D.; et al. Systemic effects of periodontitis treatment in patients with type 2 diabetes: A 12 month, single-centre, investigator-masked, randomised trial. *Lancet Diabetes Endocrinol.* **2018**, *6*, 954–965. [CrossRef]
12. Kapellas, K.; Mejia, G.; Bartold, P.M.; Skilton, M.R.; Maple-Brown, L.J.; Slade, G.D.; O'Dea, K.; Brown, A.; Celermajer, D.S.; Jamieson, L.M. Periodontal therapy and glycaemic control among individuals with type 2 diabetes: Reflections from the PerioCardio study. *Int. J. Dent. Hyg.* **2017**, *15*, e42–e51. [CrossRef] [PubMed]
13. Kiran, M.; Arpak, N.; Unsal, E.; Erdogan, M.F. The effect of improved periodontal health on metabolic control in type 2 diabetes mellitus. *J. Clin. Periodontol.* **2005**, *32*, 266–272. [CrossRef] [PubMed]
14. Masi, S.; Orlandi, M.; Parkar, M.; Bhowruth, D.; Kingston, I.; O'Rourke, C.; Virdis, A.; Hingorani, A.; Hurel, S.J.; Donos, N.; et al. Mitochondrial oxidative stress, endothelial function and metabolic control in patients with type II diabetes and periodontitis: A randomised controlled clinical trial. *Int. J. Cardiol.* **2018**, *271*, 263–268. [CrossRef] [PubMed]
15. Moeintaghavi, A.; Arab, H.R.; Bozorgnia, Y.; Kianoush, K.; Alizadeh, M. Non-surgical periodontal therapy affects metabolic control in diabetics: A randomized controlled clinical trial. *Aust. Dent. J.* **2012**, *57*, 31–37. [CrossRef]
16. Sun, W.L.; Chen, L.L.; Zhang, S.Z.; Wu, Y.M.; Ren, Y.Z.; Qin, G.M. Inflammatory cytokines, adiponectin, insulin resistance and metabolic control after periodontal intervention in patients with type 2 diabetes and chronic periodontitis. *Intern. Med. (Tokyo, Japan)* **2011**, *50*, 1569–1574. [CrossRef]
17. Higgins, J.P.; Green, S. *Cochrane Handbook for Systematic Reviews of Interventions*; John Wiley & Sons: Hoboken, NJ, USA, 2008.
18. Sbordone, L.; Ramaglia, L.; Gulletta, E.; Iacono, V. Recolonization of the subgingival microflora after scaling and root planing in human periodontitis. *J. Periodontol.* **1990**, *61*, 579–584. [CrossRef]
19. Pejcic, A.; Kesic, L.; Brkic, Z.; Pesic, Z.; Mirkovic, D. Effect of periodontal treatment on lipoproteins levels in plasma in patients with periodontitis. *South. Med. J.* **2011**, *104*, 547–552. [CrossRef]

20. Oz, S.G.; Fentoglu, O.; Kilicarslan, A.; Guven, G.S.; Tanriover, M.D.; Aykac, Y.; Sozen, T. Beneficial effects of periodontal treatment on metabolic control of hypercholesterolemia. *South. Med. J.* **2007**, *100*, 686–692. [CrossRef]
21. Feingold, K.R.; Staprans, I.; Memon, R.; Moser, A.; Shigenaga, J.; Doerrler, W.; Dinarello, C.; Grunfeld, C. Endotoxin rapidly induces changes in lipid metabolism that produce hypertriglyceridemia: low doses stimulate hepatic triglyceride production while high doses inhibit clearance. *J. Lipid Res.* **1992**, *33*, 1765–1776.
22. Fentoglu, O.; Bozkurt, F.Y. The bi-directional relationship between periodontal disease and hyperlipidemia. *Eur. J. Dent.* **2008**, *2*, 142.
23. Cutler, C.W.; Eke, P.; Arnold, R.R.; Van Dyke, T.E. Defective neutrophil function in an insulin-dependent diabetes mellitus patient. A case report. *J. Periodontol.* **1991**, *62*, 394–401. [CrossRef]
24. Stratton, I.M.; Adler, A.I.; Neil, H.A.W.; Matthews, D.R.; Manley, S.E.; Cull, C.A.; Hadden, D.; Turner, R.C.; Holman, R.R. Association of glycaemia with macrovascular and microvascular complications of type 2 diabetes (UKPDS 35): Prospective observational study. *BMJ* **2000**, *321*, 405–412. [CrossRef]
25. Borgnakke, W.S. Does treatment of periodontal disease influence systemic disease? *Dent. Clin.* **2015**, *59*, 885–917. [CrossRef]
26. Teeuw, W.J.; Gerdes, V.E.; Loos, B.G. Effect of periodontal treatment on glycemic control of diabetic patients: A systematic review and meta-analysis. *Diabetes Care* **2010**, *33*, 421–427. [CrossRef]
27. Iwamoto, Y.; Nishimura, F.; Nakagawa, M.; Sugimoto, H.; Shikata, K.; Makino, H.; Fukuda, T.; Tsuji, T.; Iwamoto, M.; Murayama, Y. The effect of antimicrobial periodontal treatment on circulating tumor necrosis factor-alpha and glycated hemoglobin level in patients with type 2 diabetes. *J. Periodontol.* **2001**, *72*, 774–778. [CrossRef]
28. Thompson, P.D.; Panza, G.; Zaleski, A.; Taylor, B. Statin-associated side effects. *J. Am. Coll. Cardiol.* **2016**, *67*, 2395–2410. [CrossRef]
29. Feingold, K.R.; Grunfeld, C. Cholesterol Lowering Drugs. *MDText* **2000**.

9

New Functions of Classical Compounds against Orofacial Inflammatory Lesions

Norifumi H. Moritani [1], Emilio Satoshi Hara [2] and Satoshi Kubota [3,*]

1 Department of Oral and Maxillofacial Reconstructive Surgery, Okayama University Graduate School of Medicine, Dentistry and Pharmaceutical Sciences, Okayama 700-8558, Japan; hachi70@md.okayama-u.ac.jp
2 Department of Biomaterials, Okayama University Graduate School of Medicine, Dentistry and Pharmaceutical Sciences, Okayama 700-8558, Japan; gmd421209@s.okayama-u.ac.jp
3 Department of Biochemistry and Molecular Dentistry, Okayama University Graduate School of Medicine, Dentistry and Pharmaceutical Sciences, Okayama 700-8558, Japan
* Correspondence: kubota1@md.okayama-u.ac.jp

Abstract: Anti-inflammatory agents have been widely used to ameliorate severe inflammatory symptoms of a number of diseases, and such therapeutics are particularly useful for diseases with intolerable pain without significant mortality. A typical example of this is a disease known as stomatitis; although stomatitis itself is not a life-threatening disease, it severely impairs the individual's quality of life, and thus a standard therapeutic strategy for it has already been established. The topical application of a bioactive agent is quite easy, and a strong anti-inflammatory agent can be used without significant adverse effects. In contrast, natural products with relatively mild bioactivity are used for systemic intervention. However, new aspects of classical drugs used in these established therapeutic methods have recently been discovered, which is expanding the utility of these compounds to other oral diseases such as osteoarthritis of temporomandibular joints (TMJ-OA). In this review article, after summarizing the general concept and pathobiology of stomatitis, its established therapeutics are explained. Thereafter, recent advances in the research into related compounds, which is uncovering new biological functions of the agents used therein, are introduced. Indeed, regenerative therapeutics for TMJ-OA may be developed with the classical compounds currently being used.

Keywords: stomatitis; recurrent aphthous stomatitis; oral lichen planus; CCN2; glucocorticoids; alkaloids

---

1. Introduction

The oral cavity is a biological apparatus that enables the intake of food, drink, and air, thus enabling the intake of the most basic elements needed to support the development, growth, and maintenance of human bodies. Therefore, inflammatory lesions in the oral area are always deleterious to human health, impairing all of the biological activities of the cells constituting an individual. The most common inflammatory diseases in the oral region are those in, or around the teeth. Endodontic inflammation is where there is designated pulpitis, the acute form of which usually yields intolerable pain. However, owing to its poor regeneration potential, recovery of the affected pulp tissue can hardly be expected [1]. As such, a major intervention used to terminate pulpitis is a pulpectomy, which is the removal of the dental pulp under local anesthesia without anti-inflammatory treatment. In contrast, periodontitis is usually chronic and occasionally even asymptomatic. Needless to say, inflammatory responses of the host are critically involved in the etiology of periodontitis [2,3]. However, since periodontitis is based on the infection of a number of oral bacteria, the principal therapeutic methods against periodontitis have been the regulation of bacterial infection. For a better clinical outcome, the utilization of desiccants has recently been proposed [4], and acceleration of periodontal tissue regeneration by laser treatment has also been attempted [5,6]. In addition, the osseous drilling protocol has been regarded as critical for dental implants, rather than inflammation control [7]; therefore, anti-inflammatory molecules are not major agents in the treatment of these dental diseases.

Food intake can be more severely affected by stomatitis as any contact with the affected oral mucosa will cause great pain to the affected individual. Additionally, since it depends on mastication that is performed by the collaborative movement of temporomandibular joints (TMJ), osteoarthritis (OA) of the TMJ strongly restricts its quality and quantity. As will be mentioned in the next section, stomatitis is characterized by prominent inflammatory responses that have no apparent relationship with bacterial infection [8,9]. Notably, in contrast to the dental pulp, the regeneration potential of oral mucosa is quite high; as such, anti-inflammatory compounds have been widely used for the treatment of stomatitis to promptly redeem the individual's food intake ability. In this article, starting from the review of stomatitis and related disorders, established therapeutics using classical compounds are summarized. Then, we report on the recent research topics that unveiled the possible utilities of a few such classical compounds in the treatment of the OA of TMJ for which no fundamental therapeutics have yet to be established. In particular, CCN family protein 2 (CCN2), a profibrotic protein involved in inflammation and tissue regeneration [10], has been found to mediate the novel biological effects therein. As such, we believe that the consideration of CCN2-mediated effects is critical in developing new therapeutic methods against inflammation.

2. Stomatitis and Oral Mucosal Diseases

Stomatitis is a term commonly used to describe the inflammation of oral mucosa. The names of several stomatitis-related conditions are listed in Table 1. Among them, the most commonly recognized type of stomatitis is aphthous stomatitis. Aphthous stomatitis is where there are painful ulcers that are clearly defined as shallow, round, or oval, with a necrotic center covered by yellowish-tan pseudomembranes, and surrounded by an erythematous halo. An example of aphthous stomatitis is shown in Figure 1. The term "aphtha" refers to the clinical condition and is not the name of the disease; the appropriate disease name is recurrent aphthous stomatitis (RAS). As above-mentioned, stomatitis is a generic name for the inflammation of oral mucosa, and is also known as oral mucosal disease.

Table 1. Stomatitis-related conditions.

Disease Names
aphthous stomatitis
recurrent aphthous stomatitis (RAS) (synonym: recurrent aphthous ulcer)
herpetic stomatitis
catarrhal stomatitis
drug-induced stomatitis
radiation-induced stomatitis
gangrenous stomatitis
nicotinic stomatitis
angular stomatitis (synonym: angular cheilitis)
denture-related stomatitis

Oral mucosal diseases have numerous conditions such as those listed in Table 1. However, as we cannot present all such diseases, we have at least tried to classify oral mucosal diseases by their clinical manifestations, as shown in Table 2. Furthermore, the classification of the diseases listed in Table 2, according to etiology, is shown in Table 3. The oral mucosal diseases listed in Tables 1–3 pose a number of treatment challenges to clinicians such as: (1) few treatment opportunities being presented at clinics; (2) the cause being largely unknown; (3) symptomatic treatment is the mainstay of treatment, and not causal therapy, where a radical cure is difficult to achieve; and (4) that an efficacious therapy has not yet been established. It is probably recognized that the above-mentioned representative diseases are RAS and oral lichen planus (OLP).

Table 2. Oral mucosal disease; classification by clinical manifestations.

Major Symptoms	Diseases
bulla/vesicle	herpetic stomatitis, herpes zoster, pemphigus, pemphigoid, epidermolysis bullosa hereditaria
erythema, erosion	erythroplakia, drug-induced stomatitis, radiation-induced stomatitis, angular stomatitis, oral candidiasis, OLP
ulcer	RAS, Behçet's disease, gangrenous stomatitis, denture-related stomatitis
white spot/patch	leukoplakia, OLP, nicotinic stomatitis
pigmentation	Peutz–Jeghers syndrome, melanin pigmentation
atrophic disease	glossitis with anemia (e.g., Hunter's glossitis)

RAS, recurrent aphthous stomatitis; OLP, oral lichen planus.

Table 3. Oral mucosal disease; classification by etiology.

Etiology	Diseases
Congenital or developmental anomalies	epidermolysis bullosa hereditaria, Peutz–Jeghers syndrome
Physical or chemical cause	drug-induced stomatitis, radiation-induced stomatitis, nicotinic stomatitis, denture-related stomatitis
Bacterial infection	angular stomatitis, gangrenous stomatitis
Mycotic infection	oral candidiasis, angular stomatitis
Viral infection	herpetic stomatitis, herpes zoster
Allergic disease	drug-induced stomatitis, Quincke's edema
Autoimmune disease	pemphigus, pemphigoid
Precancerous lesion	erythroplakia, leukoplakia
Unidentified or complex cause	RAS, Behçet's disease, OLP

RAS, recurrent aphthous stomatitis; OLP, oral lichen planus.

2.1. *Recurrent Aphthous Stomatitis (RAS)*

RAS is also known as recurrent aphtha or recurrent aphthous ulcers. RAS occurs as single or multiple recurrences of aphtha occurring irregularly in the oral mucosa (Figure 1). The etiology of RAS is scientifically unclear, but we here show the conditions that are regarded as the etiology of RAS (Table 4). Since the etiology is unknown, its diagnosis is entirely based on history and clinical criteria, and no laboratory procedures exist to confirm the diagnosis.

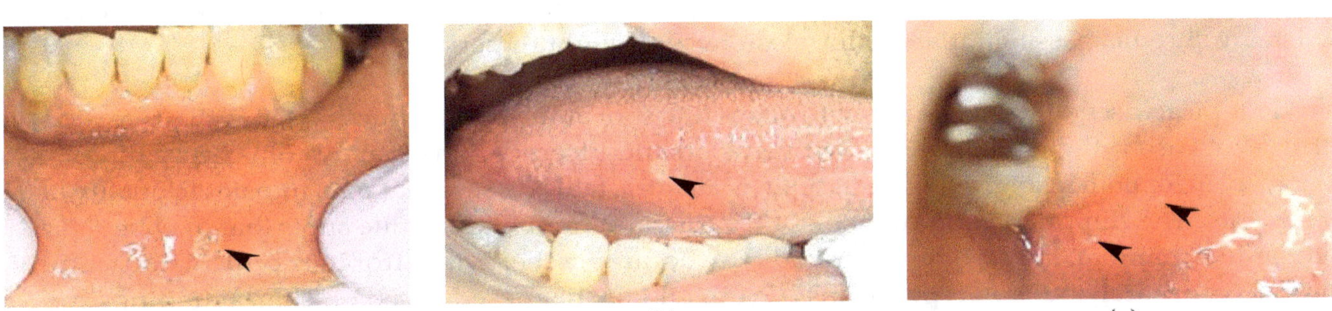

(a) (b) (c)

Figure 1. Aphthous stomatitis that occurs in a patient with recurrent aphthous stomatitis (RAS). Images are of the same patient and were taken on the same day. (**a**) Lower labial mucosa. (**b**) Right margin of the tongue. (**c**) Right hard palate mucosa (black arrowheads).

Table 4. Proposed etiology of RAS.

Heredity/Genetic Factor
Local trauma such as sharp food and tooth-brushing
Adverse effect of drugs
Deficiency such as iron, zinc, vitamin B12, and folate
Smoking
Virus
Bacteria
Allergy
Hormonal change
Stress
Inflammatory digestive system disease
Immunological abnormality
Cardinal symptom of Behçet's disease
Food hypersensitivity

Generally, the RAS ulcer is resolved spontaneously after a few days or up to 10 days, so the ulcer can be left untreated. However, the RAS ulcer may lead to difficulty in speaking, eating, and swallowing and, thus, may negatively affect the patient's quality of life. As a result, topical therapies for the treatment of ulcers such as steroid ointment or mouthwash are often used. These therapies are directed at palliating symptoms and promoting the rapid healing of the RAS ulcer. However, there is no curative therapy to prevent the recurrence of ulcers, and all available treatment modalities only reduce the frequency or severity of the lesions. Although many causative factors have been proposed, the pathogenesis of RAS is still unknown, and a fundamental treatment for the disease has not been established. RAS is a cardinal symptom of Behçet's disease, which is a systemic inflammatory disorder and is associated with a four-symptom complex of the oral mucosa, genitalia, eyes, and skin [8,9]. RAS occurs in Behçet's disease in all cases and in the whole oral mucosa. Therefore, in the medical examination of patients with RAS, Behçet's disease should be suspected, and a diagnosis to rule it out is necessary.

Behçet's disease has been proposed to be caused by allergy, virus, and autoimmune-related mechanisms, but the exact etiology is still unknown. As for treatment, systemic therapies such as corticosteroid, immunosuppressant, anti-inflammatory, and anti-fibrinolysis medicines are used [11].

2.2. *Oral Lichen Planus (OLP)*

Oral lichen planus (OLP) is a relatively common diagnosis of oral lesions and has a prevalence of approximately 2% among oral mucosal diseases. OLP presents as reticular or plaque-like white lesions, which are chronic, passing inflammatory lesions with slight hyperkeratosis.

In typical cases, OLP occurs as a reticular white spot at the buccal mucosa (Figure 2). Occasionally, OLP occurs as erythematous lesions with erosion and ulcers. As these symptoms cause discomfort, contact pain, or both in affected subjects, OLP is an intractable disease that may impair the quality of life of patients. The clinical manifestation of OLP varies and presents as white spots that may be reticular, plaque-like, papular, linear, or circular and may occur together with atrophic erythematous, erosive, ulcerative, or rarely bullous-type lesions [12,13]. OLP is diagnosed based on clinical findings such as the previously mentioned pathognomonic gross appearance and the histopathological examination of lesional tissues by biopsy. Pathognomonic histopathological findings are shown in Figure 3. Predisposing factors are not clear yet, but some implicated etiological triggers or aggravating factors of OLP are shown in Table 5 [14–16].

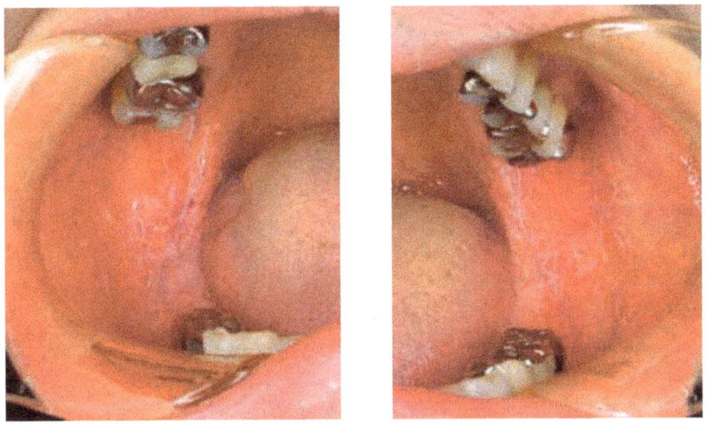

Figure 2. Oral lichen planus (OLP) in a patient, which occurred on both sides of the buccal mucosa with a white and papuloreticular lesion.

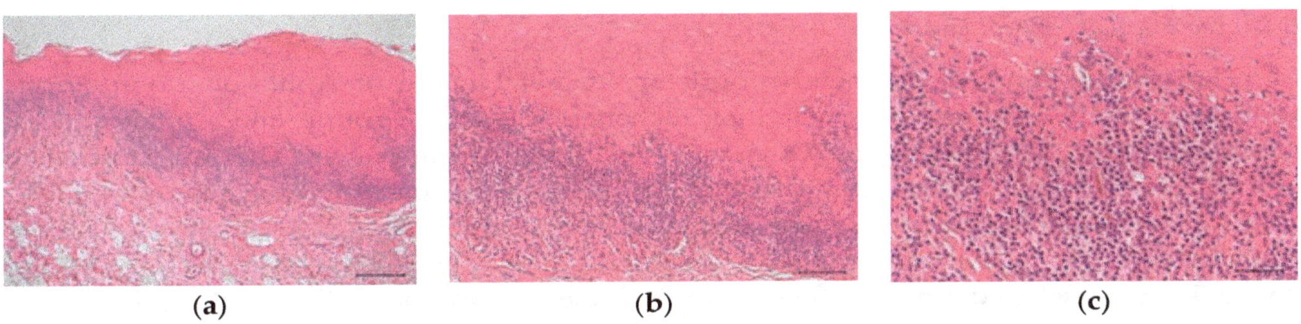

Figure 3. Hematoxylin and eosin (H&E) staining of an OLP tissue section. (**a**) Low power photomicrograph. Hyperkeratosis is presented on the surface of the epithelium and a band-like infiltrate of lymphocytes immediately subjacent to the epithelium. Scale bar: 100 μm. (**b**) Medium power photomicrograph. The rete ridge has a saw-toothed shape. Scale bar: 50 μm. (**c**) High power photomicrograph. Migration of lymphocytes into the lower epithelium is observed with liquefaction degeneration of the basal layer. The epithelial spinous cell layer directly contacts the infiltrating lymphocytes. Scale bar: 25 μm.

Table 5. Proposed etiology of OLP.

Adverse Drug Reaction
Intraoral dental metal and filler
Intraoral cosmetics including preservatives, aromatic substances
Overwork and stress
Smoking
Hepatitis (hepatitis C in particular)
Oral candidiasis
Herpetic infection
Immunological abnormality

3. Topical or Systemic Therapeutic Agents for RAS and OLP

As the same therapeutic agents are used for RAS and OLP, we mainly describe the medications used in this review (Figure 4). We consider that understanding the mechanism of action of the therapeutic agents for RAS and OLP might contribute to elucidating their etiology.

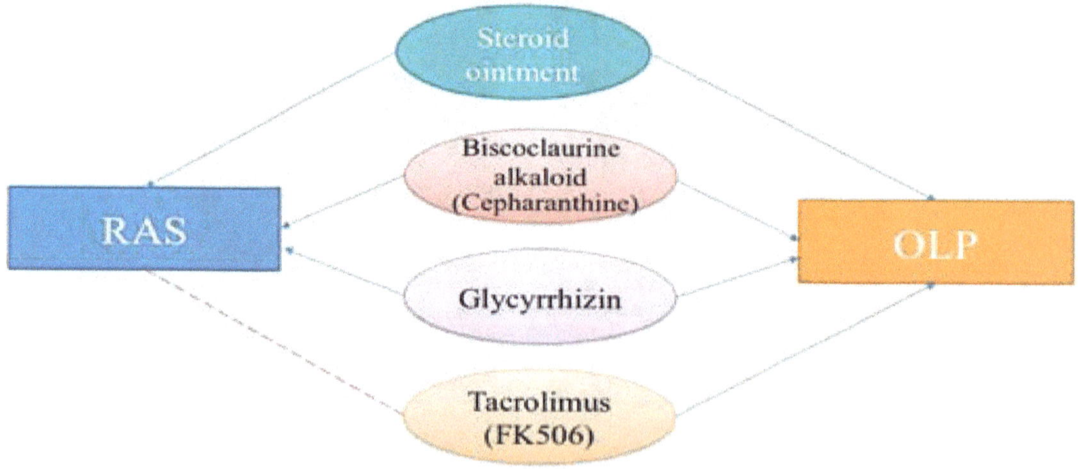

Figure 4. Therapeutic topical and systemic agents for recurrent aphthous stomatitis (RAS) and oral lichen planus (OLP). Blue lines with arrowheads: effective. Red dashed lines: probably effective.

3.1. *Glucocorticoids (Topical Use)*

In Japan, Dexaltin oral ointment (proprietary name) 1 mg/g or Aphtasolon oral ointment (proprietary name) 0.1% are the major topical therapies used. Dexaltin and Aphtasolon 1.0 g both contain 1.0 mg dexamethasone (Dex), which is the active component. Dex is a corticosteroid glucocorticoid (GCs) and GCs are the most commonly used anti-inflammatory and immunosuppressive drugs. Topical GCs were introduced into medicine approximately 50 years ago. Corticosteroid strength is classified according to their effects in the vasoconstrictor assay and Dex showed the lowest potency in the ranking of a selected group of topical corticosteroid preparations [17]. Therefore, the incidence of associated adverse effects of topical applied steroid is low, and Dex-containing steroid ointments are often used as first choice medications for oral mucosal disease. The molecular mechanisms of the action of steroids include: (1) direct combination of the steroid–steroid receptor complex and DNA sequences called the steroid-responsive element; (2) interactions between the steroid–steroid receptor complex and other transcriptional factors, and (3) non-genomic pathways. The immunosuppressive activity results from the inhibition of neutrophil tissue infiltration, macrophages, eosinophils, and basophils. The anti-inflammatory activity results from both a decrease in the production of inflammatory cytokines and an increase in the production of anti-inflammatory cytokines [18,19]. After entry into the target cells, GCs bind to the GC receptor (GR), which then translocates into the nucleus to directly or indirectly regulate gene transcription. The ligand-activated GR binds as a homodimer to consensus sequences, termed as GC response elements, in the promoter region of GC-sensitive genes to induce the transcription (transactivation) of genes such as tyrosine aminotransferase (*TAT*). An indirect negative regulation of gene expression (transrepression) is achieved by GR-protein interaction. The ligand-activated receptor binds as a monomer to transcription factors such as nuclear factor (NF)-κb and activator protein-1 (AP-1) to inhibit the activity of many proinflammatory transcription factors. This transrepression is considered the key mechanism behind the anti-inflammatory activity of GCs.

3.1.1. RAS

It is generally recognized that topical agents such as steroid ointments are the first treatment choice for RAS. Corticosteroids used in patients with RAS are intended to restrict the inflammatory process associated with the formation of aphthous stomatitis. Corticosteroids may act directly on T lymphocytes in the local environment and alter the response of effector cells to participants of immunopathogenic events. Neutrophils are also found in the surrounding tissue of the RAS ulcers at a marked concentration. The production of oxygen radicals by these neutrophils in RAS has been found to be similar to that in the controls [20].

3.1.2. OLP

The topical use of steroids has been the standard treatment for OLP. In local legion sites of the OLP, oral steroid ointments suppress inflammatory changes and inhibit immune reactions. Therefore, oral steroid ointments are often used as first choice medications for OLP. However, the long-term, repeated application of steroid ointments may be associated with side effects such as candidiasis mainly, which requires attention [21].

3.2. *Biscoclaurine Alkaloid (BA) and Cepharanthine (CEP)*

Cepharanthine is an alkaloid extracted from the plant *Stephania cepharantha* Hayata, which is naturally found in the woods of southern Formosa, which is now in Taiwan. CEP is a member of a class of compounds known as biscoclaurine alkaloids (BAs). Alkaloids have long attracted the attention of pharmacologists and clinicians owing to their resemblance to polypeptides and their physiological action. It has been widely used in Japan to treat a number of acute and chronic diseases. CEP inhibits tumor necrosis factor (TNF)-α-mediated NF-κB stimulation, plasma membrane lipid peroxidation, and platelet aggregation, and suppresses cytokine production. CEP is recognized to exhibit reactive oxygen species (ROS)-scavenging properties and a protective effect against some of the responses mediated by pro-inflammatory cytokines including TNF-α, interleukin (IL)-1β, and IL-6 [22,23]. In addition, it has been reported that CEP has anti-allergic actions, stabilizes the biological membrane, augments the action of cortical hormones, and improves the peripheral circulation. In Japan, indications for CEP include radiation-induced leukopenia, alopecia areata, and alopecia pityrodes (Cepharanthine package insert, 2018). CEP has not demonstrated significant safety issues, and its side effects have been very rarely reported [22]. In addition, it is available for long-term treatment, and the treatment effect is persistent. Therefore, CEP is often used for OLP.

3.2.1. RAS

RAS has been reported to apparently be related to the excessive generation of ROS including O_2^- [24]. It has been reported that when CEP 3 g (30 mg per day as alkaloid extracted from the plant *S. cepharantha*) was administered daily in three divided doses after each meal for seven cases of RAS patients, the results showed a percent improvement of 71.4% and a response rate of 85.7% [25].

3.2.2. OLP

It has been reported that the administration of BA effectively reduced the generation of O_2^-, one of the most potent reactive oxygen intermediates, and diminished the clinical symptoms of OLP [26]. When CEP was administered to patients with OLP, a significant suppression of O_2^- generation by peripheral blood neutrophils was found as symptoms were improved (such as ulcers, redness, and contact pain of the oral mucosa). Therefore, O_2^- excess generation of the OLP lesion was inhibited by the administration of CEP, and those symptoms were thought to be relieved. Moreover, it has been reported that the rate of plasma inflammatory cytokine production (such as TNF-α, IL-1β, IL-6, and granulocyte-colony stimulating factor (G-CSF)) was unchanged by CEP administration [24,27].

In addition, previous studies have reported improved microcirculation induced by the vasodilatory effect of CEP [28]. Furthermore, in previous studies, CEP 3 g (30 mg/day as the alkaloid extracted from the plant *S. cepharantha*) was administered daily in three divided doses after each meal to 12 patients with OLP [25]. The results indicated a percentage improvement and response rate of 75.0% for each [25]. These reports suggest that the suppression of O_2^- generation by peripheral blood neutrophils may be closely related to the improvement of symptoms of RAS and OLP.

3.3. Glycyrrhizin (GL)

In Japan, glycyrrhizin (GL) is an established treatment for improving liver function in patients with viral hepatitis [29]. GL, which is a triterpenoid saponin isolated from the root of licorice (*Glycyrrhiza glabra*), is a compound consisting of a single glycyrrhetic acid (GA) molecule linked with two glucuronic acid molecules. GL exhibits multiple biological and pharmacological activities such as anti-inflammatory, anti-allergic, and antiviral [e.g., against herpes simplex virus (HSV), Varicella zoster, influenza, hepatitis C virus (HCV), and human immunodeficiency virus (HIV)] effects [30,31]. The mechanism of action of GL is not completely understood. However, a number of recent studies have indicated a number of distinct GL-binding functional proteins (GBFPs) as essential mediators, which are involved in the GL-induced anti-inflammatory effect. These proteins include arachidonate cascade-related enzymes [secretory phospholipase A_2 ($sPLA_2$), 5-lipoxygenase (5-Lox), and cyclooxygenase-2 (Cox-2), inducible nitric oxide synthase (iNOS), and the high mobility group box-1 protein (HMGB1)] [32]. One tablet of glycyron contains 25 mg glycyrrhizic acid as the main ingredient. In Japan, indication for GL includes stomatitis, the improvement of liver function abnormality in chronic hepatitis, eczema, dermatitis, alopecia areata, and strophulus infantum (Glycyron, package insert, 2018).

3.3.1. RAS

Apparently, no previous study has reported the effect of GL on RAS. According to the Glycyron package insert (2018), when glycyron tablets are orally administered at a dose of nine tablets daily for 12 consecutive weeks, it is more than effective at 82.3%. Licorice, the name given to the roots and stolons of Glycyrrhiza species, has been used since ancient times as a traditional herbal remedy [33]. Some reports on the effect of licorice for controlling pain and reducing the healing time of aphthous ulcerations have been published [34–36]. However, these studies suggest that additional research is required to arrive at conclusions on the potential benefits of licorice in RAS [33]. Therefore, it is suggested that GL has a certain effect on RAS because of an effect that occurs in stomatitis (oral mucosal disease).

3.3.2. OLP

Hasizume reported that when glycyron tablets were orally administered at a dose of six tablets daily for almost three consecutive months for OLP affecting the bilateral buccal mucosa with alcoholic chronic hepatitis, the symptoms were remitted [37]. In addition, Glycyrrhizin (GL) was used to treat chronic liver dysfunction in nine patients with OLP who were positive for HCV antibody and HCV RNA. GL was administered intravenously at a dose of 40 mL (0.2% solution) daily for four consecutive weeks, and the results showed that 66.7% of patients with OLP improved clinically [38].

3.4. Tacrolimus (FK506: Topical Use)

Tacrolimus, also called FK506, is a macrolide immunosuppressant produced by *Streptomyces tsukubaensis*, which has similar effects to those of cyclosporin A. It acts by inhibiting calcineurin, a ubiquitous calcium-dependent protein phosphatase that is responsible for immune responses [39]. Tacrolimus was formulated as an ointment for atopic dermatitis that is used commonly and seems effective as a second choice for treating OLP, which is refractory to other standard treatments [40]. Since the relationship between tacrolimus and cancer development has been reported in only a few cases, clinicians must be careful in selecting tacrolimus as a second-line treatment for OLP [41]. In RAS and OLP, immunopathy is regarded as one of the onset triggers. Therefore, if tacrolimus is effective for OLP, it is also expected that there is enough efficacy for RAS. However, tacrolimus is thought to have limited applicability for aphthous treatment as steroidal external preparations have a lower-risk than tacrolimus external preparations.

3.5. *Desiccants (Topical Use)*

Although not used in Japan, desiccants have been used for the treatment of RAS in the US and other countries. A typical desiccant cocktail contains sulfonic acid and other highly reactive agents, which destroys the attached cells [4]. Destruction of nerve endings results in the prompt relief of pain, which is followed by the regeneration of the destroyed tissue. Thus, the mechanism of action of desiccants can be regarded as the chemical removal of lesions, which is not related to the etiology of RAS. Nowadays, the utility of a desiccant in the treatment of periodontitis is being recognized [4].

4. Role of CCN Family 2 (CCN2) in Inflammation

Steroid hormone derivatives counteract inflammatory responses by inhibiting the action of proinflammatory transcription factors. In addition to this action, these molecules are known to activate the transcription of the *CCN2*, which encodes protein that is critical in wound healing. Therefore, while repressing the inflammatory response, glucocorticoids also promote the last stage of inflammation to reconstruct the damaged tissues.

The protein, CCN2 is a classical member of the CCN family, consisting of six members in mammals. CCN stands for the first letters of the initial names of its three founding members: cysteine-rich 61 (Cyr61/CCN1), connective tissue growth factor (CTGF/CCN2), and nephroblastoma-overexpressed (NOV/CCN3). CCN2 is composed of an insulin-like growth factor binding protein-like (I), von Willebrand factor type C repeat (V), thrompospondin 1 type 1 repeat (T), and C-terminal cystine-knot (C) modules. Multiple interactions via these modules with a variety of biomolecules in the microenvironment yield pleiotropic and context-dependent biological outcomes, which usually induce harmonized tissue development and regeneration [42–44]. Indeed, CCN2 is expressed at particular stages during the development of a variety of tissues and organs. After development and growth, CCN2 is transiently induced upon tissue injury and repair, and the tissue regeneration potential of CCN2 is also indicated [45,46]. CCN2 appears to play a pivotal role to proceed with inflammatory stages.

As illustrated in Figure 5a, *CCN2* expression is differentially regulated by inflammatory mediators. Tumor necrosis factor-α (TNF-α) and nitric oxide repress *CCN2* expression in a variety of cells, whereas histamine contrarily induces it [10]. Moreover, CCN2 itself may enhance the gene expression of inflammatory cytokines in several types of cells. It is indicated that a processed CT module fragment of CCN2 is responsible for its inflammatory actions [47]. Such an apparently complex regulatory network around CCN2 during inflammation suggests that *CCN2* is precisely regulated in order to appear upon the initiation of the last stage of inflammation. Once the CCN2 protein is produced, this molecule starts reconstructing the damaged tissues under the direct interaction with other growth factors and their receptors. As a result, the production of matrix metalloproteinases (MMPs) as well as the extracellular matrix (ECM) components, is enhanced, which are then utilized for tissue reconstruction, as summarized in Figure 5b. Of note, MMP-3 was found to go back into the nuclei of producers to further enhance *CCN2* expression in chondrocytes, representing the collaborative action of CCN2 and MMP-3 [48,49].

After tissue repair, *CCN2* expression should be turned off immediately in order to avoid continuous tissue remodeling and excessive ECM production leading to fibrosis, a typical outcome of chronic inflammation [50–53]. Indeed, *CCN2* overexpression is commonly observed in fibrotic disorders in a variety of organs. Therefore, turning CCN2 production on and off are key for terminating acute and chronic inflammation, respectively. If we could turn on and off the CCN2 production by medication, we would thus be able to successfully control the inflammation and regeneration of affected tissues in a harmonized manner.

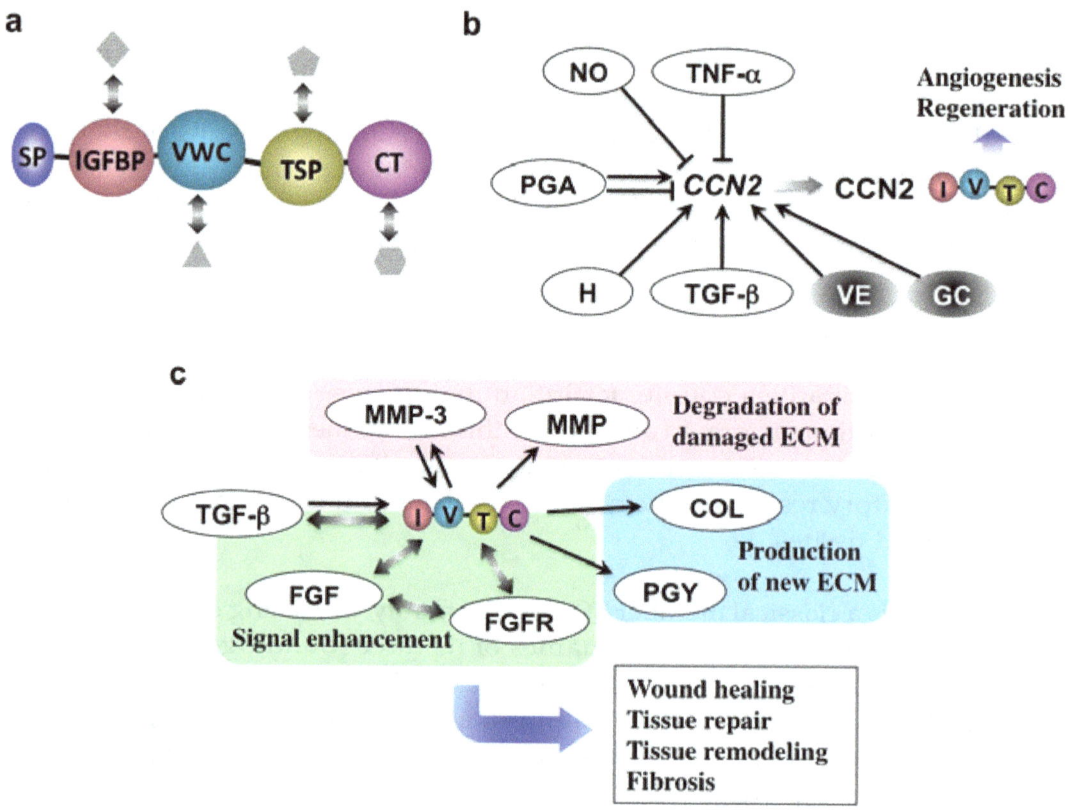

Figure 5. (**a**) Molecular structure of CCN2. Following the signal peptide for secretion (SP), insulin-like growth factor binding protein-like (IGFBP), von Willebrand factor type C repeat (VWC), thrombospondin type I repeat (TSP), and C-terminal cystine knot (CT) modules are connected in tandem. Interaction with multiple co-factors (objects in grey) that support the function of CCN2 is also illustrated. (**b**) CCN2 inducers and repressors. TNF-α, tumor necrosis factor alpha; NO, nitric oxide; PGA, prostaglandin; H, histamine; TGF-β, transforming growth factor beta; VE, vitamin E; GC, glucocorticoid. (**c**) Molecular action of CCN2. MMP, MMPs other than MMP-3; COL, collagen; PGY, proteoglycan; ECM, extracellular matrix; FGFR, fibroblast growth factor receptor; FGF, fibroblast growth factor. Arrows and T-bars indicate induction and repression, respectively. Bidirectional arrows denote direct molecular interactions.

5. Novel Utility of Particular Glucocorticoid and Alkaloid in Orofacial Disorders

5.1. Fluocinolone Acetonide

Due to their enhanced medical utility, most of the ointments used for stomatitis contain synthetic GCs with fluoride introduction at the position of C9 in the steroid nucleus (Figure 6). Dex is the most popular active ingredient, whereas triamcinolone acetonide (TA) is also employed. Another related compound, fluocinolone acetonide (FA) is commonly used in the field of dermatology in the form of an oil or paste, and its effectiveness and safety are also indicated in the treatment of stomatitis [54]. For a long time, the pharmacological effects of these synthetic glucocorticoids were believed to be basically the same. However, surprisingly, screening of the Food and Drug Administration (FDA) of the United States-approved small molecules rediscovered FA as a special molecule with novel biological potential to regenerate cartilage.

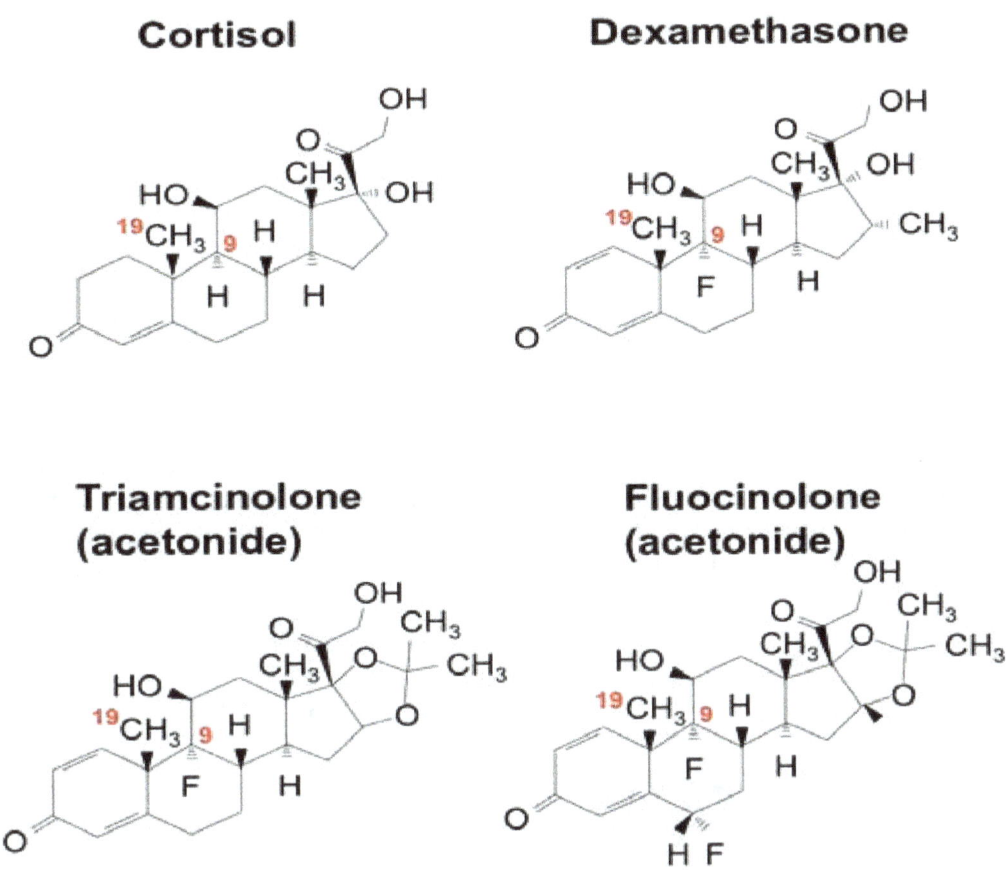

Figure 6. Chemical structures of glucocorticoids. The positions of C9 and C19 are indicated in red.

FA dramatically enhanced the chondrogenesis from mesenchymal stem cells in vitro when it was combined with transforming growth factor (TGF)-β3. Furthermore, analysis in vivo revealed the ability of FA to regenerate damaged articular cartilage in collaboration with TGF-β3 [55]. TGF-β3, as a member of the TGF-β superfamily, is known to enhance extracellular matrix deposition mainly through the canonical signaling pathway mediated by secondary messengers termed Smads. The observed effect of FA was shown to be mediated by the mammalian target of the rapamycin (mTOR)-AKT signaling pathway as well as by the interaction with the Smad pathway and GR activation. This collaboration is highly member-specific, since FA combined with BMP-2, another member of TGF-β superfamily, did not show such an effect. Similarly, articular cartilage regeneration in vivo was not effectively exerted by the combination of TGF-β3 and either TA or Dex. A structural comparison between these three compounds suggests a structural–functional relationship between corticosteroids and the extra functionality to regenerate cartilage in collaboration with TGF-β3 (Figure 7a) [55]. Obviously, the fluoride modification at C16 adds a structural property to enable the unusual collaboration of FA with TGF-β. It should also be noted that FA is able to strongly induce *CCN2* expression in ATDC5 chondrogenic cells, which may result in the modification of TGF-β signaling via direct molecular interaction between these molecules (Figure 7b). Since CCN2 itself regenerates articular cartilage, involvement of this protein in the outcome of FA-TGF-β3 collaboration is strongly suspected (Figure 8).

In the field of orofacial medicine, TMJ dysfunction based on osteoarthritis is one of the major complications that affects proper mastication. However, there are currently no therapeutics for regenerating damaged TMJ cartilage that has been established. However, FA has already been widely approved and is being used in clinics, meaning that its clinical application for recovering damaged TMJ cartilage is now expected, although particular care should be taken to avoid possible side effects as a glucocorticoid.

a

		Dex	TA	FA
Structure	C16 modification	CH_3	OH	OH
	C9 modification	-	-	F
Chondrocytic phenotype in vitro		-	↑	↑↑
Chondrogenesis in vitro		-	-	↑↑
Regeneration in vivo		-	-	↑

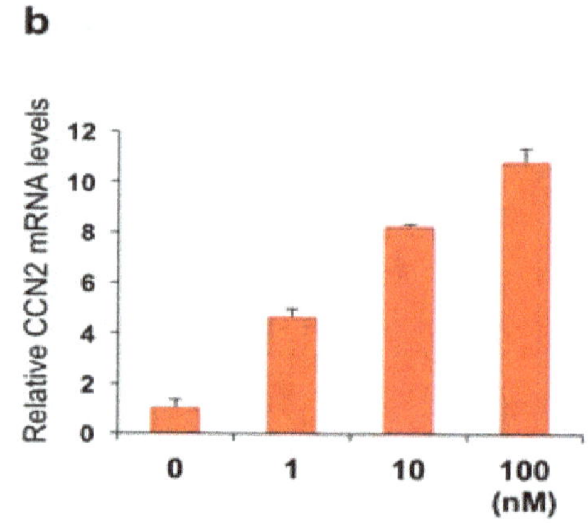

Figure 7. (**a**) Structural–functional relationship of three glucocorticoids. TA, triamcinolone acetonide; FA, fluocinolone acetonide. (**b**) Induction of CCN2 in ATDC5 chondrogenic cells by FA. ATDC5 cells in monolayer culture were treated with different concentrations (1–100 nM: horizontal axis) of FA for 24 h, and analyzed for expression levels of CCN2 mRNA.

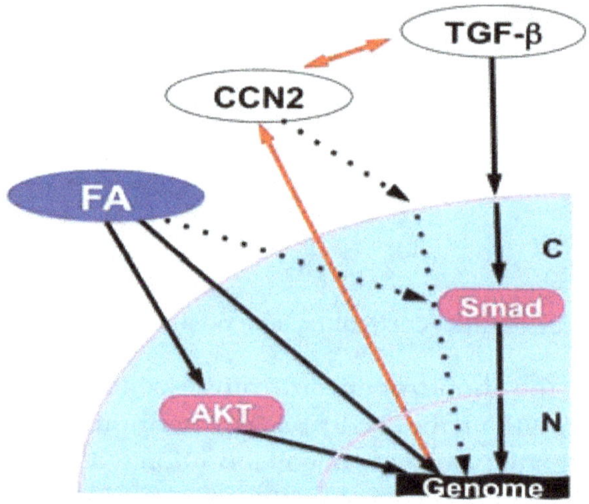

Figure 8. Possible cartilage regeneration mechanism by FA in collaboration with TGF-β. N, Nucleus; C, cytoplasm; FA, fluocinolone acetonide.

5.2. *Harmine*

As a related attempt to study small molecules that enhance cartilage regeneration, Hara et al. also screened an orphan ligand library based on the ability to induce CCN2 expression. Among the 84 compounds screened, harmine, one of the β-carboline alkaloids, was found to be a potent inducer of CCN2 in the human chondrocytic cell line (Figure 9a). Harmine is a natural product that can be extracted from a plant named *Peganum harmala*, which has been used in folk medicine in a number of countries for thousands of years [56]. Later scientific studies showed an anti-depressant effect of this alkaloid via inhibiting monoamine oxidase activity and its vasorelaxant-like effect by blocking voltage-gated calcium channels. One should take these functions into account upon its clinical application to avoid possible adverse effects. The family of β-carboline alkaloids is composed of several members; however, harmine was confirmed to be the only one that could exert this novel effect to induce CCN2 expression (Figure 9b). Further investigation confirmed harmine's ability to enhance chondrogenesis with the elevated gene expression of chondrocytic marker genes, as well as that of CCN2, in culture. Interestingly, enhanced production of SOX-9, which is a master transcription factor of chondrogenesis, was found to be stronger than that of CCN2. Therefore, harmine enhances chondrogenesis by inducing both CCN2 and SOX-9, which subsequently promotes the production of cartilaginous ECM components [57].

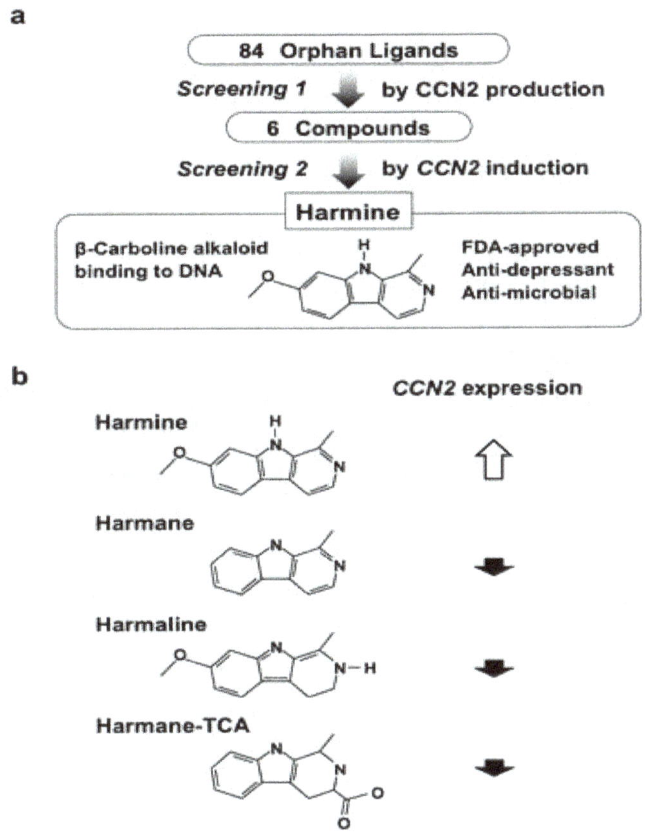

Figure 9. (**a**) Screening procedure employed for the re-discovery of harmine; (**b**) chemical structures and CCN2 inducing the activity of β-carboline alkaloids.

In addition to this novel discovery, the anti-inflammatory effect of this compound was surprisingly also indicated in the same study. Indeed, harmine was shown to protect chondrocytes from the catabolic effects conferred by an inflammatory cytokine, TNF-α (Figure 10) [57]. Therefore, therapeutic use of this compound in OA, including that of TMJ, could well be considered. Also, such a molecular function of this particular alkaloid, counteracting inflammatory response and enhancing regenerative activity, is reminiscent of that of glucocorticoids. Thus, harmine may be an effective agent for the treatment of stomatitis as well, which ought to be examined in future studies.

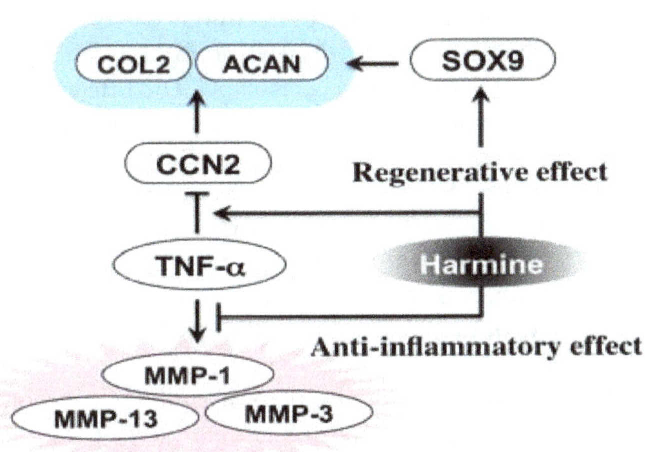

Figure 10. Molecular activity of harmine counteracting the inflammatory degradation of cartilage. COL2, type II collagen; ACAN, aggrecan; MMP, matrix metalloproteinase.

6. Conclusive Remarks

Inflammation in the oral region representative of stomatitis is not typically fatal but is highly painful, and thus strongly impairs an individual's quality of life. Therefore, symptomatic, rather than fundamental treatment has been the major therapeutic strategy for these kinds of diseases. As such, glucocorticoids and alkaloids have commonly been employed to ameliorate local and systemic inflammatory responses for a long time, without significant advances in therapeutics and etiological research. However, recent research on these classical compounds is unveiling their utility in the regenerative therapy of damaged connective tissue, including intractable cartilage defects. These research outcomes also emphasize the close and delicate relationship between inflammation and tissue regeneration, in which CCN2 may be pivotally involved. Further investigation of other classical anti-inflammatory compounds may uncover unexpected molecular functions in those molecules as well, and the research outcome may be of help in exploring novel comprehensive therapeutics to terminate excessive inflammation and promote harmonized tissue regeneration in oral inflammatory lesions.

Author Contributions: N.H.M. and S.K. wrote the paper; E.S.H. contributed the data and proofread the manuscript.

References

1. Hayama, T.; Kamio, N.; Okabe, T.; Muromachi, K.; Matsushima, K. Kallikrein Promotes Inflammation in Human Dental Pulp Cells via Protease-Activated Receptor-1. *J. Cell. Biochem.* **2016**, *117*, 1522–1528. [CrossRef] [PubMed]
2. Takashiba, S.; Naruishi, K.; Murayama, Y. Perspective of cytokine regulation for periodontal treatment: Fibroblast biology. *J. Periodontol.* **2003**, *74*, 103–110. [CrossRef] [PubMed]
3. Yamamoto, T.; Ugawa, Y.; Kawamura, M.; Yamashiro, K.; Kochi, S.; Ideguchi, H.; Takashiba, S. Modulation of microenvironment for controlling the fate of periodontal ligament cells: The role of Rho/ROCK signaling and cytoskeletal dynamics. *J. Cell Commun. Signal.* **2018**, *12*, 369–378. [CrossRef] [PubMed]
4. Isola, G.; Matarese, G.; Williams, R.C.; Siciliano, V.I.; Alibrandi, A.; Cordasco, G.; Ramaglia, L. The effects of a desiccant agent in the treatment of chronic periodontitis: A randomized, controlled clinical trial. *Clin. Oral Investig.* **2018**, *22*, 791–800. [CrossRef] [PubMed]
5. Isola, G.; Matarese, G.; Lo Giudice, G.; Briguglio, F.; Alibrandi, A.; Crupi, A.; Cordasco, G.; Ramaglia, L. A New Approach for the Treatment of Lateral Periodontal Cysts with an 810-nm Diode Laser. *Int. J. Periodontics Restor. Dent.* **2017**, *37*, e120–e129. [CrossRef] [PubMed]
6. Matarese, G.; Ramaglia, L.; Cicciù, M.; Cordasco, G.; Isola, G. The Effects of diode laser therapy as an adjunct to scaling and root planing in the treatment of aggressive periodontitis: A 1-Year randomized controlled clinical trial. *Photomed. Laser Surg.* **2017**, *35*, 702–709. [CrossRef] [PubMed]
7. Marheineke, N.; Scherer, U.; Rücker, M.; von See, C.; Rahlf, B.; Gellrich, N.C.; Stoetzer, M. Evaluation of accuracy in implant site preparation performed in single- or multi-step drilling procedures. *Clin. Oral Investig.* **2018**, *22*, 2057–2067. [CrossRef] [PubMed]
8. Natah, S.S.; Konttinen, Y.T.; Enattah, N.S.; Ashammakhi, N.; Sharkey, K.A.; Hayrinen-Immonen, R. Recurrent aphthous ulcers today: A review of the growing knowledge. *Int. J. Oral Maxillofac. Surg.* **2004**, *33*, 221–234. [CrossRef] [PubMed]
9. Femiano, F.; Lanza, A.; Buonaiuto, C.; Gombos, F.; Nunziata, M.; Piccolo, S.; Cirillo, N. Guidelines for diagnosis and management of aphthous stomatitis. *Pediatr. Infect. Dis. J.* **2007**, *26*, 728–732. [CrossRef] [PubMed]
10. Kular, L.; Pakradouni, J.; Kitabgi, P.; Laurent, M.; Martinerie, C. The CCN family: A new class of inflammation modulators? *Biochimie* **2011**, *93*, 377–388. [CrossRef] [PubMed]

11. Mat, M.C.; Sevim, A.; Fresko, I.; Tuzun, Y. Behcet's disease as a systemic disease. *Clin. Dermatol.* **2014**, *32*, 435–442. [CrossRef] [PubMed]
12. Kovac-Kovacic, M.; Skaleric, U. The prevalence of oral mucosal lesions in a population in Ljubljana, Slovenia. *J. Oral Pathol. Med.* **2000**, *29*, 331–335. [CrossRef] [PubMed]
13. Pentenero, M.; Broccoletti, R.; Carbone, M.; Conrotto, D.; Gandolfo, S. The prevalence of oral mucosal lesions in adults from the Turin area. *Oral Dis.* **2008**, *14*, 356–366. [CrossRef] [PubMed]
14. Ismail, S.B.; Kumar, S.K.; Zain, R.B. Oral lichen planus and lichenoid reactions: Etiopathogenesis, diagnosis, management and malignant transformation. *J. Oral Sci.* **2007**, *49*, 89–106. [CrossRef] [PubMed]
15. Gupta, S.; Jawanda, M.K. Oral Lichen Planus: An Update on Etiology, Pathogenesis, Clinical Presentation, Diagnosis and Management. *Indian J. Dermatol.* **2015**, *60*, 222–229. [CrossRef] [PubMed]
16. Alrashdan, M.S.; Cirillo, N.; McCullough, M. Oral lichen planus: A literature review and update. *Arch. Dermatol. Res.* **2016**, *308*, 539–551. [CrossRef] [PubMed]
17. Schäcke, H.; Schottelius, A.; Döcke, W.D.; Strehlke, P.; Jaroch, S.; Schmees, N.; Rehwinkel, H.; Hennekes, H.; Asadullah, K. Dissociation of transactivation from transrepression by a selective glucocorticoid receptor agonist leads to separation of therapeutic effects from side effects. *Proc. Natl. Acad. Sci. USA* **2004**, *101*, 227–232. [CrossRef] [PubMed]
18. Lowenberg, M.; Stahn, C.; Hommes, D.W.; Buttgereit, F. Novel insights into mechanisms of glucocorticoid action and the development of new glucocorticoid receptor ligands. *Steroids* **2008**, *73*, 1025–1029. [CrossRef] [PubMed]
19. Stahn, C.; Lowenberg, M.; Hommes, D.W.; Buttgereit, F. Molecular mechanisms of glucocorticoid action and selective glucocorticoid receptor agonists. *Mol. Cell. Endocrinol.* **2007**, *275*, 71–78. [CrossRef] [PubMed]
20. Ueta, E.; Umazume, M.; Yamamoto, T.; Osaki, T. Leukocyte dysfunction in oral mucous membrane diseases. *J. Oral Pathol. Med.* **1993**, *22*, 120–125. [CrossRef] [PubMed]
21. Thongprasom, K.; Dhanuthai, K. Steriods in the treatment of lichen planus: A review. *J. Oral Sci.* **2008**, *50*, 377–385. [CrossRef] [PubMed]
22. Rogosnitzky, M.; Danks, R. Therapeutic potential of the biscoclaurine alkaloid, cepharanthine, for a range of clinical conditions. *Pharmacol. Rep.* **2011**, *63*, 337–347. [CrossRef]
23. Akamatsu, H.; Komura, J.; Asada, Y.; Niwa, Y. Effects of cepharanthin on neutrophil chemotaxis, phagocytosis, and reactive oxygen species generation. *J. Dermatol.* **1991**, *18*, 643–648. [CrossRef] [PubMed]
24. Harada, T.; Kingetsu, A.; Nariai, Y.; Yoshimura, H. Effects of biscoclaurine alkaloids on clinical symptoms and superoxide anion generation from peripheral blood neutrophils in patients with oral lichen planus. *Asian J. Oral Maxillofac. Surg.* **2001**, *13*, 117–124.
25. Shinnoki, S.; Morita, N.; Sumiyoshi, M.; Kawashima, N.; Wada, T.; Miyata, K.; Sakamoto, T. Effect of Cepharanthin on intractable oral mucosal disease (oral lichen planus, recurrent aphthous stomatitis). *Dent. Outlook* **1992**, *80*, 1223–1234.
26. Harada, T.; Mishima, K.; Obara, S.; Yoshimura, Y. Effects of radiation therapy on superoxide anion generation from peripheral blood neutrophils in oromaxillary cancer patients: A preliminary report of radiation-induced oral mucositis. *Asian J. Oral Maxillofac. Surg.* **1996**, *8*, 9–14.
27. Harada, T.; Nariai, Y.; Yoshimura, Y. Effects of biscoclaurine alkaloids (Cepharanthin) on patients with oral lichen planus. Study on superoxide anion generation from peripheral blood neutrophils and plasma cytokine levels in patients. *Oral. Ther. Pharm.* **2004**, *23*, 46–53.
28. Asano, M.; Ohkubo, C.; Sasaki, A.; Sawanobori, K.; Nagano, H. Vasodilator effects of cepharanthine, a biscoclaurine alkaloid, on cutaneous microcirculation in the rabbit. *J. Ethnopharmacol.* **1987**, *20*, 107–120. [PubMed]
29. Abe, N.; Ebina, T.; Ishida, N. Interferon induction by glycyrrhizin and glycyrrhetinic acid in mice. *Microbiol. Immunol.* **1982**, *26*, 535–539. [CrossRef] [PubMed]
30. Pompei, R.; Laconi, S.; Ingianni, A. Antiviral properties of glycyrrhizic acid and its semisynthetic derivatives. *Mini Rev. Med. Chem.* **2009**, *9*, 996–1001. [CrossRef] [PubMed]
31. Patrick, L. Hepatitis C: Epidemiology and review of complementary/alternative medicine treatments. *Altern. Med. Rev.* **1999**, *4*, 220–238. [PubMed]
32. Ohtsuki, K. The anti-inflammatory molecular mechanism of glycyrrhizin. *Minophagen Med. Rev.* **2010**, *55*, 95–118.

33. Messier, C.; Epifano, F.; Genovese, S.; Grenier, D. Licorice and its potential beneficial effects in common oro-dental diseases. *Oral Dis.* **2012**, *18*, 32–39. [CrossRef] [PubMed]
34. Moghadamnia, A.A.; Motallebnejad, M.; Khanian, M. The efficacy of the bioadhesive patches containing licorice extract in the management of recurrent aphthous stomatitis. *Phytother. Res.* **2009**, *23*, 246–250. [CrossRef] [PubMed]
35. Martin, M.D.; Sherman, J.; van der Ven, P.; Burgess, J. A controlled trial of a dissolving oral patch concerning glycyrrhiza (licorice) herbal extract for the treatment of aphthous ulcers. *Gen. Dent.* **2008**, *56*, 206–210. [PubMed]
36. Das, S.K.; Das, V.; Gulati, A.K.; Singh, V.P. Deglycyrrhizinated liquorice in aphthous ulcers. *J. Assoc. Phys. India* **1989**, *37*, 647.
37. Hashizume, K. A case of the oral lichen planus with alcoholic chronic hepatitis patients improved by glycyron tablets. *Minophagen Med. Rev.* **2007**, *52*, 352–354.
38. Nagao, Y.; Sata, M.; Suzuki, H.; Tanikawa, K.; Itoh, K.; Kameyama, T. Effectiveness of glycyrrhizin for oral lichen planus in patients with chronic HCV infection. *J. Gastroenterol.* **1996**, *31*, 691–695. [CrossRef] [PubMed]
39. Graef, I.A.; Mermelstein, P.G.; Stankunas, K.; Neilson, J.R.; Deisseroth, K.; Tsien, R.W.; Crabtree, G.R. L-type calcium channels and GSK-3 regulate the activity of NF-ATc4 in hippocampal neurons. *Nature* **1999**, *401*, 703–708. [CrossRef] [PubMed]
40. Shichinohe, R.; Shibaki, A.; Nishie, W.; Tateishi, Y.; Shimizu, H. Successful treatment of severe recalcitrant erosive oral lichen planus with topical tacrolimus. *J. Eur. Acad. Dermatol. Venereol.* **2006**, *20*, 66–68. [CrossRef] [PubMed]
41. Morita, M.; Asoda, S.; Tsunoda, K.; Soma, T.; Nakagawa, T.; Shirakawa, M.; Shoji, H.; Yagishita, H.; Nishikawa, T.; Kawana, H. The onset risk of carcinoma in patients continuing tacrolimus topical treatment for oral lichen planus: A case report. *Odontology* **2017**, *105*, 262–266. [CrossRef] [PubMed]
42. Jun, J.I.; Lau, L.F. Taking aim at the extracellular matrix: CCN proteins as emerging therapeutic targets. *Nat. Rev. Drug Discov.* **2011**, *10*, 945–963. [CrossRef] [PubMed]
43. Kubota, S.; Takigawa, M. The CCN family acting throughout the body: Recent research developments. *Biomol. Concepts* **2013**, *4*, 477–494. [CrossRef] [PubMed]
44. Perbal, B. The concept of the CCN protein family revisited: A centralized coordination network. *J. Cell Commun. Signal.* **2018**, *12*, 3–12. [CrossRef] [PubMed]
45. Kubota, S.; Takigawa, M. The role of CCN2 in cartilage and bone development. *J. Cell Commun. Signal.* **2011**, *5*, 209–217. [CrossRef] [PubMed]
46. Abd El Kader, T.; Kubota, S.; Nishida, T.; Hattori, T.; Aoyama, E.; Janune, D.; Hara, E.S.; Ono, M.; Tabata, Y.; Kuboki, T.; et al. The regenerative effects of CCN2 independent modules on chondrocytes in vitro and osteoarthritis models in vivo. *Bone* **2014**, *59*, 180–188. [CrossRef] [PubMed]
47. Rodrigues-Díez, R.; Rodrigues-Díez, R.R.; Rayego-Mateos, S.; Suarez-Alvarez, B.; Lavoz, C.; Stark Aroeira, L.; Sánchez-López, E.; Orejudo, M.; Alique, M.; Lopez-Larrea, C.; et al. The C-terminal module IV of connective tissue growth factor is a novel immune modulator of the Th17 response. *Lab. Investig.* **2013**, *93*, 812–824. [CrossRef] [PubMed]
48. Eguchi, T.; Kubota, S.; Kawata, K.; Mukudai, Y.; Uehara, J.; Ohgawara, T.; Ibaragi, S.; Sasaki, A.; Kuboki, T.; Takigawa, M. Novel transcription-factor-like function of human matrix metalloproteinase 3 regulating the CTGF/CCN2 gene. *Mol. Cell. Biol.* **2008**, *28*, 2391–2413. [CrossRef] [PubMed]
49. Muromachi, K.; Kamio, N.; Narita, T.; Annen-Kamio, M.; Sugiya, H.; Matsushima, K. MMP-3 provokes CTGF/CCN2 production independently of protease activity and dependently on dynamin-related endocytosis, which contributes to human dental pulp cell migration. *J. Cell. Biochem.* **2012**, *113*, 1348–1358. [CrossRef] [PubMed]
50. Leask, A. CCN2: A bona fide target for anti-fibrotic drug intervention. *J. Cell Commun. Signal.* **2011**, *5*, 131–133. [CrossRef] [PubMed]
51. Abd El Kader, T.; Kubota, S.; Janune, D.; Nishida, T.; Hattori, T.; Aoyama, E.; Perbal, B.; Kuboki, T.; Takigawa, M. Anti-fibrotic effect of CCN3 accompanied by altered gene expression profile of the CCN family. *J. Cell Commun. Signal.* **2013**, *7*, 11–18. [CrossRef] [PubMed]
52. Kubota, S.; Takigawa, M. Cellular and molecular actions of CCN2/CTGF and its role under physiological and pathological conditions. *Clin. Sci.* **2015**, *128*, 181–196. [CrossRef] [PubMed]

53. Toda, N.; Mori, K.; Kasahara, M.; Koga, K.; Ishii, A.; Mori, K.P.; Osaki, K.; Mukoyama, M.; Yanagita, M.; Yokoi, H. Deletion of connective tissue growth factor ameliorates peritoneal fibrosis by inhibiting angiogenesis and inflammation. *Nephrol. Dial. Transplant.* **2018**, *33*, 943–953. [CrossRef] [PubMed]
54. Buajeeb, W.; Pobrurksa, C.; Kraivaphan, P. Efficacy of fluocinolone acetonide gel in the treatment of oral lichen planus. *Oral Surg. Oral Med. Oral Pathol. Oral Radiol. Endodontol.* **2000**, *89*, 42–45. [CrossRef]
55. Hara, E.S.; Ono, M.; Pham, H.T.; Sonoyama, W.; Kubota, S.; Takigawa, M.; Matsumoto, T.; Young, M.F.; Olsen, B.R.; Kuboki, T. Fluocinolone Acetonide Is a Potent Synergistic Factor of TGF-β3-Associated Chondrogenesis of Bone Marrow-Derived Mesenchymal Stem Cells for Articular Surface Regeneration. *J. Bone Miner. Res.* **2015**, *30*, 1585–1596. [CrossRef] [PubMed]
56. Moloudizargari, M.; Mikaili, P.; Aghajanshakeri, S.; Asghari, M.H.; Shayegh, J. Pharmacological and therapeutic effects of *Peganum harmala* and its main alkaloids. *Pharmacogn. Rev.* **2013**, *7*, 199–212. [CrossRef] [PubMed]
57. Hara, E.S.; Ono, M.; Kubota, S.; Sonoyama, W.; Oida, Y.; Hattori, T.; Nishida, T.; Furumatsu, T.; Ozaki, T.; Takigawa, M.; et al. Novel chondrogenic and chondroprotective effects of the natural compound harmine. *Biochimie* **2013**, *95*, 374–381. [CrossRef] [PubMed]

10

QSAR Prediction Model to Search for Compounds with Selective Cytotoxicity Against Oral Cell Cancer

Junko Nagai [1], Mai Imamura [1], Hiroshi Sakagami [2] and Yoshihiro Uesawa [1,*]

1 Department of Medical Molecular Informatics, Meiji Pharmaceutical University, 2-522-1 Noshio, Kiyose, Tokyo 204-8588, Japan; nagai-j@my-pharm.ac.jp (J.N.); y151038@std.my-pharm.ac.jp (M.I.)
2 Meikai University Research Institute of Odontology (M-RIO), 1-1 Keyakidai, Sakado, Saitama 350-0283, Japan; sakagami@dent.meikai.ac.jp
* Correspondence: uesawa@my-pharm.ac.jp

Abstract: Background: Anticancer drugs often have strong toxicity against tumours and normal cells. Some natural products demonstrate high tumour specificity. We have previously reported the cytotoxic activity and tumour specificity of various chemical compounds. In this study, we constructed a database of previously reported compound data and predictive models to screen a new anticancer drug. **Methods**: We collected compound data from our previous studies and built a database for analysis. Using this database, we constructed models that could predict cytotoxicity and tumour specificity using random forest method. The prediction performance was evaluated using an external validation set. **Results**: A total of 494 compounds were collected, and these activities and chemical structure data were merged as database for analysis. The structure-toxicity relationship prediction model showed higher prediction accuracy than the tumour selectivity prediction model. Descriptors with high contribution differed for tumour and normal cells. **Conclusions**: Further study is required to construct a tumour selective toxicity prediction model with higher predictive accuracy. Such a model is expected to contribute to the screening of candidate compounds for new anticancer drugs.

Keywords: quantitative structure-activity relationship; machine learning; random forest; natural products; tumour-specificity

---

1. Introduction

Various anticancer drugs are used to treat oral cancer; however, most of these drugs also affect normal cells. Damage to normal cell induces several adverse effects, one of these is oral mucositis (OM). OM of patients who receiving cancer therapy makes difficult to eat and to deprive volition of treatment. OM is an inflammation induced by various factors such as trauma, viruses and bacterial infections, genetic factors, stress, vitamin deficiency, and chemotherapy [1,2]. The mechanism of detail is still not well known; however, toxicity to normal cells is one of the causes. In addition, many anticancer drugs are toxic to normal cells and have low selectivity for tumour cells. For these reasons, anticancer drugs which have low toxicity on normal cells are urgently needed.

Compounds which are highly tumour-specific exist in natural products. Previously, we reported cytotoxic activity against human oral squamous cell carcinoma (OSCC) cell lines and human oral normal cells using a variety of natural and synthesized organic compounds with chromone and azulene, which are present in various natural products, as the mother nucleus [3]. We have recently reported that many anticancer drugs induce keratinocyte toxicity by inducing apoptosis [4]. However, very few reports have been published [5] about the exploration of new synthetic substances that show low keratinocyte toxicity except of our studies (Table 1).

Table 1. Urgency of manufacturing new anticancer drugs with low keratinocyte toxicity (data obtained from SciFinder® [5] on 5 February 2019)

Search Terms	Number of Total Reports (A)	Number of Our Reports (B)	% (B/A) × 100
OSCC	8951 (100)	141	1.6
OSCC + Anticancer Drug	335 (3.70)	60	17.9
OSCC + Anticancer Drug + Tumour-Specificity	50 (0.56)	40	80.0
OSCC + Anticancer Drug + Tumour-Specificity + Newly Synthesized	2 (0.02)	2	100.0
OSCC + Anticancer Drug + Keratinocyte Toxicity	5 (0.06)	4	80.0
OSCC + anticancer drug + QSAR	27 (0.30)	25	92.6
OSCC + Anticancer Drug + QSAR+ Newly Synthesized	3 (0.03)	3	100.0

Based on the notion that similar structures have similar activity, the relationship between chemical structure and activity is referred to as the structure-activity relationship (SAR). Currently, using information about chemical structure which called "descriptor" that is structural, physicochemical and quantum chemical variety of characteristics, data were calculated and used for relation analysis. Conventionally, multiple regression analysis, which is a standard statistical approach, has been employed to analyse the relationship between the characteristic amount and activity of such drugs. Recently, machine-learning methods have been applied to such analyses due to their high prediction performance, and the quantitative structure activity relationship (QSAR) model is used to screen lead compounds in drug discovery research [6–8].

We have also studied the properties of compounds relative to cytotoxicity activity using QSAR analysis of compound and cytotoxic activity reported in the literature [3]. However, we could not employ high performance analysis methods due to the limited number of compounds evaluated in each study.

Thus, in this study, we gathered compound data from our previous reports and developed a database with a sufficient number of compounds to facilitate the use of a more advanced prediction method than single regression analysis. We attempted to construct a prediction model to search for compounds with high cytotoxic activity and tumour specificity score, using the collected data of cytotoxic activity of various compounds against tumour and normal cells.

To construct the prediction model, random forest (RF; one of the machine learning method) [9,10], was adopted, expecting the collection of sufficient numbers of compounds for QSAR analysis.

2. Materials and Methods

2.1. Data Collection and Preparation

We collected our original articles published up to May 2018 (with the exception of literature reviews), and compound and cytotoxicity data were extracted from the collected articles. All OSCC and normal human oral cells were incubated at 2 × 103/96-microwell and incubated for 48 h to produce near confluent cells (approximately half of the plate covered by cells) so that cells can further grow. Cells were then treated with various conditions of samples for 48 h. Controls contains the same concentration of DMSO, and subtracted from the experimental values to correct for DMSO cytotoxicity. Relative viable cell numbers were determined by MTT method. The conditions of cytotoxic assays were the same for all experiments we have done in our previous publications [11–49].

Cytotoxicity data were used as a ratio of mean 50% cytotoxic concentration (CC_{50}) against OSCC cell lines (HSC-2, HSC-3, and HSC-4) and human oral normal cells (human gingival fibroblast, HGF;

human pulp cells, HPC; human periodontal ligament fibroblast, and HPLF), and these CC_{50} were converted to $-\log CC_{50}$ (pCC_{50}), which is a negative common logarithm.

The tumour cell selective toxic index (selectivity index; SI) was defined as the ratio of the mean CC_{50} of OSCC cell lines to the mean CC_{50} of the human oral normal cells, and the SI was calculated for all individual compounds.

2.2. Chemical Structure Data Acquisition and Descriptor Calculation

The collected compounds were drawn using MarvinSketch 18.10.0 (ChemAxon, Budapest, Hungary) [50] and then converted to SMILES that is a form of a line notation based on graph theory, to obtain numerical data from the chemical structure.

The compound data were dealt with using the integrated computational chemistry system Molecular Operating Environment (MOE) version 2018.0101 (Chemical Computing Group Inc., Quebec, Canada) [51] as follows; salts were removed, structure optimization was calculated, and load partial charges were obtained. The structural data were converted to a 3D format by MOE using "Rebuild 3D" and structural optimization was realized by force field calculation (amber-10: EHT).

From this compound data, we calculated 2D and 3D descriptors using MOE and Dragon (version 7.0.2, Kode srl., Pisa, Italy) [52], respectively. Descriptors were treated independently by the software. Standard deviations were calculated with each descriptor; in cases where the value was zero, the descriptor was excluded. These descriptor data calculated by MOE and Dragon were merged for each compound.

2.3. Preparation of Data Table

The cytotoxic activity and descriptor data were merged to a data table for analysis. The compounds in this data table were checked for duplication by using SMILES. Compounds that had one SMILES to several cytotoxic activity data from different articles adopted the mean pCC_{50}.

2.4. Construction of Prediction Models by RF

The data table was randomly split (2:1 ratio) into a training set and an external validation set [53].

Eight structure-toxicity relationship prediction models were constructed by RF using the training set. The response variables of eight prediction models were three pCC_{50} against each OSCC cell line, three pCC_{50} against each human oral normal cell, the mean pCC_{50} against OSCC cell lines (mean tumour cell), and the mean pCC_{50} against human oral normal cells (i.e., the mean normal cell).

In the same manner, a tumour cell selective toxicity prediction model in which the response variable was the SI was constructed by using RF. Construction of prediction models by RF was performed "Bootstrap Forest" [54] in statistical software JMP® Pro. 13.1.0 (SAS Institute Inc., Cary, NC, USA) [55].

To construct the prediction model, changing parameter settings and largest coefficient of determination prediction model that was selected. Figure 1 shows the procedures from Sections 2.1–2.4.

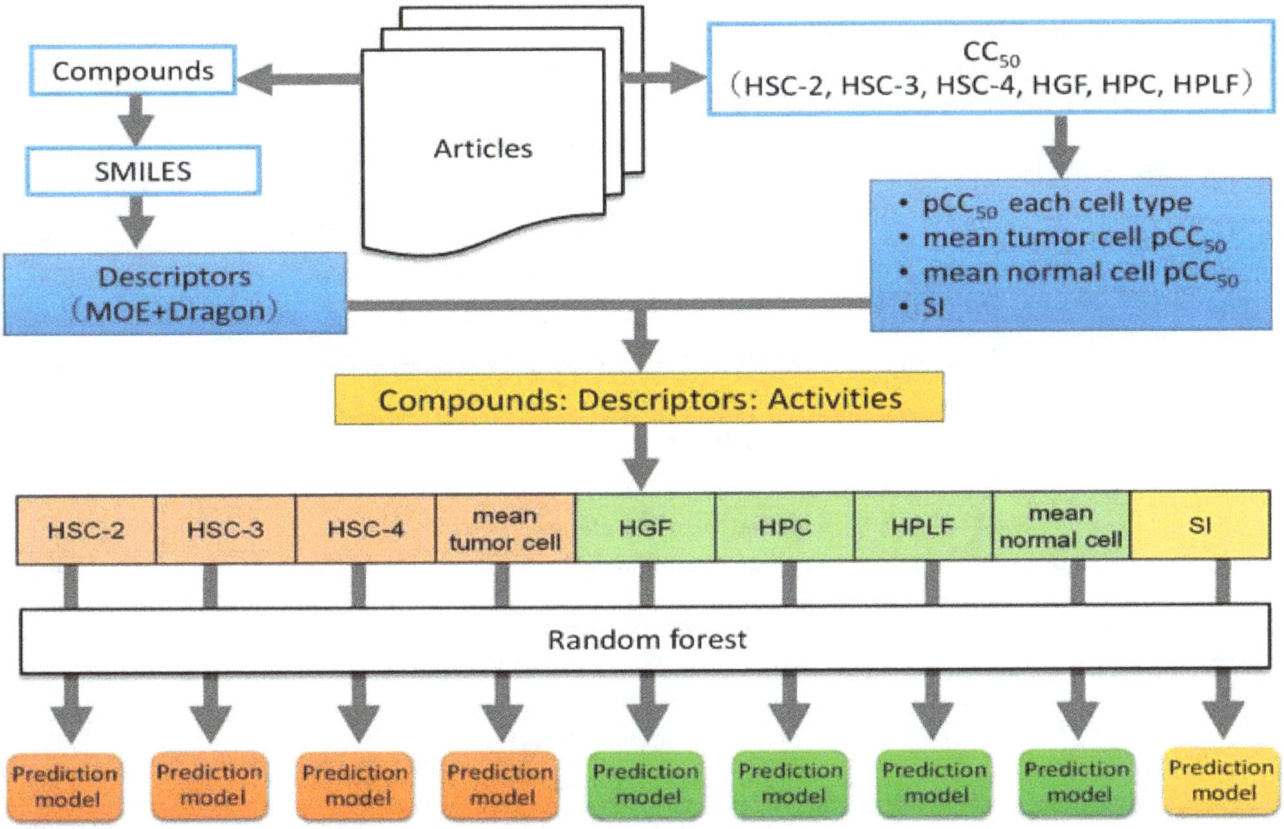

Figure 1. Schematic diagram of data collection and analysis.

3. Results

3.1. Data Collection

We obtained 498 compounds from 39 articles [11–49]. After eliminating duplicate compounds by SMILES, 494 compounds were analysed. Table 2 shows the articles and number of extracted compounds. These 494 compounds belong to the compound groups developed from various natural products, having skeletons shown in Table 2. SMILES data of these compounds are provided in Supplementary Materials (Table S1).

Table 2. Number of compounds and basic skeleton extracted from articles.

No.	Number of Compounds	Basic Skeleton	Ref.
1	9	Isoflavones and Isoflavanones	[9]
2	3	Three β-Diketones	[10]
3	6	Styrylchromones	[11]
4	3	Nocobactins NA-a, NA-b and Their Ferric Complexes	[12]
5	5	Betulinic Acid and Its Derivatives	[13]
6	2	Berberines	[14]
7	20	Coumarin and Its Derivatives	[15]
8	1	Mitomycin C, Bleomycin and Peplomycin	[16]
9	13	4-Trifluoromethylimidazole Derivatives	[17]
10	15	Phenoxazine Derivatives	[18]

Table 2. *Cont.*

No.	Number of Compounds	Basic Skeleton	Ref.
11	7	Vitamin K_2 Derivatives	[19]
12	2	4-Trifluoromethylimidazoles	[20]
13	10	Phenoxazines	[21]
14	18	Vitamin K_2 Derivatives and Prenylalcohols	[22]
15	10	3-Formylchromone Derivatives	[23]
16	12	5-Trifluoromethyloxazole Derivatives	[24]
17	19	1,2,3,4-Tetrahydroisoquinoline Derivatives	[25]
18	19	1,2,3,4Tetrahydroisoquinoline Derivatives	[26]
19	12	Dihydroimidazoles	[27]
20	24	Tropolones	[28]
21	24	Trihaloacetylazulenes	[29]
22	22	Trihaloacetylazulene Derivatives	[30]
23	10	Licorice Flavonoids	[31]
24	4	1,2,3,4-Tetrahydroisoquinoline Derivatives	[32]
25	19	2-Aminotropones	[33]
26	12	Phenylpropanoid Amides	[34]
27	12	Piperic Acid Amides	[35]
28	15	3-Styrylchromones	[36]
29	16	3-Styryl-2*H*-chromenes	[37]
30	18	Oleoylamides	[38]
31	17	3-Benzylidenechromanones	[39]
32	18	Licorice Root Extracts	[40]
33	15	Chalcones	[41]
34	11	Piperic Acid Esters	[42]
35	17	Aurones	[43]
36	24	2-Azolylchromones	[44]
37	10	Cinnamic Acid Phenetyl Esters	[45]
38	10	Azulene Amide Derivatives	[46]
39	10	Alkylaminoguaiazulenes	[47]

Descriptors were calculated from each software MOE and Dragon, subsequently excluded in case of the value is constant. After cleaning, 3750 descriptors were remained and used for analyses (319 descriptors calculated by MOE and 3431 descriptors calculated by Dragon).

Figure 2a shows applicability domain (AD). AD is the range of molecular properties or structures for which the model is considered to be applicable [56]. This scatter plot shows the result of principal component analysis using descriptors. The horizontal axis is the first principal component, and the vertical axis is the second principal component. Training set and test set compounds distribute as well balanced.

Moreover, to indicate detailed properties of these compounds, scatter plot of molecular weight (MW) and octanol-water partitioning coefficient (logP) is shown in Figure 2b. These compounds showed characteristic distribution of MW from 114.2 to 1125.8 (median 297.9); and logP from −1.53 to 13.9 (median 3.46).

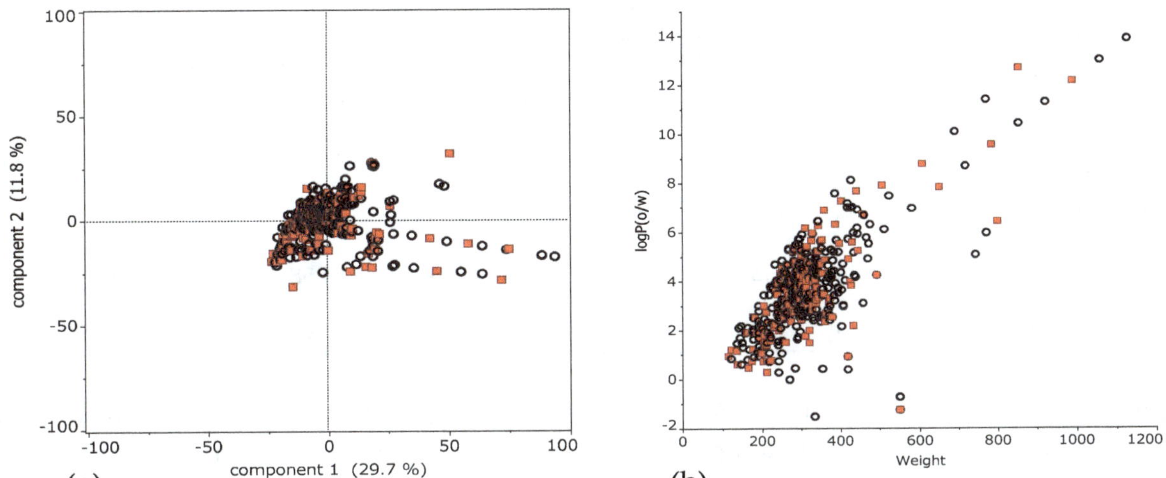

(a) (b)

Figure 2. Chemical space of 494 compounds. (**a**) Applicability domain (AD) of 494 compounds. Scatter plot of principal component analysis using descriptors. The horizontal axis is the first principal component, and the vertical axis is the second principal component. These percentage are eigenvalue that represent a partition of the total variation in the multivariate sample. Each dot represents a compound; black circle is the training set and red square is the external validation set. (**b**) The horizontal axis is molecular weight (MW) and the vertical axis is octanol-water partitioning coefficient (logP). Here, each dot represents a compound; black is the training set and red is the external validation set.

3.2. Construction of Prediction Models by RF

Several prediction models were built by parameter turning. Here, the model that demonstrated the largest value was selected. The prediction accuracy and parameters of each model are shown in Table 3. These models were evaluated by using parameters as follows; R^2, root-mean-square error (RMSE), out of bag (OOB) RMSE, maximum absolute value of the residue, mean absolute error (MAE). The OOB RMSE is computed as the square root of the sum of squared errors divided by the number of OOB observations. OOB observations are training observations that are not used to construct a tree in RF. MAE is a mean of error at a model which the value is the closer to zero indicates the model is the higher accuracy.

Table 3. Parameters of each model by random forest

Parameters	Tumour Cells				Normal Cells				SI
	HSC-2	HSC-3	HSC-4	Mean	HGF	HPC	HPLF	Mean	
Number of Tree	100	300	100	100	100	100	100	100	300
Number of Term	952	1000	952	952	952	952	952	952	1000
Number of Maximum Split at Tree	100	1000	2000	2000	2000	2000	2000	2000	2000
Minimum Node Size	3	5	5	5	5	5	3	5	5
Seed Value	29	36	44	77	93	91	730	9045	124
Number of Tree	23	8	21	20	9	4	34	12	8
Number of Term at a Split	1000	1000	952	952	952	952	952	952	1000
R^2 (Training Set)	0.904	0.847	0.868	0.876	0.862	0.815	0.908	0.858	0.817
R^2 (External Validation Set)	0.564	0.568	0.631	0.563	0.554	0.659	0.515	0.576	0.404

Table 3. *Cont.*

Parameters	Tumour Cells				Normal Cells				SI
	HSC-2	HSC-3	HSC-4	Mean	HGF	HPC	HPLF	Mean	
RMSE (External Validation Set)	0.480	0.496	0.496	0.473	0.435	0.372	0.442	0.397	0.340
OOB RMSE	0.808	0.778	0.742	0.760	0.593	0.587	0.618	0.573	0.579
Maximum Absolute Value of the Residue	2.052	1.875	1.424	1.408	1.347	1.758	1.331	1.582	1.188
Mean Absolute Error	0.236	0.255	0.232	0.216	0.216	0.199	0.240	0.198	0.191

Figure 3 shows scatter plots of each RF model obtained using the training and external validation sets, the measured pCC_{50}, the predicted pCC_{50}, the predicted SI, and the observed SI.

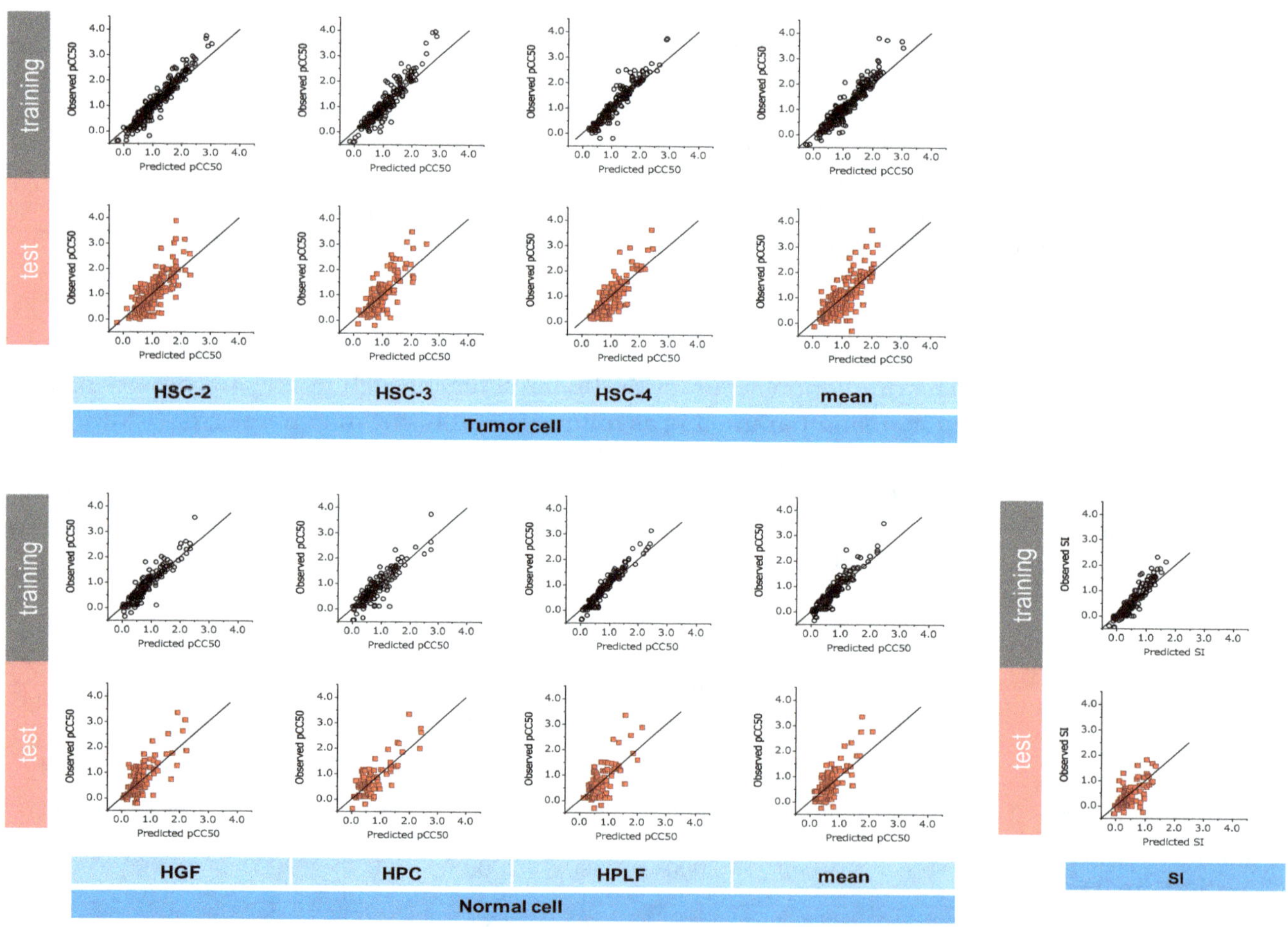

Figure 3. Scatter plot of training set and external validation set. In scatter plots of tumour and normal cell, the horizontal axis is the predicted pCC_{50}, and the vertical axis is the observed pCC_{50} of tumour and normal cell. In scatter plot of SI, the horizontal axis is the predicted SI, and the vertical axis is the observed SI. Each dot represents a compound; black circle is the training set and red square is the external validation set.

The model that demonstrated the greatest R^2 value with the external validation set was the normal cell HPC model ($R^2 = 0.659$, RMSE = 0.372), and the SI model ($R^2 = 0.404$, RMSE = 0.340) demonstrated the smallest R^2 value.

3.3. *Large Contribution Descriptor for Prediction Model*

Table 4 shows the top five contributing descriptors for the RF prediction model. Importance of descriptor were evaluated "LogWorth" in JMP® Pro software. "LogWorth" is calculated as negative common logarithm of p-value. This p-value is calculated in a complex manner that takes into account the number of different ways splits can occur. This calculation is very fair compared to the unadjusted p-value [57]. In the structure-toxicity relationship prediction model, most descriptors were classified into groups representing the topological shape. Note that descriptors meaning lipophilicity were observed in the tumour cell model, and electric charge descriptors were observed in the normal cell model. Topological or 3D shape descriptors were selected in the tumour cell selective toxicity prediction model.

Table 4. Top five contributing descriptors for random forest prediction model.

Cell Type		Descriptor	Meaning
Tumour Cells	HSC-2	vsurf_D7	Lipophilicity
		vsurf_D2	Lipophilicity
		GCUT_SMR_0	Topological shape
		CATS2D_07_LL	Lipophilicity
		SpMin2_Bh(e)	Topological shape and electric state
	HSC-3	SssNH	Topological shape and electric state
		b_max1len	Topological shape
		Mor13s	3D shape and electric state
		Mor15s	3D shape and electric state
		F01[C-C]	Topological shape
	HSC-4	SpMax_L	Topological shape
		SpAD_EA(dm)	Topological shape and dipole moment
		ATSC2s	Topological shape and electric state
		vsurf_D7	Lipophilicity
		ATSC5s	Topological shape and electric state
	Mean	logP(o/w)	Lipophilicity
		vsurf_D2	Lipophilicity
		vsurf_D6	Lipophilicity
		P_VSA_ppp_L	Topological shape and lipophilicity
		SssNH	Topological shape and electric state
Normal Cells	HGF	GCUT_SLOGP_0	Topological shape
		F10[C-N]	Topological shape
		SssNH	Topological shape and electric state
		SpMin2_Bh(s)	Topological shape
		GCUT_SMR_0	Topological shape
	HPC	VE1_B(p)	Topological shape and polarizability
		b_max1len	Topological shape
		CATS3D_10_PL	3D shape and electric state
		h_pKb	Topological shape and electric state
		SpMin1_Bh(p)	Topological shape and polarizability

Table 4. *Cont.*

Cell Type		Descriptor	Meaning
Normal Cells	HPLF	P_VSA_e_3	Topological shape and electric state
		GCUT_SLOGP_0	Topological shape
		F10[C-N]	Topological shape
		SssNH	Topological shape and electric state
		h_pavgQ	Topological shape and electric state
	Mean	h_pstrain	Topological shape and electric state
		h_pavgQ	Topological shape and electric state
		b_max1len	Topological shape
		SssNH	Topological shape and electric state
		F10[C-N]	Topological shape
SI		TDB08p	3D shape and polarizability
		F06[C-N]	Topological shape
		PEOE_VSA+1	Topological shape and electric state
		R5u+	3D shape and size
		RDF035m	3D shape and size

4. Discussion

From our previous articles, 494 compounds and activity data were obtained. As reported in previous studies, compounds with higher tumour specificity than existing anticancer drugs are present among these 494 compounds. For example, in a study of 3-Styryl-2*H*-chromenes, several compounds showed higher tumour specificity than doxorubicin (at most approximately 4.8 times higher specificity) [39].

In this study, we constructed a database of seed compounds for anticancer drugs, including a sufficient number of compounds for analysis.

Regarding cell type, the structure-toxicity relationship prediction models demonstrated the maximum R^2 value for cytotoxic activity against normal cells. If toxicity against normal cells can be predicted accurately, it is hoped that such prediction models can be applied to the estimation of side effects caused by cytotoxicity against normal cells, such as OM, hematotoxicity alopecia and so on. In contrast, with the training set, the R^2 values were greater than 0.9. In addition, the R^2 values of all structure-toxicity relationship prediction models obtained with the external validation set were greater 0.5.

We consider that the structure responsible for lipophilicity or a combination of lipophilicity and another characteristic descriptors may contribute to cytotoxic activity prediction because lipophilicity was tend to observed in the tumour cell models and not in the normal cell models. Relationship of between lipophilicity and cytotoxicity against tumour cell might be considered that penetration mechanism of compounds into tumour cell is one of the reason, however, further study is needed.

We expect that these findings will be useful relative to examining prediction models in future. In construct to structure-toxicity relationship prediction model, the R^2 results of the tumour cell selective toxicity prediction models were less than 0.5.

In light of these results, further study is required to construct a tumour cell selective toxicity prediction model. With the RF method, the meaning of the top five contributing descriptors tended to differ from the structure-toxicity relationship and tumour cell selective toxicity prediction models.

These results indicate that tumour cell selective toxicity prediction is difficult to realize using the methods employed in the cytotoxic activity prediction model.

Thus, further study involving other methods, parameter tuning, and so on is required to construct a tumour cell selective toxicity prediction model with high prediction accuracy. Superior anticancer drugs require both strong cytotoxicity against tumour cells and selectivity to tumour cells, therefore cytotoxic activity prediction model is needed.

In this study, we constructed prediction models that can estimate cytotoxicity and tumour selective toxicity based on cytotoxic activity data derived from various compounds. The RF machine learning method constructed models with higher prediction accuracy.

In future, using our findings as reference, we would like to construct a high-performance prediction model that can be used to search for candidate compounds for a new anticancer drug.

5. Conclusions

In this study, we constructed a database of different compounds with structure and cytotoxic activity data derived from various compounds reported in previous studies. With this database, cytotoxicity and tumour cell selective toxicity prediction models were constructed by RF method. It was found that the structure-toxicity relationship prediction model tended to demonstrate greater R^2 values.

In future, we expect that collecting addition compound data and investigating various model construction methods will help realize a prediction model with good prediction accuracy, which would facilitate the search for candidate compounds for anticancer drugs.

Author Contributions: J.N., M.I. performed QSAR analysis; H.S. performed cytotoxicity assay; Y.U. organized the review.

Acknowledgments: The authors acknowledge Yoshiaki Sugita and Koichi Takao for the supply of chromones, and Meikai University School of Dentistry for the support for the research.

Abbreviations

HGF	Human gingival fibroblast
HPC	Human pulp cell
HPLF	Human periodontal fibroblast
Log P	Octanol-water partitioning coefficient
MOE	Molecular Operating Environment
OM	Oral mucositis
OOB	Out-of-bag
OSCC	Oral squamous cell carcinoma
pCC_{50}	$-\log CC_{50}$, a negative common logarithm
QASR	Quantitative structure-activity relationship
R^2	Coefficient of determination
RF	Random forest
RMSE	Root-mean-square error
SAR	Structure-activity relationship

References

1. Sonis, S.T. Mucositis: The impact, biology and therapeutic opportunities of oral mucositis. *Oral Oncol.* **2009**, *45*, 1015–1020. [CrossRef] [PubMed]
2. Yoshino, F.; Yoshida, A.; Nakajima, A.; Wada-Takahashi, S.; Takahashi, S.S.; Lee, M.C. Alteration of the redox state with reactive oxygen species for 5-fluorouracil-induced oral mucositis in hamsters. *PLoS ONE* **2013**, *8*, e82834. [CrossRef] [PubMed]

3. Sugita, Y.; Takao, K.; Uesawa, Y.; Sakagami, H. Search for New Type of Anticancer Drugs with High Tumor Specificity and Less Keratinocyte Toxicity. *Anticancer Res.* **2017**, *37*, 5919–5924. [PubMed]
4. Sakagami, H.; Okudaira, N.; Masuda, Y.; Amano, O.; Yokose, S.; Kanda, Y.; Suguro, M.; Natori, T.; Oizumi, H.; Oizumi, T. Induction of apoptosis in human oral keratinocyte by doxorubicin. *Anticancer Res.* **2017**, *37*, 1023–1029.
5. SciFinder®. Available online: https://www.cas.org/products/scifinder (accessed on 5 February 2019).
6. Wolfgang, S.; Dina, R. QSAR/QSPR. In *Applied Chemoinformatics*; Thomas, E., Johann, G., Eds.; Wiley-VCH: Weinheim, Germany; Berlin, Germany, 2018; pp. 9–13.
7. Guohui, S.; Tengjiao, F.; Xiaodong, S.; Yuxing, H.; Xin, C.; Lijiao, Z.; Ting, R.; Yue, Z.; Rugang, Z.; Yongzhen, P. In Silico Prediction of O^6-Methylguanine-DNA Methyltransferase Inhibitory Potency of Base Analogs with QSAR and Machine Learning Methods. *Molecules* **2018**, *23*, 2892.
8. Tengjiao, F.; Guohui, S.; Lijiao, Z.; Xin, C.; Rugang, Z. QSAR and Classification Study on Prediction of Acute Oral Toxicity of N-Nitroso Compounds. *Int. J. Mol. Sci.* **2018**, *19*, 3015.
9. Breiman, L. Random forests. *Mach. Learn.* **2001**, *45*, 5–32. [CrossRef]
10. Svetnik, V.; Liaw, A.; Tong, C.; Culberson, J.C.; Sheridan, R.P.; Feuston, B.P. Random forest: A classification and regression tool for compound classification and QSAR modeling. *J. Chem. Inf. Comput. Sci.* **2003**, *43*, 1947–1958. [CrossRef]
11. Shirataki, Y.; Wakae, M.; Yamamoto, Y.; Hashimoto, K.; Satoh, K.; Ishihara, M.; Kikuchi, H.; Nishikawa, H.; Minagawa, K.; Motohashi, N.; et al. Cytotoxicity and radical modulating activity of isoflavones and isoflavanones from sophora species. *Anticancer Res.* **2004**, *24*, 1481–1488.
12. Ishihara, M.; Sakagami, H. Re-evaluation of cytotoxicity and iron chelation activity of three β-diketones by semiempirical molecular orbital method. *In Vivo* **2005**, *19*, 119–124.
13. Momoi, K.; Sugita, Y.; Ishihara, M.; Satoh, K.; Kikuchi, H.; Hashimoto, K.; Yokoe, I.; Nishikawa, H.; Fujisawa, S.; Sakagami, H. Cytotoxic activity of styrylchromones against human tumor cell lines. *In Vivo* **2005**, *19*, 157–164. [PubMed]
14. Sakagami, H.; Ishihara, M.; Hoshino, Y.; Ishikawa, J.; Mikami, Y.; Fukai, T. Cytotoxicity of nocobactins NA-a, NA-b and their ferric complexes assessed by semiempirical molecular orbital method. *In Vivo* **2005**, *19*, 277–282. [PubMed]
15. Ishihara, M.; Sakagami, H.; Liu, W.K. Quantitative structure-cytotoxicity relationship analysis of betulinic acid and its derivatives by semi-empirical molecular-orbital method. *Anticancer Res.* **2005**, *25*, 3951–3956. [PubMed]
16. Inoue, K.; Kulsum, U.; Chowdhury, SA.; Fujisawa, S.; Ishihara, M.; Yokoe, I.; Sakagami, H. Tumor-specific cytotoxicity and apoptosis-inducing activity of berberines. *Anticancer Res.* **2005**, *25*, 4053–4060. [PubMed]
17. Ishihara, M.; Yokote, Y.; Sakagami, H. Quantitative structure-cytotoxicity relationship analysis of coumarin and its derivatives by semiempirical molecular orbital method. *Anticancer Res.* **2006**, *26*, 2883–2886. [PubMed]
18. Sasaki, M.; Okamura, M.; Ideo, A.; Shimada, J.; Suzuki, F.; Ishihara, M.; Kikuchi, H.; Kanda, Y.; Kunii, S.; Sakagami, H. Re-evaluation of tumor-specific cytotoxicity of mitomycin c, bleomycin and peplomycin. *Anticancer Res.* **2006**, *26*, 3373–3380.
19. Ishihara, M.; Kawase, M.; Sakagami, H. Quantitative structure-activity relationship analysis of 4-trifluoromethylimidazole derivatives with the concept of absolute hardness. *Anticancer Res.* **2007**, *27*, 4047–4052.
20. Ishihara, M.; Kawase, M.; Westman, G.; Samuelsson, K.; Motohashi, N.; Sakagami, H. Quantitative structure-cytotoxicity relationship analysis of phenoxazine derivatives by semiempirical molecular-orbital method. *Anticancer Res.* **2007**, *27*, 4053–4058. [PubMed]
21. Ishihara, M.; Sakagami, H. QSAR of molecular structure and cytotoxic activity of vitamin K_2 derivatives with concept of absolute hardness. *Anticancer Res.* **2007**, *27*, 4059–4064.
22. Takekawa, F.; Nagumo, T.; Shintani, S.; Hashimoto, K.; Kikuchi, H.; Katayama, T.; Ishihara, M.; Amano, O.; Kawase, M.; Sakagami, H. Tumor-specific cytotoxic activity and type of cell death induced by 4-trifluoromethylimidazoles in human oral squamous cell carcinoma cell lines. *Anticancer Res.* **2007**, *27*, 4065–4070.
23. Suzuki, F.; Hashimoto, K.; Ishihara, M.; Westman, G.; Samuelsson, K.; Kawase, M.; Motohashi, N.; Sakagami, H. Tumor-specificity and type of cell death induced by phenoxazines. *Anticancer Res.* **2007**, *27*, 4233–4238. [PubMed]

24. Sakagami, H.; Hashimoto, K.; Suzuki, F.; Ishihara, M.; Kikuchi, H.; Katayama, T.; Satoh, K. Tumor-specificity and type of cell death induced by vitamin K_2 derivatives and prenylalcohols. *Anticancer Res.* **2008**, *28*, 151–158. [PubMed]
25. Ishihara, M.; Sakagami, H. Quantitative structure-cytotoxicity relationship analysis of 3-formylchromone derivatives by a semiempirical molecularorbital method with the concept of absolute hardness. *Anticancer Res.* **2008**, *28*, 277–282.
26. Ishihara, M.; Kawase, M.; Sakagami, H. Quantitative structure-cytotoxicity relationship analysis of 5-trifluoromethyloxazole derivatives by a semiempirical molecular-orbital method with the concept of absolute hardness. *Anticancer Res.* **2008**, *28*, 997–1004.
27. Ishihara, M.; Hatano, H.; Kawase, M.; Sakagami, H. Estimation of relationship between the structure of 1, 2, 3, 4-tetrahydroisoquinoline derivatives determined by a semiempirical molecular-orbital method and their cytotoxicity. *Anticancer Res.* **2009**, *29*, 2265–2272.
28. Hatano, H.; Takekawa, F.; Hashimoto, K.; Ishihara, M.; Kawase, M.; Qing, C.; Qin-Tao, W.; Sakagami, H. Tumor-specific cytotoxic activity of 1, 2, 3, 4-tetrahydroisoquinoline derivatives against human oral squamous cell carcinoma cell lines. *Anticancer Res.* **2009**, *29*, 3079–3086.
29. Takekawa, F.; Sakagami, H.; Ishihara, M. Estimation of relationship between structure of newly synthesized dihydroimidazoles determined by a semiempirical molecular-orbital method and their cytotoxicity. *Anticancer Res.* **2009**, *29*, 5019–5022. [PubMed]
30. Ishihara, M.; Wakabayashi, H.; Motohashi, N.; Sakagami, H. Quantitative structure-cytotoxicity relationship of newly synthesized tropolones determined by a semiempirical molecular-orbital method (PM5). *Anticancer Res.* **2010**, *30*, 129–134.
31. Ishihara, M.; Wakabayashi, H.; Motohashi, N.; Sakagami, H. Quantitative structure–cytotoxicity relationship of newly synthesized trihaloacetylazulenes determined by a semi-empirical molecular-orbital method (PM5). *Anticancer Res.* **2011**, *31*, 515–520.
32. Ishihara, M.; Wakabayashi, H.; Motohashi, N.; Sakagami, H. Estimation of relationship between the structure of trihaloacetylazulene derivatives determined by a semiempirical molecular–orbital method (PM5) and their cytotoxicity. *Anticancer Res.* **2010**, *30*, 837–842. [PubMed]
33. Ohno, H.; Araho, D.; Uesawa, Y.; Kagaya, H.; Ishihara, M.; Sakagami, H.; Yamamoto, M. Evaluation of cytotoxicity and tumor-specificity of licorice flavonoids based on chemical structure. *Anticancer Res.* **2013**, *33*, 3061–3068.
34. Uesawa, Y.; Mohri, K.; Kawasc, M.; Ishihara, M.; Sakagami, H. Quantitative structure–activity relationship (QSAR) analysis of tumor-specificity of 1, 2, 3, 4-tetrahydroisoquinoline derivatives. *Anticancer Res.* **2011**, *31*, 4231–4238. [PubMed]
35. Sekine, S.; Shimodaira, C.; Uesawa, Y.; Kagaya, H.; Kanda, Y.; Ishihara, M.; Amano, O.; Sakagami, H.; Wakabayashi, H. Quantitative structure–activity relationship analysis of cytotoxicity and anti-uv activity of 2-aminotropones. *Anticancer Res.* **2014**, *34*, 1743–1750.
36. Shimada, C.; Uesawa, Y.; Ishihara, M.; Kagaya, H.; Kanamoto, T.; Terakubo, S.; Nakashima, H.; Takao, K.; Saito, T.; Sugita, Y.; et al. Quantitative structure–cytotoxicity relationship of phenylpropanoid amides. *Anticancer Res.* **2014**, *34*, 3543–3548.
37. Shimada, C.; Uesawa, Y.; Ishihara, M.; Kagaya, H.; Kanamoto, T.; Terakubo, S.; Nakashima, H.; Takao, K.; Miyashiro, T.; Sugita, Y.; et al. Quantitative structure–cytotoxicity relationship of piperic acid amides. *Anticancer Res.* **2014**, *34*, 4877–4884.
38. Shimada, C.; Uesawa, Y.; Ishii-Nozawa, R.; Ishihara, M.; Kagaya, H.; Kanamoto, T.; Terakubo, S.; Nakashima, H.; Takao, K.; Sugita, Y.; et al. Quantitative structure–cytotoxicity relationship of 3-styrylchromones. *Anticancer Res.* **2014**, *34*, 5405–5412.
39. Uesawa, Y.; Sakagami, H.; Ishihara, M.; Kagaya, H.; Kanamoto, T.; Terakubo, S.; Nakashima, H.; Yahagi, H.; Takao, K.; Sugita, Y. Quantitative structure–cytotoxicity relationship of 3-styryl-2*H*-chromenes. *Anticancer Res.* **2015**, *35*, 5299–5308. [PubMed]
40. Sakagami, H.; Uesawa, Y.; Ishihara, M.; Kagaya, H.; Kanamoto, T.; Terakubo, S.; Nakashima, H.; Takao, K.; Sugita, Y. Quantitative structure–cytotoxicity relationship of oleoylamides. *Anticancer Res.* **2015**, *35*, 5341–5355. [PubMed]
41. Uesawa, Y.; Sakagami, H.; Kagaya, H.; Yamashita, M.; Takao, K.; Sugita, Y. Quantitative structure-cytotoxicity relationship of 3-benzylidenechromanones. *Anticancer Res.* **2016**, *36*, 5803–5812. [CrossRef]

42. Fukuchi, K.; Okudaira, N.; Adachi, K.; Odai-Ide, R.; Watanabe, S.; Ohno, H.; Yamamoto, M.; Kanamoto, T.; Terakubo, S.; Nakashima, H.; et al. Antiviral and antitumor activity of licorice root extracts. *In Vivo* **2016**, *30*, 777–786. [CrossRef]
43. Sakagami, H.; Masuda, Y.; Tomomura, M.; Yokose, S.; Uesawa, Y.; Ikezoe, N.; Asahara, D.; Takao, K.; Kanamoto, T.; Terakubo, S.; et al. Quantitative structure–cytotoxicity relationship of chalcones. *Anticancer Res.* **2017**, *37*, 1091–1098.
44. Sakagami, H.; Uesawa, Y.; Masuda, Y.; Tomomura, M.; Yokose, S.; Miyashiro, T.; Murai, J.; Takao, K.; Kanamoto, T.; Terakubo, S.; et al. Quantitative structure–cytotoxicity relationship of newly synthesized piperic acid esters. *Anticancer Res.* **2017**, *37*, 6161–6168.
45. Uesawa, Y.; Sakagami, H.; Ikezoe, N.; Takao, K.; Kagaya, H.; Sugita; Y. Quantitative structure–cytotoxicity relationship of aurones. *Anticancer Res.* **2017**, *37*, 6169–6176.
46. Sakagami, H.; Okudaira, N.; Uesawa, Y.; Takao, K.; Kagaya, H.; Sugita, Y. Quantitative structure–cytotoxicity relationship of 2-azolylchromones. *Anticancer Res.* **2018**, *38*, 763–770.
47. Uesawa, Y.; Sakagami, H.; Okudaira, N.; Toda, K.; Takao, K.; Kagaya, H.; Sugita, Y. Quantitative structure–cytotoxicity relationship of cinnamic acid phenetyl esters. *Anticancer Res.* **2018**, *38*, 817–823. [CrossRef] [PubMed]
48. Wada, T.; Maruyama, R.; Irie, Y.; Hashimoto, M.; Wakabayashi, H.; Okudaira, N.; Uesawa, Y.; Kagaya, H.; Sakagami, H. In vitro anti-tumor activity of azulene amide derivatives. *In Vivo* **2018**, *32*, 479–486. [PubMed]
49. Uehara, M.; Minemura, H.; Ohno, T.; Hashimoto, M.; Wakabayashi, H.; Okudaira, N.; Sakagami, H. In vitro antitumor activity of alkylaminoguaiazulenes. *In Vivo* **2018**, *32*, 541–547. [PubMed]
50. Marvin. Available online: https://chemaxon.com/products/marvin (accessed on 15 November 2018).
51. MOE. Available online: http://www.chemcomp.com/MOE-Molecular_Operating_Environment.htm (accessed on 15 November 2018).
52. Dragon. Available online: https://chm.kode-solutions.net/products_dragon.php (accessed on 15 November 2018).
53. Paola, G. Principles of QSAR models validation: Internal and external. *QSAR Comb. Sci.* **2007**, *26*, 694–701.
54. SAS Institute Inc. Chapter 6 Bootstrap Forest. In *JMP® 13 Predictive and Specialized Modeling*, 2nd ed.; SAS Institute Inc.: Cary, NC, USA, 2017; pp. 107–122.
55. JMP®. Available online: https://www.jmp.com/en_us/home.html (accessed on 15 November 2018).
56. Wolfgang, S.; Dina, R. Applicability domain and model acceptability critera. In *Applied Chemoinformatics*; Thomas, E., Johann, G., Eds.; Wiley-VCH: Weinheim, Germany; Berlin, Germany, 2018; pp. 41–43.
57. SAS Institute Inc. Chapter 5 Partition Models. In *JMP® 13 Predictive and Specialized Modeling*, 2nd ed.; SAS Institute Inc.: Cary, NC, USA, 2017; pp. 104–106.

11

Periodontal Disease in Patients Receiving Dialysis

Yasuyoshi Miyata [1,*], Yoko Obata [2], Yasushi Mochizuki [1,3], Mineaki Kitamura [2,3], Kensuke Mitsunari [1], Tomohiro Matsuo [1], Kojiro Ohba [1], Hiroshi Mukae [4], Tomoya Nishino [2], Atsutoshi Yoshimura [5] and Hideki Sakai [1,3]

1 Department of Urology, Nagasaki University Graduate School of Biomedical Sciences, Nagasaki 852-8501, Japan
2 Department of Nephrology, Nagasaki University Hospital, Nagasaki 852-8501, Japan
3 Division of Blood Purification, Nagasaki University Hospital, Nagasaki 852-8501, Japan
4 Department of Respiratory Medicine, Unit of Basic Medical Sciences, Nagasaki University Graduate School of Biomedical Sciences, Nagasaki 852-8591, Japan
5 Department of Periodontology and Endodontology, Nagasaki University Graduate School of Biomedical Sciences, Nagasaki 852-8501, Japan
* Correspondence: yasu-myt@nagasaki-u.ac.jp

Abstract: Chronic kidney disease (CKD) is characterized by kidney damage with proteinuria, hematuria, and progressive loss of kidney function. The final stage of CKD is known as end-stage renal disease, which usually indicates that approximately 90% of normal renal function is lost, and necessitates renal replacement therapy for survival. The most widespread renal replacement therapy is dialysis, which includes peritoneal dialysis (PD) and hemodialysis (HD). However, despite the development of novel medical instruments and agents, both dialysis procedures have complications and disadvantages, such as cardiovascular disease due to excessive blood fluid and infections caused by impaired immunity. Periodontal disease is chronic inflammation induced by various pathogens and its frequency and severity in patients undergoing dialysis are higher compared to those in healthy individuals. Therefore, several investigators have paid special attention to the impact of periodontal disease on inflammation-, nutrient-, and bone metabolism-related markers; the immune system; and complications in patients undergoing dialysis. Furthermore, the influence of diabetes on the prevalence and severity of manifestations of periodontal disease, and the properties of saliva in HD patients with periodontitis have been reported. Conversely, there are few reviews discussing periodontal disease in patients with dialysis. In this review, we discuss the available studies and review the pathological roles and clinical significance of periodontal disease in patients receiving PD or HD. In addition, this review underlines the importance of oral health and adequate periodontal treatment to maintain quality of life and prolong survival in these patients.

Keywords: periodontal disease; peritoneal dialysis; hemodialysis; immune response; diabetes

---

1. Introduction

Chronic kidney disease (CKD) is defined as a specific, irreversible loss of functional nephrons characterized by progression towards end-stage renal disease (ESRD). The loss of renal function is the most severe form of CKD. In general, when renal function decreases below approximately 10% of normal efficiency, renal replacement therapy is necessary to maintain survival.

Dialytic therapy, mainly peritoneal dialysis (PD) and hemodialysis (HD), are common renal replacement therapies that are used worldwide. Both techniques are performed to remove excessive fluids, electrolytes, and uremic toxins. PD uses the peritoneum as the membrane through which fluids and substances are exchanged with the blood. Solute clearance occurs by solute diffusion from the plasma into a dialysate or ultrafiltration is driven by the osmotic gradient between the hyperosmotic dialysate and the plasma. In contrast, in HD, the transfer between blood and dialysis fluid is performed using a dialyzer membrane. Furthermore, PD has been reported to have the advantage of maintaining residual renal function (RRF) and achieving better outcomes than HD during the first few years of treatment [1]. Other benefits include greater effectiveness in improving quality of life (QoL) and better tolerability in patients with decreased cardiac function. However, PD is less efficient at removing wastes from the body than HD, and the presence of the catheter presents a risk of peritonitis due to the possibility of microbial entry into the abdomen.

Periodontal disease is an oral, chronic infectious, and inflammatory disease caused predominantly by gram-negative anaerobic bacteria, and is characterized by the destruction of tooth-supporting tissues, including the alveolar bone and connective tissues of the periodontium [2,3]. Currently, there is a general agreement that the prevalence of periodontal disease in patients undergoing dialysis is higher than that in healthy individuals. In fact, Borawski et al. [4] reported a marked increase in periodontitis in CKD patients, including patients undergoing predialysis, PD, and HD, compared with the general population. Conversely, when the prevalence and severity of periodontal disease are stratified according to PD or HD treatment, the observed rate was as high as 42.6% in continuous ambulatory PD (CAPD) patients [5]. Moreover, Cengiz et al. [6] reported that the prevalence of moderate to severe periodontitis was 67.3% in CAPD patients. However, in contrast to these results, there have been several reports indicating that PD patients and healthy individuals show a similar prevalence of periodontitis [7,8]. Surprisingly, a recent report suggested that 106 of 107 HD patients (99.1%) exhibit some form of periodontitis [9], and another study also showed that only one of 103 HD patients evaluated had a healthy periodontium [10]. Even if such reports are excluded, many studies have reported that over half of HD patients exhibit periodontitis [11–14]. Furthermore, most periodontal parameters in HD patients were reported to be significantly higher than those in age-matched control subjects and healthy individuals [15–17]. Thus, many investigators have shown that periodontal disease is an important issue in patients with PD and HD.

In this review, we searched for the literature on "periodontal disease" or "periodontitis" and "peritoneal dialysis" or "hemodialysis" using PubMed. We subsequently excluded studies without clinical and laboratory data, and prioritized the most recent studies and those with comparative analyses. We also discuss periodontal indices, the biochemical profile of the blood, and the molecular mechanisms involved in periodontal disease in patients with PD. We focus on the impact of periodontal disease on pathological mechanisms including inflammation, the immune response, and bone metabolism in HD patients. In addition, we compare the severity of periodontal disease, periodontal parameters, and oral health-related conditions in HD patients with diabetic and non-diabetic nephropathies.

2. Peritoneal Dialysis

2.1. Impact of Periodontal Disease

In this review, different measures of the severity of periodontal disease are discussed. These measures and their criteria are familiar essentially to dentists. Therefore, we present a summary of some representative measures Table 1 [4].

There have been several studies to date indicating that longer duration of CAPD is associated with the severity of periodontitis [5,6]. In addition, the severity of periodontitis correlated positively with levels of inflammatory parameters (high-sensitivity C-reactive protein (hs-CRP), serum ferritin, and white blood cell count) and atherosclerotic risk factors (serum low-density lipoprotein cholesterol, lipoprotein (a), and homocysteine) [5,6]. Conversely, periodontal health status showed a significant negative correlation with serum albumin and blood urea nitrogen (BUN) levels, which suggest poor nutritional status [6]. In contrast to HD, the timing of blood sampling did not have a significant impact in CAPD. Therefore, we believe that periodontal conditions affect the inflammatory and nutritional parameters in PD patients' blood samples.

Table 1. Criteria for representative periodontal measures.

Plaque Index	
0	No plaque in the gingival area
1	A film of plaque adhering to the free gingival margin and adjacent area of the tooth; may be recognized only by running a probe across the tooth surface
2	Moderate accumulation of soft deposits within the gingival pocket and on the gingival margin and/or adjacent tooth surface; can be seen by the naked eye
3	Abundance of soft material within the gingival pocket and/or on the gingival margin and adjacent tooth surface
Papillary Bleeding Index	
0	No bleeding on probing
1	Single ecchymosis of the gingiva on probing
2	Multiple ecchymoses or minor single spot extravasation from the gingiva on probing
3	Bleeding into the pocket immediately after probe insertion
4	Intensive extra pocket bleeding on probing
Gingival Index	
0	Normal gingiva
1	Mild inflammation, slight change in color, slight edema, no bleeding on palpation
2	Moderate inflammation, redness, edema, glazing, bleeding on palpation
3	Severe inflammation, marked redness and edema, ulceration, tendency to spontaneous bleeding
Community Periodontal Index	
0	Healthy gingiva
1	Bleeding observed, directly or by using mouth mirror, after probing
2	Calculus detected during probing, but all the black band on the probe visible
3	Pocket 4–5 mm (gingival margin within the black band on the probe)
4	Pocket 6 mm or more (black band on the probe not visible)
X	Excluded sextant (less than two teeth present)

Hepatocyte growth factor (HGF) is known to play important roles in embryogenesis, morphogenesis, wound repair, and tissue regeneration [18]. Oshima et al. reported that these pleiotropic properties of HGF might be involved in the development and progression of periodontal diseases [19–21]. Previously, Wilczynska-Borawska et al. [22] showed that there was no difference in HGF levels in the saliva of HD, PD, and chronic renal failure patients, although the levels in the saliva of periodontitis patients were higher than those in the healthy population. In PD patients specifically, significant and positive correlations between HGF levels in the saliva and plaque index (PI), papillary bleeding index (PBI), and gingival index (GI) have been reported. Similar to blood sampling, the timing of saliva collection may not be a factor influencing HGF levels in patients on PD. Thus, HGF might contribute to the development of periodontal disease in PD patients. However, the molecular mechanism involved in the pathogenesis of periodontal disease in PD patients remains to be clarified. Herein, we hoped to clarify the precise mechanisms of pathogenesis and progression of periodontal diseases.

2.2. *Impact of Periodontal Care and Treatment*

Several studies have investigated the effects of periodontal therapy in PD patients [5,22]. Briefly, treatment of periodontal disease improved periodontal status, inflammatory markers, and nutrition status [5]. Tasdemir et al. [23] investigated the effects of periodontal therapy on inflammation markers in PD patients with diabetic nephropathy, diabetic patients without CKD, and in the healthy population, since it has been reported that diabetes mellitus (DM) is one of the risk factors of periodontitis, and that periodontal inflammation causes poor glycemic control. The authors demonstrated that all inflammatory markers including tumor necrosis factor (TNF)-α, pentraxin-3 (PTX-3), interleukin (IL)-6, and hs-CRP in blood samples were significantly higher in PD patients with diabetic nephropathy than in the other two groups, and TNF-α was reduced after 3 months of periodontal treatment in all patients [23]. Conversely, PTX-3, IL-6, and hs-CRP levels were decreased after periodontal treatment only in PD patients with diabetic nephropathy [23]. Thus, the authors speculated that periodontal disease is a major source of inflammation in CAPD patients with diabetes [23]. Conversely, in a study evaluating the clinical impact of PD on oral health, Keles et al. [23] reported that the degree of halitosis was significantly reduced by PD therapy. As a potential underlying mechanism, the authors speculated that a decrease in BUN levels and an increase in salivary flow rates (SFR) resulting from adequate PD treatment might be associated with the improvement of halitosis, as high BUN levels and low SFRs have been reported to play important roles in the severity of halitosis [24]. Thus, periodontal care and treatment are useful for ameliorating a variety of the inflammatory manifestations in diabetic nephropathy patients, and for partially relieving symptoms caused by periodontal diseases. However, further studies in non-diabetic patients, with a focus on periodontal disease-related symptoms, are necessary before drawing definitive conclusions.

3. Hemodialysis

3.1. *Correlations with Blood Test Indices*

As mentioned above, HD is a form of renal replacement therapy, whereby toxins, waste, and excessive proteins and electrolytes, such as urea, potassium, and excess fluids are removed from the blood. This enables HD to improve QoL and prolong survival in patients with ESRD. Unfortunately, bacterial infection is common in patients with HD, and is a major cause of death because of the suppression of immunological function, increasing incidence of diabetes, and deterioration of nutritional status [25–27]. In HD patients, periodontal disease induces not only local inflammation but also systematic inflammatory responses [28–30]. In a QoL analysis of HD patients, 5 of 8 indices of the SF-36 health scale (physical functioning, role physical, vitality, social functioning, and mental health) were significantly lower in patients with severe periodontitis ($p < 0.05$) compared to those with no/mild periodontitis [14]. Thus, many studies have investigated the relationships between the prevalence and/or severity of periodontal disease and serum levels of inflammation-related factors in HD patients. Moreover, periodontal disease may also affect nutritional and bone loss parameters in HD patients [10,31]. Based on these reports, several researchers and clinicians have paid special attention to the relationship between periodontal disease and changes in systemic conditions, including inflammation, nutrition, and bone metabolism, resulting from HD. Therefore, we have reviewed the data on serum levels of CRP, albumin, calcium, phosphorus, parathyroid hormone (PTH), and other hematological parameters in HD patients. However, we should note the fact that the timing of blood sampling is not clearly defined in almost all of the previous reports. In general, routine blood sampling is performed at the initiation of HD. However, if it is performed at the time of a dental consultation, sampling at the initiation of HD is not possible. In real-world settings, the overall management of patients and supervision of HD is performed by nephrologists or urologists. Therefore, blood sampling can be assumed to have been performed at the initiation of HD.

3.1.1. Serum CRP Levels

Serum CRP levels in HD patients with advanced periodontitis have been reported to be significantly higher ($p < 0.05$) than in those without periodontitis [32]. Furthermore, other investigators have shown that serum CRP levels were decreased following periodontal therapy ($p = 0.001$) in HD patients with periodontal disease [30]. Moreover, the number of teeth was negatively associated with serum CRP level in patients with HD ($r = -0.23$, $p < 0.05$) [10]. These results support the notion that serum CRP levels may reflect the inflammatory status of periodontal tissues, and that the serum CRP level is a useful marker of treatment success in HD patients with periodontal disease. In contrast to these findings, in 154 patients on HD, the mean serum CRP level in those with severe periodontitis was reported to be similar to that in those without periodontitis (9.27 and 11.90 mg/dL, respectively; $p = 0.28$) [33]. In addition, the same study found no significant difference in serum CRP levels ($p = 0.23$) between HD patients with no/mild periodontitis ($n = 100$) and moderate/severe periodontitis ($n = 68$). This non-significant relationship between serum CRP levels and severity of periodontal disease was supported by other investigators [10,12]. Moreover, salivary CRP levels in HD patients were reported to be significantly higher compared to both controls and patients with CKD not receiving HD [34]. Thus, there are contrasting opinions regarding the pathological significance of serum CRP levels in HD patients with periodontal disease.

Conversely, a study measuring hs-CRP levels showed that the median (interquartile range) serum level in HD patients with no, mild, moderate, and severe periodontitis was 1.96 (0.79–8.17), 2.72 (0.87–6.91), 4.19 (1.92–10.47), and 4.42 (2.46–13.4), respectively, showing a significant positive correlation ($p = 0.008$) [35]. Likewise, serum hs-CRP levels have been reported to be a significant and independent predictor for the development of periodontal disease in a multivariate model that included DM, frequency of teeth brushing, and various serum markers in HD patients [36]. Based on these results, we felt that hs-CRP was a better marker of the severity of periodontal disease and progression of the disease in HD patients than CRP.

Regarding changes in serum CRP level following treatment of periodontal disease in HD patients, conflicting results have been reported. For example, one report showed that serum CRP levels were significantly decreased ($p = 0.001$) after periodontal treatment in 41 patients receiving HD [30]. Similar results have also been reported in 77 HD patients treated with non-surgical methods [12]. In contrast, other investigators have reported that serum CRP levels in HD patients with treated chronic periodontitis ($n = 43$) were similar ($p = 0.634$) to untreated patients ($n = 30$) [37]. Conversely, a study measuring hs-CRP showed that serum levels were significantly decreased ($p < 0.001$) by the treatment of periodontal diseases, including non-surgical and surgical methods (mean/SD: 3.8/21.9 to 0.6/5.9 mg/L) [38]. As mentioned above, there is the possibility that hs-CRP levels are a better indicator of the inflammatory status caused by periodontal disease in HD patients. However, it should be noted that not only periodontal diseases but also other factors are recognizable as sources of inflammation in patients with HD [39,40]. Further studies with more detailed analyses and larger populations are necessary to determine the pathological significance and value of CRP or hs-CRP levels as biomarkers in HD patients with periodontal disease. A summary of these results is shown in Table 2.

Table 2. Relationships between serum C-reactive protein level and periodontal disease.

n	Correlation with Periodontal Disease and Its Severity	Author/Year/Ref
253 *	Positively correlated with periodontitis severity	Chen/2006/[35]
44	Higher in advanced periodontitis versus non-cases	Franek/2006/[32]
154	Not different between non-cases and periodontitis	Kshirsagar/2007/[33]
253 *	Positively correlated with periodontitis severity	Chen/2011/[11]
77	Not correlated with periodontitis severity	Yazdi/2013/[12]
136 *	Higher in periodontal disease versus non-cases	Hou/2017/[36]
128	Not different between healthy/gingivitis and periodontitis	Cholewa/2018/[10]
211	Higher in periodontal disease versus non-cases	Iwasaki/2018/[41]

* High-sensitive C-reactive protein; Ref: Reference.

3.1.2. Serum Albumin Levels

Evaluation of nutritional status in HD patients is important because hypo-albuminemia is known as a predictive factor of worse mobility and mortality [42,43]. Many investigators have paid special attention to the relationship between periodontal disease and serum albumin levels. Kshirsagar et al. reported that the mean/SD serum albumin levels in HD patients with and without periodontitis ($n = 35$ and 119, respectively) were 3.83/0.41 and 3.99/0.53 mg/dL, respectively, although this difference did not reach statistical significance ($p = 0.06$) [33]. However, their study also showed that severe periodontitis was significantly associated with low serum albumin levels in univariate logistic regression analysis (odds ratio = 3.23, 95% confidential interval [CI]; 1.16–8.96, $p = 0.02$) [33]. In addition, the same significant correlation was confirmed by multivariate analysis models including clinical features and laboratory data [33]. A positive association between periodontitis and hypo-albuminemia was confirmed by other investigators [13]. Furthermore, several reports have demonstrated that serum albumin levels were negatively associated with representative parameters of periodontal health status including plaque index ($r = -0.26$, $p < 0.01$), ($r = -0.28$, $p < 0.01$), periodontal disease index ($r = -0.29$, $p < 0.01$), and pocket depth ($r = -0.20$, $p < 0.05$) [10,35], and a multivariate analysis showed that the serum albumin level is an independent predictor of the periodontal disease index (relative ratio = −0.47, CI = −0.91 to 0.03, $p = 0.036$) [35]. Moreover, serum albumin levels in HD patients with treated chronic periodontitis were significantly lower ($p = 0.023$) than in untreated patients [37]. Thus, periodontal disease seems to decrease serum albumin level in patients with HD. This negative correlation can be explained by various reasons, including protein energy malnutrition, consistent inflammation, and reduced oral intake [33]. However, in patients with HD, there is no general agreement on this relationship, and the detailed mechanism is not fully understood. In fact, a recent report indicated that serum albumin levels were not significantly different between dentate HD patients and edentulous patients ($p = 0.761$), or patients with healthy periodontium or gingivitis and those with periodontitis ($p = 0.601$) [10].

In contrast to these findings, HD patients with moderate-severe periodontitis exhibited higher serum albumin levels (mean/SD; none or mild periodontitis: 3.7/0.4 g/dL and moderate or severe periodontitis: 3.9/0.4 g/dL) [44]. In addition, another report suggested that serum albumin levels increased following treatment of periodontal diseases (mean/SD: 3.15/0.30 to 3.38/0.37 g/dL) in 30 patients with HD [38]. We have no clear answer for these differing findings. However, besides nutritional status, serum albumin levels are regulated by various pathological conditions including aortic calcification, peptic ulcer diseases, and body fat mass [45–47]. Furthermore, we should note the method of statistical analysis used for each study. Briefly, one study showed that the frequency of patients with hypo-albuminemia (<3.6 g/dL) was not significantly associated with periodontitis in HD patients [14,41], the same group also showed that serum albumin levels in HD patients with periodontitis was significantly lower ($p = 0.01$) compared to patients without periodontitis [41]. This information is shown in Table 3.

Table 3. Relationships between serum albumin levels and periodontal disease.

n	Correlation with Periodontal Disease and Its Severity	Author/Year/Ref
253	Negatively correlated with periodontitis severity	Chen/2006/[35]
154	No difference between non-patients and periodontitis patients	Kshirsagar/2007/[33]
154	Lower in severe periodontitis versus no periodontitis	Kshirsagar/2007/[33]
253	Negatively correlated with periodontitis severity	Chen/2011/[11]
96	Lower in periodontal disease versus no periodontal disease	Rodrigues/2014/[13]
188	Not correlated with periodontitis severity	Iwasaki/2016/[14]
1355	Positively correlated with periodontitis severity	Ruospo/2017/[44]
57	Lower in periodontitis versus gingivitis cases	Naghsh/2017/[48]
128	No difference between healthy/gingivitis and periodontitis	Cholewa/2018/[10]

3.1.3. Calcium, Phosphorus, Alkaline Phosphatase, and PTH

Secondary hyper-parathyroidism and 1,25-dihydroxy vitamin D3 deficiency are common and important complications in HD patients. Furthermore, they can lead to bone fracture and arthropathy via the reduction in bone density, and changes in serum calcium, and phosphorus, while PTH levels play important roles in pathogenesis and progression of HD-related complications. However, there is a report indicating that alkaline phosphatase is a useful marker for the diagnosis of periodontal disease [49]. Therefore, we will discuss the relationship between periodontal disease and serum levels of calcium, phosphorus, alkaline phosphatase, and PTH in patients with HD.

As shown in Table 3, to our knowledge, all reports that have investigated changes in serum calcium levels by periodontitis in HD patients showed no significant difference [10,13,36,48]. In contrast, a cross-sectional study reported that higher calcium intake (584.5–1478.5 mg/day) was inversely associated with probing pocket depth (PPD) > 4 mm (adjusted odds ratio; 0.53, 95% CI; 0.30–0.94, $p = 0.03$) compared to a lower intake group (230.7–393.4 mg/day) [50]. Based on this result, supplementation with calcium might be useful to prevent periodontal disease in HD patients [36].

However, we must consider the fact that the study population comprised young women with a mean age of 31.5 years and normal renal function [50].

Regarding phosphorus in HD patients, the mean/SD serum levels in healthy/gingivitis patients (5.87/1.59 mg/dL) showed a trend towards being higher than in moderate/severe periodontitis (5.29/1.68 mg/dL) patients; however, this difference did not reach statistical significance ($p = 0.084$) [10]. In addition, several investigators have shown that serum phosphorus levels in periodontal disease are not significantly different compared to non-gingivitis groups [36,48]. However, in contrast to these results, other investigators showed that serum phosphorus levels in HD patients with periodontitis (mean/SD; 5.02/1.19 mg/dL) were significantly lower ($p = 0.024$) than in patients without periodontitis (6.25/1.72 mg/dL) [13]. In addition, serum phosphorus levels have been reported to be positively correlated with clinical attachment loss (CAL; $r = 0.47$, $p = 0.037$) [48]. However, the above study also showed that serum phosphorus levels were not associated with other periodontal parameters, such as PD, PI, GI, or bleeding on probing [48]. Conversely, serum phosphorus levels in patients with untreated chronic periodontitis (6.1/1.2 mg/dL) have been reported to be similar ($p = 0.221$) to those of treated patients (6.5/1.2 mg/dL) [37]. Although further studies are necessary, it appears that serum phosphorus levels might not influence periodontal disease in HD patients based on the calcium and PTH levels observed (see below).

Several studies have reported that periodontal disease had no significant correlation with serum PTH levels in HD patients [10,35,36,51]. In addition, alveolar bone loss was not correlated to serum PTH level in 35 HD patients with secondary hyper-parathyroidism [51]. Finally, the authors speculated that secondary hyper-parathyroidism and increased serum PTH levels played minimal roles in periodontal disease and periodontal indices in HD patients, a speculation that we also find plausible.

Conversely, as shown in Table 3, several reports have shown no significant correlation between serum levels of alkaline phosphatase and periodontal diseases [10,13]. In addition, serum alkaline phosphatase levels in HD patients with untreated chronic periodontitis (mean/SD: 134/145 mg/dL) showed a trend towards higher levels than in treated patients (117/70 mg/dL); however, this difference was not statistically significant ($p = 0.687$) [37]. Thus, there is no evidence that periodontal disease affects serum alkaline phosphatase levels. Unfortunately, there is little information on changes in serum bone-specific alkaline phosphatase levels related to periodontal disease in HD patients. In an animal model, experimental periodontitis was reported to affect serum levels of bone-specific alkaline phosphatase [52]. Thus, there is a possibility that bone-specific alkaline phosphatase reflects periodontal bone loss and/or its metabolism in patients with HD. These results are shown in Table 4.

Table 4. Correlations of alkaline phosphatase, calcium, parathyroid hormone, and phosphorous with periodontal disease in patients receiving hemodialysis.

	n	Correlation with Periodontal Disease or Its Severity	Author/Year/Ref
ALP	96	Not different between no disease and periodontal disease	Rodrigues/2014/[13]
	128	Not different between no disease and periodontal disease	Cholewa/2018/[10]
Ca	96	Not different between no disease and periodontal disease	Rodrigues/2014/[13]
	136	Not different between no disease and periodontal disease	Hou/2017/[36]
	57	Not different between gingivitis and periodontitis	Naghsh/2017/[48]
	128	Not different between healthy/gingivitis and periodontitis	Cholewa/2018/[10]
PTH	35	Not correlated with periodontal indices	Frankenthal/2002/[51]
	253	Not correlated with periodontitis severity	Chen/2006/[35]
	136	Not different between no disease and periodontal disease	Hou/2017/[36]
	128	Not different between healthy/gingivitis and periodontitis	Cholewa/2018/[10]
P	96	Lower in periodontal disease versus no disease	Rodrigues/2014/[13]
	136	Not different between no disease and periodontal disease	Hou/2017/[36]
	57	Not different between gingivitis and periodontitis	Naghsh/2017/[48]
	128	Not different between healthy/gingivitis and periodontitis	Cholewa/2018/[10]

ALP; alkaline phosphatase, Ca; calcium, PTH; parathyroid hormone, P; phosphorous.

3.1.4. Hematological Data

Several investigators have reported that there was no significant correlation between periodontitis and hematological data, such as white blood cell and platelet counts, and hematocrit [11,13,28,35,48]. However, others have found that the presence of periodontal disease was positively correlated with white blood cell count ($p < 0.001$), but not with hemoglobin levels or platelet count [36]. Such increases in white blood cell count might be due to local and/or systematic inflammation. However, to our knowledge, a significant correlation between periodontal disease and white blood cell counts was found in only one study [36]. In addition, the number of white blood cells in the gingival crevicular fluid of HD patients with periodontal disease (mean/SD: 6.05/1.81 k/μL) was significantly lower ($p < 0.001$) than that in a control group (7.02/1.30 k/μL) [53]. Based on these findings, the impact of inflammation on circulating white blood cell counts in HD patients with periodontal disease can be considered minimal.

Periodontal treatment has also been reported to significantly increase hemoglobin levels, from 9.4 g/dL to 10.6 g/dL ($p = 0.009$) [30]. In addition, hemoglobin levels in HD patients receiving periodontal treatment (11.7/1.5 mg/dL) were significantly higher ($p = 0.039$) when compared to untreated patients (10.9/1.6 mg/dL) [37]. Thus, anemia might be associated with periodontal disease in HD patients. In general, various factors can affect the anemic status of HD patients, including administration of recombinant erythropoietin and iron, nutrition, inflammation, and dialysis dose. Regarding iron deficiency-related markers, serum ferritin levels have been reported to be positively associated with periodontitis severity in 253 HD patients [35]. However, interpretation of this finding is difficult because serum ferritin levels are recognized to be not only a marker of bone marrow iron stores but also inflammation [54,55]. In addition, the role of inflammation and serum ferritin levels in HD patients also depends on iron sufficiency [56]. Conversely, other reports have shown that serum transferrin levels in HD patients with periodontitis (mean/SD; 211.7/68.2 mg/dL) were similar ($p = 0.11$) to those without periodontitis (263.8/81.4 mg/dL) [13]. Thus, the impact of iron metabolism and storage on anemia caused by periodontal disease in HD patients is not fully understood and we believe that further studies are necessary to reach a definitive conclusion [48].

3.2. *Correlation with Duration of HD*

Various physiological functions and pathological conditions are mediated by long term HD [56–60]. Regarding periodontitis, the lack of a significant correlation between severity of the disease and the duration of HD has been reported in 103 HD patients [10]. Likewise, no significant relationships between HD duration and the prevalence and/or severity of periodontal disease have been reported by other investigators [9,11,14,41,61]. Furthermore, one report indicated that periodontal indices, such as PI, GI, and PPD, in HD patients were similar to those in healthy controls, and these values showed no variation during the first 5 years of HD [16]. However, that study also demonstrated that a significant increase in these values was detected during the second 5-year period, and a significantly greater increase was observed after 10 years [16]. In short, their results showed that these periodontal indices worsened with longer duration of HD. In addition, another report showed that GI and PPD scores were significantly higher in subgroups receiving HD for 3 or more years ($p \leq 0.001$ and < 0.001, respectively), and were positively correlated with HD duration ($r = 0.48$; $p < 0.001$ and $r = 0.48$; $p < 0.001$, respectively) [15]. Furthermore, another study confirmed the correlation between duration of HD and GI or PPD ($r = 0.27$; $p = 0.008$ or r = 0.39, $p < 0.001$, respectively) [62]. Thus, several reports have indicated a positive correlation between longer dialysis duration and periodontal disease-related parameters in HD patients [15,16,35,44], and a multivariate analysis model including age, DM, smoking status, and serum albumin level confirmed these findings [35].

Conversely, there have been conflicting results regarding the relationship between HD duration and decayed, missing, and filled teeth (DMFT). In short, although Bayrakter et al. reported that HD duration was positively correlated with missing ($r = 0.26$, $p = 0.024$), but not with decayed, filled teeth, or the DMFT index, Sekiguchi et al. found that HD duration was correlated with decayed teeth ($r = 0.42$, $p < 0.001$) and the DMFT index ($r = 0.28$, $p = 0.006$), but not with missing and filled teeth [15,62]. Thus, the relationship between the prevalence and/or severity of periodontitis and duration of HD is still under debate. This discrepancy may be due to differences in patient backgrounds and lifestyle habits, as various factors including age, diabetes, and smoking status, may have affected the pathogenesis and progression of periodontitis [35]. Furthermore, negligence of oral hygiene and a period of pre-dialysis with CKD are the main causes of higher prevalence and severity of periodontitis in HD patients rather than uremic conditions [10]. Conversely, a study has also reported that the duration of HD was not associated with specific microbiota or biofilms in 52 HD patients [63]. In this review, we would like to emphasize that duration of HD is one of the most powerful predictors of HD-induced complications and survival. Finally, more detailed investigations considering factors such as patient background, lifestyle habits, microbiota, complications, quantity, and method of HD are important to further clarify this issue.

3.3. Correlation with an Immune Response

A variety of immune cells, such as monocytes and dendritic cells, in periodontal tissues recognize and/or phagocytose bacteria, and subsequently secret various inflammatory mediators including ILs, TNF-α, vascular endothelial growth factor, and matrix metalloproteinase [33,64,65]. Furthermore, intervention studies have shown that treatment of periodontal disease decreased systemic levels of IL-6 and CRP [29]. Thus, the above evidence suggests that periodontal disease may mediate the immune response in patients receiving HD.

It has been suggested that a weak immune response underlies the increased incidence and rapid progression of periodontitis in patients with HD [66]. In short, the immune system in HD patients, especially those with DM-induced ESRD, might be unable to fend off the bacteria. In addition to this immune vulnerability, deteriorated dental and oral status due to greater plaque accumulation, dental calculus, salivary urea concentration, and salivary pH levels have been suggested to be related the high frequency of periodontal diseases [66,67]. Furthermore, poor oral hygiene due to gingival bleeding and decreased SFR compared to healthy persons is likely to be associated with persistent inflammation of periodontal tissues in HD patients [61,63,66,68,69]. In fact, a study with a large population (n = 4205 adults) showed that poorer dental health was positively associated with early all-cause death and cardiovascular diseases [70]. Finally, this chronic inflammation and consistent bacterial infection under weak immune responses is speculated to contribute to spreading of bacteria from the focal periodontal tissues into the bloodstream, and to the subsequent systematic inflammation in patients with HD.

The cytokine levels in the periodontium of HD patients have been previously investigated [53]. In that study, TNF-α and IL-8 were measured in the gingival fluids of 43 HD patients. The results showed that gingival fluid levels of TNF-α in HD patients (31.4/1.41 pg/mL) was nearly ten times as high as those in healthy controls (3.06/0.15; $p < 0.001$) [53]. A similar significant difference in IL-8 levels was also detected (90.98/94.03 and 35.05/16.86 pg/mL, respectively; $p < 0.001$) [53]. Furthermore, TNF-α levels in the gingival crevicular fluids were positively associated with PI, GI, and PPD ($p < 0.001$) in HD patients, and similar positive correlations were also detected between IL-8, and PI ($p = 0.002$), GI ($p = 0.002$), and PPD ($p = 0.012$) [53]. Based on these observations, TNF-α and IL-8 expression in the periodontal pocket is speculated to play crucial roles in the pathogenesis, development, and immune response to periodontal disease in HD patients. Nevertheless, there is no general agreement on the relationship between periodontal disease and gingival crevicular fluid levels of TNF-α and IL-8 in patients with normal renal function. In short, the levels of these cytokines in patients with periodontal disease were significantly higher than in healthy controls [71]; however, other investigators have shown that gingival crevicular fluid levels of TNF-α and IL-8 in periodontitis patients were similar to non-periodontitis patients [72,73]. Indeed, both of TNF-α and IL-8 levels in the gingival crevicular fluids of HD patients with periodontitis were reportedly not significantly different compared to patients with gingivitis ($p = 0.213$ and 0.823, respectively) [53]. However, we should also note that IL-1ra, IL-6, and interferon-γ levels in gingival crevicular fluids were significantly correlated to serum levels, whereas TNF-α and IL-8 were not identified in the serum of periodontitis patients with normal renal function, [74]; however, similar analyses have not been performed in HD patients to date. Thus, the pathological roles of TNF-α and IL-8 in periodontal disease in HD patients are not fully understood. The immune system is regulated by numerous cytokines, growth factors, and immune response-related molecules. However, unfortunately, immune function in the context of periodontal disease in HD patients is only partially understood. We strongly suggest that more detailed studies are necessary to understand the pathological characteristics of periodontal disease in patients undergoing dialysis.

3.4. *Correlation with Cardiovascular Diseases, Metabolic Syndromes, and Pneumonia*

There is a general agreement that the most important comorbidities and/or causes of death in HD patients are cardiovascular disease and DM [11,37,75]. Therefore, in this section, we reviewed the impact of periodontal disease on cardiovascular diseases in HD patients. In addition, we also reported findings regarding metabolic syndrome and pneumonia because of their frequency and significant contributions to mortality in patients with HD. DM was also discussed in the following section.

3.4.1. Cardiovascular Disease

Kaplan–Meier survival analyses have shown that cardiovascular disease-free survival rates in HD patients with moderate/severe periodontitis (defined as 2 or more teeth with at least 6 mm of inter-proximal attachment loss) were significantly worse ($p = 0.01$) compared to those with no/mild periodontitis [3]. In addition, a multivariate analysis model including age, center, sex, dialysis vintage, smoking status, cause of ESRD, DM, and hypertension demonstrated that moderate/severe periodontitis was an independent predictor of cardiovascular diseases in HD patients (hazard ratio = 5.0, 95% CI; 1.2–19.1, $p = 0.02$) compared to no/mild periodontitis [3]. However, the study also showed that periodontitis does not play a significant role in all-cause mortality among patients with HD (hazard ratio = 1.8 and 95% CI; 0.7–4.5) [3]. In contrast, other investigators showed that periodontal disease was significantly associated with risks of both cardiovascular-related and all-cause mortality [11]. Briefly, Kaplan–Meier survival curves showed that the cumulative survival rates in HD patients with severe periodontitis were significantly worse ($p < 0.001$) than in HD patients with no/mild or moderate periodontitis [11]. In addition, they found that the overall mortality rates in the no/mild ($n = 104$), moderate ($n = 98$), and severe periodontitis ($n = 51$) groups were 24.0%, 41.8%, and 70.6%, respectively, a statistically significant difference ($p < 0.001$) [11]. Interestingly, this study also showed that in a multivariate analysis model including age, serum levels of albumin, hs-CRP, the Charlson Comorbidity index score, education level, and history of smoking, severe periodontitis was an independent risk factor for all-cause mortality (hazard ratio = 1.83, 95% CI; 1.04–3.24, $p < 0.05$), but not cardiovascular-related diseases (hazard ratio = 1.95, 95% CI; 0.90–4.23, $p = 0.09$) [11]. To summarize, while a prior study had demonstrated that periodontitis is closely associated with mortality from cardiovascular disease, but not with all-cause mortality, the latter study showed opposing results.

A contrasting opinion regarding how periodontitis affects the risk for all-cause and cardiovascular mortality in patients on HD has been raised [44]. In short, the risk of all-cause and cardiovascular disease morality in HD patients with moderate-severe periodontitis was lower (hazard ratio = 0.74, CI = 0.61–0.90 and 0.67, 0.51–0.88, respectively) compared to those with none/mild periodontitis [44]. Importantly, these analyses were performed in propensity-matched cohorts.

3.4.2. Metabolic Syndromes and Pneumonia

Poor oral heath was reported to be associated with metabolic syndrome in 312 HD patients [76]. Briefly, HD patients with metabolic syndrome ($n = 145$) had a higher score compared to those without metabolic syndrome ($n = 108$) in terms of PI (mean/SD; 2.23/0.05 vs. 2.03/0.06; $p = 0.01$), GI (1.63/0.07 vs. 1.33/0.08; $p = 0.003$), and PDI (4.35/0.10 vs. 3.84/0.14; $p = 0.002$) [76]. In addition, they found that metabolic syndrome was positively associated with the severity of periodontitis ($p = 0.002$), and multivariate analysis also showed that moderate or severe periodontitis was an independent risk factor for metabolic syndrome in HD patients (odds ratio; 2.74, 95% CI; 1.29–5.79, $p = 0.008$) [76]. Furthermore, other investigators have compared periodontal indices in HD patients with and without metabolic syndrome [77]. The authors found that bone resorption in the metabolic syndrome group (mean/SD: 1.99/0.39 mm) was significantly higher than in the non-metabolic syndrome group (1.45/0.12 mm) [77]. In addition, PPD showed significant differences between the metabolic syndrome and non-metabolic syndrome groups (mean/SD: 2.73/0.47 and 2.17/0.18, respectively; $p < 0.05$).

Conversely, the cumulative incidence of pneumonia mortality in HD patients with periodontal disease was found to be significantly higher than in HD patients without periodontal disease ($p < 0.01$) [41]. Interestingly, another report showed contrasting findings where intensive treatment of periodontal disease led to a reduced risk of acute and sub-acute pneumonia (hazard ratio; 0.77, 95% CI; 0.65–0.78, $p < 0.001$) in patients with HD [78]. Incidentally, this study also demonstrated that periodontal disease treatment in HD patients was associated with a lower risk of endocarditis (hazard ratio; 0.54, 95% CI; 0.35–0.84, $p < 0.01$) and osteomyelitis (hazard ratio; 0.77, 95% CI; 0.62–0.96, $p < 0.05$) [78]. Thus, periodontal disease is speculated to have played an important role in the pathogenesis and mortality due to metabolic syndrome and pneumonia in HD patients.

3.5. *Diabetic and Non-Diabetic Nephropathy*

Currently, there is a general agreement that DM is a major cause of dialysis. In other words, many patients with dialysis have been receiving treatment for DM for a long time. Conversely, DM is considered to be one of the major causes of periodontal diseases [79,80]. It has been speculated that HD patients with DM have higher risk of periodontal diseases compared to those without DM. Unfortunately, few studies on the prevalence and severity of periodontal disease in HD patients with DM have been performed, and there is no systematic review on this issue to date.

3.5.1. Comparison of the Prevalence

In Japan, a cross-sectional study composed of HD patients with DM ($n = 29$), HD patients with chronic kidney nephropathy (CGN; $n = 69$), and a control group ($n = 106$) was performed. The study showed that mean/SD number of teeth present in HD patients with DM (17.9/9.8) was significantly lower ($p < 0.05$) compared to those with CGN (24.1/6.8) and the control group (25.3/5.8) [81]. In addition, the same study showed that the percentage of sites with bleeding on probing in HD patients with DM (22.2%) was significantly higher ($p < 0.05$) than in those with CGN (15.9%) and in controls (9.3%) [81]. The authors indicated that the reason for this difference in periodontal conditions between HD patients with DM and those with CGN were unclear; however, they speculated that various factors, such as healthy behavior, social, economic, and environmental status, and mental and systemic conditions, might influence the oral status in these patients [81]. Furthermore, the authors found that the SFR and total score of xerostomia in HD patients with DM or those with CGN were significantly different than those of the control group; however, these periodontitis-related parameters were similar between DM and CGN patients [81]. Thus, the oral health status in patients with renal dysfunction was worse than that of individuals with normal renal function, albeit with similarities observed between HD patients with DM or GCN. Interestingly, they showed that smoking status was significantly associated with the number of teeth in HD patients with DM. Smoking is a well-known risk factor for periodontitis and teeth loss, and it is also associated with development of DM. [82,83]. Thus, smoking played an important role, both directly and indirectly, in the oral health of HD patients with DM [81].

In contrast, the prevalence of moderate or severe periodontitis in HD patients with DM (74/76 patients = 97.4%) was reported to be similar to that of those without DM (51/53 ones = 96.2%), and the severity of periodontitis was not significantly associated with DM status ($p = 0.71$) [84]. In addition, this study showed that various periodontal findings, such as the PBI, PPD, CAL, and bleeding on probing, showed no significant differences in HD patients with and without DM ($p = 0.72$, 0.40, 0.58, and 0.79, respectively) [84]. Thus, the impact of diabetes on the prevalence and/or severity of periodontal disease in HD patients must be clarified by further investigations.

Interestingly, the prevalence of a variety of bacteria differed between HD patients with and without DM (*Capnocytophaga* species $p = 0.02$; *Eubacterium nodatum*, $p = 0.02$; *Parvimonas micra*, $p = 0.03$, *Porphyromonas gingivalis*, $p = 0.02$) [84]. However, the authors could not definitively conclude on the relationships between periodontitis and DM in patients with HD due to several limitations; for example, the plaque index was not assessed, the mean age of patients was different, and the study was performed across multiple centers. However, they concluded that DM has no decisive influence on periodontal conditions in HD patients [84]. Nevertheless, we should consider that their study population included HD patients with well-controlled DM (mean/SD hemoglobin A1c level = 6.3/2.7).

3.5.2. Objective and Subjective Manifestations

The first comparative study of oral health, dental conditions, and periodontal status in HD patients with and without DM was reported in 2005 [85]. Regarding objective manifestations, the study showed that the percentage of HD patients with DM exhibiting uremic odor (12/43 patients; 27.9%) was significantly lower ($p = 0.018$) compared to those without DM (42/85 patients; 49.4%). However, a similar significant difference was not found in tongue coating, mucosa petechia, or ecchymosis [85]. Conversely, other investigators found that all of these objective manifestations, including uremic odor, did not differ significantly between HD patients with ($n = 46$) and without DM ($n = 54$) [86]. Nevertheless, another report showed that uremic odor, tongue coating, and mucosa petechia were significantly different between the two patient groups ($p = 0.044$, 0.026, and 0.008, respectively) [87].

Another report using a visual analogue scale to assess subjective symptoms, including dry mouth (xerostomia), taste change (dysgeusia), and tongue/mucosa pain, showed that HD patients with DM had significantly higher scores than those without DM ($p = 0.040$, 0.004, and 0.018, respectively) [85]. This was in contrast to findings indicating that DM status in HD patients was significantly associated with dysgeusia ($p = 0.008$), but not with dry mouth or mucosal pain [87]. Thus, these 2 studies showed that taste change (dysgeusia) in HD patients differed significantly among patients with and without DM; however, another report showed that the frequency of dysgeusia was similar [86]. In addition, no significant relationships with regard to diabetic status or xerostomia have been reported by other studies [81,87]. Thus, there is no general agreement concerning differences in objective and subjective manifestations of HD patients with and without DM.

3.5.3. The Community Periodontal Index and DMFT Index

As mentioned above, the DMFT index has been commonly used to determine the incidence of dental caries, while the community periodontal index (CPI) has been used to assess periodontal condition using a mouth mirror and a probe according to the World Health Organization criteria [88]. The DMFT index consists of 4 parameters (decayed, missing, fillings, and total teeth) and the CPI consists of 6 (healthy periodontium, bleeding on probing, calculus deposition, probing depth of 4 to 5 mm, probing depth of 6 mm or deeper, and 3 or more teeth missing).

We compared the DMFT index of HD patients with and without DM in Table 5. The overall DMFT score in HD patients, which was calculated as the sum of the number of decayed, missing, and filled teeth, was remarkably higher ($p = 0.001$) in DM patients (19.93/81.9) than in non-DM patients (14.26/9.19) [85]. This finding was supported by other investigators [87]. However, the overall DMFT score was not associated with DM status in HD patients (Table 5) [83,85]. Nevertheless, as shown in Table 4, one report showed that the DM status was significantly associated with each index item, while others showed opposing results [84,85,87].

Table 5. Decayed, missing, and filled teeth (DMFT) index in hemodialysis patients with and without diabetes.

Author/Year/Ref	Decay	Missing	Filled	Overall
Chuang/2005/[85]	Not significant	↑ ($p = 0.039$)	Not significant	↑ ($p = 0.001$)
Murali/2012/[86]	–	–	–	Not significant
Swapna/2013/[87]	↑ ($p < 0.001$)	Not significant	↑ ($p < 0.001$)	↑ ($p < 0.001$)
Schmalz/2017/[84]	Not significant	Not significant	Not significant	Not significant

↑ means that variables in the diabetic group were higher compared to the non-diabetic group.

Evaluating the CPI in HP patients, Chuang et al. [85] reported that there was a borderline significant difference in patients with diabetic and non-diabetic nephropathy ($p = 0.055$). Murali et al. [86] also found no significant association between DM status and CPI in HD patients. These results were obtained by using the chi-square test to compare diabetic nephropathy and CPI codes. In contrast, a different study reported that one CPI variable, probing depth of 6 mm or deeper, in the DM patients receiving HD group was significantly higher ($p = 0.015$) than in non-DM patients, whereas other codes, such as calculus deposition and probing depth of 4 to 5 mm, were not [87]. Thus, with the exception of one code (probing depth 6 mm or deeper), a significant difference in CPI scores was not found in previous studies. However, in contrast to this report, another study reported that the percentage of bleeding on probing and sites in HD patients with DM was significantly higher than in non-DM patients (mean/SD%: 13.3/22.2 versus 8.2/15.9; $p < 0.05$) [81]. However, we must note that this result was obtained using the Tukey HSD test, which is a multiple comparison test, to compare among patients on HD for diabetic nephropathy and chronic glomerulonephritis and healthy controls.

3.5.4. Properties of Saliva

Regarding SFRs in patients with HD, unstimulated and stimulated salivary flow, and buffering capacity of stimulated saliva have been reported to have no significant relationship with diabetic status ($p = 0.15$, 0.20, and 1.0, respectively) [83], which was also supported by another study [81]. However, Sung et al. [89] reported that the unstimulated whole SFR in 68 diabetic HD patients was significantly lower ($p = 0.032$) than that in 116 non-diabetic HD patients.

The salivary pH level in DM patients (mean/SD; 7.97/0.67) showed a trend ($p = 0.063$) towards being lower than that of patients without DM (8.22/0.44) [85]. Similarly, another study showed that the frequency of salivary pH >7.0 in the DM patients was lower compared to the non-DM patients (17.0% versus 34.0%, respectively; $p = 0.056$); however, the frequency of salivary pH <7.0 in both patient groups was similar (DM; 36.2% and non-DM; 34.0%; $p = 0.823$) [87]. Chi-square analysis showed that the relationship between diabetic status and salivary pH level was not significant ($p = 0.623$) [87]. In contrast, Schmalz et al. [84] reported an opposing finding, where the mean/SD salivary pH level of HD patients with DM (6.7/0.7) was significantly lower than that of non-DM patients (7.0/0.9; $p < 0.01$) [84].

As shown in Table 6, the changes in the SFR and pH level according to diabetic status are unclear. While the precise reasons underlying this discrepancy are unknown, differences in patients' backgrounds, history of chronic renal failure and HD, duration of DM, and hemoglobin A1c level may be factors. Conversely, an investigation into the relationships between periodontal condition-related parameters and glycemic control in HD patients with DM showed that tongue coating, dry mouth, and tongue/mucosal pain were significantly correlated with hemoglobin A1c levels ($p = 0.001$, 0.001, and 0.004, respectively); however, salivary pH levels were decreased with higher hemoglobin A1c levels (mean/SD pH level in hemoglobin A1c level ≤6%; 8.20/0.36, 6.1%–9%; 8.00/0.58, ≥9.1%; 7.46/1.07), but the differences were not statistically significant ($p = 0.086$) [85]. Therefore, we emphasized the importance of more detailed investigations with a larger study population to arrive at a conclusion.

Table 6. Comparison of properties of saliva in diabetic and non-diabetic patients.

Properties of Saliva	No. of DM/non-DM	Compared tonon-Diabetic Patients	Author/Year/Ref
Salivary flow rate	116/68	Lower	Sung/2006/[89]
	29/69	Not significant	Teratani/2013/[81]
	66/93	Not significant	Schmalz/2017/[84]
Salivary pH level	85/43	Not significant	Chung/2005/[85]
	47/50	Not significant	Swapna/2013/[87]
	66/93	Lower	Schmalz/2017/[84]

DM; diabetic mellitus, Ref; Reference.

3.6. *Periodontal Indices and Salivary Status with Peritoneal Dialysis*

In the above sections, we discussed the changes in periodontal indices and salivary findings in response to HD. However, several reports have shown differences in these parameters between PD and HD patients, and controls (Table 7). For example, Bayraktar et al. [90]. reported that plaque and calculus accumulation in the HD and PD groups were higher than in controls. However, gingival inflammation in PD patients was significantly lower than in HD patients [22,68,90]. Moreover, the SFR in the PD group was significantly higher than that in the HD group, although both groups had significantly lower values than the control group [68]. The reduction in the SFR has been known to increase the risk of caries [91]. In fact, the authors found that the number of filled teeth was higher in the PD group than in the HD group. Differences in the SFR might be associated with better volume status in the PD group and in the relatively more liberal fluid intake because of residual renal function. In fact, the fluid dynamics of the gingiva might influence gingival health in children undergoing PD therapy [92]. We have summarized these results in Table 6. These results seem to show that the pattern of differences in periodontal indices and salivary status between healthy controls and patients with PD was not replicated between HD and PD patients. However, the data was insufficient to draw definitive conclusions.

Table 7. Periodontal parameters in the peritoneal dialysis, hemodialysis, and healthy groups.

Variables	PD Compared in the Healthy Group		PD Compared to HD	
	Difference	Author/Years/Ref	Differences	Author/Years/Ref
GI	NS	Bayrakter/2008, 2009/[68,90]	Lower	Borawski/2007, 2008/[4,90]
PBI	NS	Bayrakter/2008, 2009/[68,90]	Lower	Borawski/2007/[4] Bayrakter/2008/[90]
PI	Higher	Borawski/2007/[4] Bayrakter/2008/[90]	NS	Bayrakter/2008, 2009 /[68,90]
CSI	Higher	Bayrakter/2008/[90]	NS	Bayrakter/2008/[90]
S-pH	Higher	Bayrakter/2009/[68]	Higher	Bayrakter/2009/[68]
SFR	NS	Bayrakter/2009/[68]	Higher	Bayrakter/2009/[68]
PPD	NS	Bayrakter/2008/[90]	NS	Bayrakter/2008/[90]

GI; gingival index, PBI; papillary bleeding index, PI; plaque index, CSI; calculus surface index, S-; salivary-, SFR; salivary flow rate, PPD; probing pocket depth, NS: not significant, Ref; reference.

4. Management of Periodontal Disease

Many investigators have suggested that correct diagnosis and appropriate treatment of periodontal disease are important not only to the improvement of oral infection and inflammation, but also to maintain systemic health in patients receiving dialysis, and that managing oral health can effectively prolong survival [15–17,23,41,61,70]. In fact, brushing the teeth twice daily led to a reduced chance of developing periodontal diseases than brushing once daily, and it was identified as an independent factor [36]. Furthermore, a lower frequency of visits to the dentist has also been reported to be positively associated with higher mortality in HD patients [37]. Conversely, this report also showed that although the mortality of HD patients with chronic periodontitis is worse than of those without, the survival rate of patients treated for chronic periodontitis was not significantly different from that of untreated patients ($p = 0.774$) [37]. Furthermore, Hou et al. emphasized that special efforts for the prevention and management of periodontal disease are important in elderly HD patients because aging is another risk factor for periodontal disease in HD patients [36]. In addition to the prevention of different complex diseases and the prolongation of survival, maintenance of oral health and treatment of periodontal disease are essential for dialysis patients waiting for renal transplantation because patients with active inflammation and/or severe periodontal disease are usually judged as unfit for transplantation.

Thus, many studies support the importance of maintenance of dental health and periodontal treatment in patients with dialysis. However, in the real world, approximately 70% of Japanese HD facilities have no registered dental clinic [93]. Consequently, collaboration with dental facilities was promoted as beneficial for maintenance and management of oral health in HD patients [93], and found support from other investigators [53]. In addition, education on preventive dental care is important to the collaboration with dentists [94]. The prevalence and severity of periodontal disease are reported to vary substantially according to country, rather than being rotted in individual patient characteristics or healthcare [75].

Thus, conscientious efforts are necessary to establish an effective management and/or treatment approach to oral health in patients receiving dialysis treatment. In addition, this system must be modified for different countries in accordance with their specific conditions, including causes of ESRD, complications, and lifestyle habits. However, we believe that such a management approach in collaboration with dentists is well worth implementing because management of oral health and periodontal disease leads to maintenance or improvement in the QoL, reduction of complications, and prolongation of survival in dialysis patients.

5. Conclusions and Future Perspectives

This review showed that periodontal diseases affect the inflammation, immune response, and nutritional status in patients on dialysis. In fact, the severity of periodontal disease was significantly associated with serum levels of CRP, albumin, and a variety of minerals. In addition, several inflammation-related cytokines and molecules, such as IL-6, Il-8, TNF-α, and PTX-3 were influenced by periodontal conditions. As a result, a significant association between periodontal disease and various pathological conditions, including cardiovascular disease, metabolic syndrome, and pneumonia, is observed. Furthermore, we showed how dialysis, especially HD, exacerbates oral conditions via disruption of salivary characteristics, such as pH and flow rate. The deterioration in oral and periodontal tissues subsequently leads to a high frequency and severity of periodontal disease. Importantly, DM plays important roles in these pathological mechanisms. These findings are summarized in Figure 1. Furthermore, based on these facts, we demonstrated that maintenance of oral health and treatment of periodontal disease are important to maintaining QoL, prevention of various pathological conditions, and prolongation of survival in patients with dialysis. Unfortunately, we found that it was difficult to conduct a focused and systematic study into the relationships between periodontal disease and dialysis-related factors. Although numerous studies have been performed, they exhibit significant heterogeneity in patient characteristics, such as age, diabetic nephropathy, duration of chronic kidney disease; and methods of dialysis, such as PD or HD, the specific machine and agents used, timing of sampling, and duration. Data on the pathological roles of periodontal disease in patients with PD in particular is insufficient for a systematic review. However, continuous technological development could enable us to identify new pathogens, determine their interactions, and assess periodontal disease-related parameters in patients on dialysis. In fact, we have developed a research strategy aimed at elucidating the molecular and immune-related mechanisms of periodontal disease in patients on dialysis using novel approaches [95,96]. We emphasized that further studies with larger populations and uniform design are required to determine the pathological significance of periodontal disease and the clinical utility of oral care in patients on dialysis.

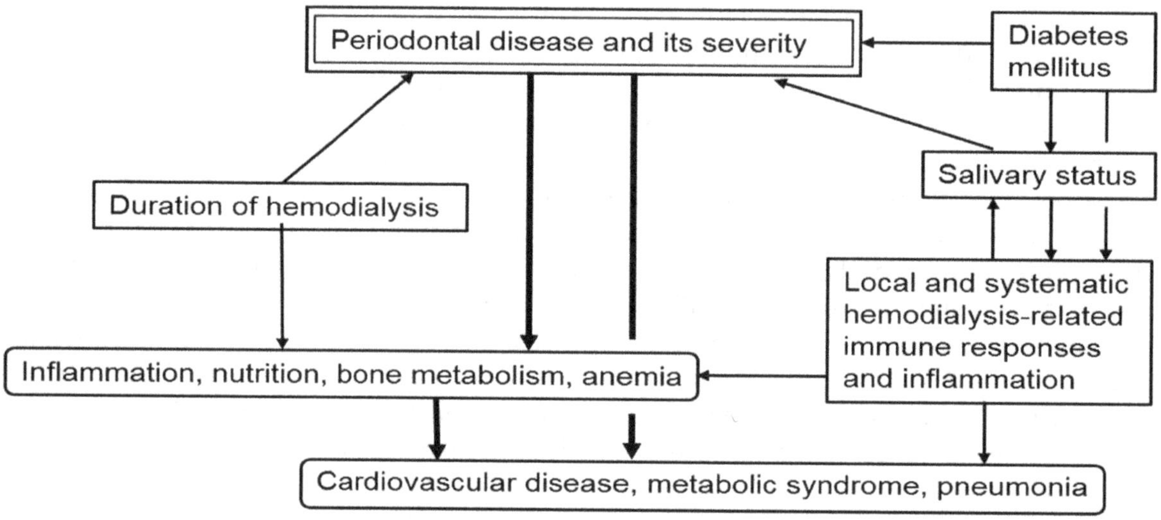

Figure 1. Schema of pathological roles played by periodontal disease in patients on hemodialysis.

Acknowledgments: We would like to thank Editage (www.editage.jp) for English language editing.

References

1. Fenton, S.S.; Schaubel, D.E.; Desmeules, M.; Morrison, H.I.; Mao, Y.; Copleston, P.; Jeffery, J.R.; Kjellstrand, C.M. Hemodialysis versus peritoneal dialysis: A comparison of adjusted mortality rates. *Am. J. Kidney Dis.* **1997**, *30*, 334–342. [CrossRef]
2. Pihlstrom, B.L.; Michalowicz, B.S.; Johnson, N.W. Periodontal diseases. *Lancet* **2005**, *366*, 1809–1820. [CrossRef]
3. Kshirsagar, A.V.; Craig, R.G.; Moss, K.L.; Beck, J.D.; Offenbacher, S.; Kotanko, P.; Klemmer, P.J.; Yoshino, M.; Levin, N.W.; Yip, J.K.; et al. Periodontal disease adversely affects the survival of patients with end-stage renal disease. *Kidney Int.* **2009**, *75*, 746–751. [CrossRef] [PubMed]
4. Borawski, J.; Wilczyńska-Borawska, M.; Stokowska, W.; Myśliwiec, M. The periodontal status of pre-dialysis chronic kidney disease and maintenance dialysis patients. *Nephrol. Dial. Transplant.* **2007**, *22*, 457–464. [CrossRef] [PubMed]
5. Kocyigit, I.; Yucel, H.E.; Cakmak, O.; Dogruel, F.; Durukan, D.B.; Korkar, H.; Unal, A.; Sipahioglu, M.H.; Oymak, O.; Gurgan, C.A.; et al. An ignored cause of inflammation in patients undergoing continuous ambulatory peritoneal dialysis: Periodontal problems. *Int. Urol. Nephrol.* **2014**, *46*, 2021–2028. [CrossRef] [PubMed]
6. Cengiz, M.I.; Bal, S.; Gökçay, S.; Cengiz, K. Does periodontal disease reflect atherosclerosis in continuous ambulatory peritoneal dialysis patients? *J. Periodontol.* **2007**, *78*, 1926–1934. [CrossRef] [PubMed]
7. Thorman, R.; Neovius, M.; Hylander, B. Clinical findings in oral health during progression of chronic kidney disease to end-stage renal disease in a Swedish population. *Scand. J. Urol. Nephrol.* **2009**, *43*, 154–159. [CrossRef]
8. Brito, F.; Almeida, S.; Figueredo, C.M.; Bregman, R.; Suassuna, J.H.; Fischer, R.G. Extent and severity of chronic periodontitis in chronic kidney disease patients. *J. Periodontal. Res.* **2012**, *47*, 426–430. [CrossRef]
9. Kim, Y.J.; Moura, L.M.; Caldas, C.P.; Perozini, C.; Ruivo, G.F.; Pallos, D. Evaluation of periodontal condition and risk in patients with chronic kidney disease on hemodialysis. *Einstein (Sao Paulo)* **2017**, *15*, 173–177. [CrossRef]
10. Cholewa, M.; Madziarska, K.; Radwan-Oczko, M. The association between periodontal conditions, inflammation, nutritional status and calcium-phosphate metabolism disorders in hemodialysis patients. *J. Appl. Oral Sci.* **2018**, *26*, e20170495. [CrossRef]

11. Chen, L.P.; Chiang, C.K.; Peng, Y.S.; Hsu, S.P.; Lin, C.Y.; Lai, C.F.; Hung, K.Y. Relationship between periodontal disease and mortality in patients treated with maintenance hemodialysis. *Am. J. Kidney Dis.* **2011**, *57*, 276–282. [CrossRef]
12. Yazdi, F.K.; Karimi, N.; Rasouli, M.; Roozbeh, J. Effect of nonsurgical periodontal treatment on C-reactive protein levels in maintenance hemodialysis patients. *Ren. Fail.* **2013**, *35*, 711–717. [CrossRef]
13. Rodrigues, V.P.; Libério, S.A.; Lopes, F.F.; Thomaz, E.B.; Guerra, R.N.; Gomes-Filho, I.S.; Pereira, A.L. Periodontal status and serum biomarkers levels in haemodialysis patients. *J. Clin. Periodontol.* **2014**, *41*, 862–868. [CrossRef]
14. Iwasaki, M.; Borgnakke, W.S.; Awano, S.; Yoshida, A.; Hamasaki, T.; Teratani, G.; Kataoka, S.; Kakuta, S.; Soh, I.; Ansai, T.; et al. Periodontitis and health-related quality of life in hemodialysis patients. *Clin. Exp. Dent. Res.* **2016**, *3*, 13–18. [CrossRef]
15. Bayraktar, G.; Kurtulus, I.; Duraduryan, A.; Cintan, S.; Kazancioglu, R.; Yildiz, A.; Bural, C.; Bozfakioglu, S.; Besler, M.; Trablus, S.; et al. Dental and periodontal findings in hemodialysis patients. *Oral Dis.* **2007**, *13*, 393–397. [CrossRef]
16. Cengiz, M.I.; Sümer, P.; Cengiz, S.; Yavuz, U. The effect of the duration of the dialysis in hemodialysis patients on dental and periodontal findings. *Oral Dis.* **2009**, *15*, 336–341. [CrossRef]
17. Altamimi, A.G.; AlBakr, S.A.; Alanazi, T.A.; Alshahrani, F.A.; Chalisserry, E.P.; Anil, S. Prevalence of periodontitis in patients undergoing hemodialysis: A case control study. *Mater. Sociomed.* **2018**, *30*, 58–61. [CrossRef]
18. Boros, P.; Miller, C.M. Hepatocyte growth factor: A multifunctional cytokine. *Lancet* **1995**, *345*, 293–295. [CrossRef]
19. Ohshima, M.; Noguchi, Y.; Ito, M.; Maeno, M.; Otsuka, K. Hepatocyte growth factor secreted by periodontal ligament and gingival fibroblasts is a major chemoattractant for gingival epithelial cells. *J. Periodontal. Res.* **2001**, *36*, 377–383. [CrossRef]
20. Ohshima, M.; Fujikawa, K.; Akutagawa, H.; Kato, T.; Ito, K.; Otsuka, K. Hepatocyte growth factor in saliva: A possible marker for periodontal disease status. *J. Oral Sci.* **2002**, *44*, 35–39. [CrossRef]
21. Ohshima, M.; Sakai, A.; Ito, K.; Otsuka, K. Hepatocyte growth factor (HGF) in periodontal disease: Detection of HGF in gingival crevicular fluid. *J. Periodontal. Res.* **2002**, *37*, 8–14. [CrossRef]
22. Wilczyńska-Borawska, M.; Borawski, J.; Bagińska, J.; Małyszko, J.; Myśliwiec, M. Hepatocyte growth factor in saliva of patients with renal failure and periodontal disease. *Ren. Fail.* **2012**, *34*, 942–951. [CrossRef]
23. Tasdemir, Z.; Özsarı Tasdemir, F.; Gürgan, C.; Eroglu, E.; Gunturk, I.; Kocyigit, I. The effect of periodontal disease treatment in patients with continuous ambulatory peritoneal dialysis. *Int. Urol. Nephrol.* **2018**, *50*, 1519–1528. [CrossRef]
24. Keles, M.; Tozoglu, U.; Uyanik, A.; Eltas, A.; Bayindir, Y.Z.; Cetinkaya, R.; Bilge, O.M. Does peritoneal dialysis affect halitosis in patients with end-stage renal disease? *Perit. Dial. Int.* **2011**, *31*, 168–172.
25. Trimarchi, H.; Dicugno, M.; Muryan, A.; Lombi, F.; Iturbe, L.; Raña, M.S.; Young, P.; Nau, K.; Iriarte, R.; Pomeranz, V.; et al. Pro-calcitonin and inflammation in chronic hemodialysis. *Medicina (B Aires)* **2013**, *73*, 411–416.
26. Guo, M.; Chen, R.; Xiang, F.; Cao, X.; Hu, J.; Lu, Z.; Gong, S.; Chen, X.; Chen, X.; Ding, X.; et al. Decreased percentage of memory B cells is independently associated with increased susceptibility to infection in patients on maintenance hemodialysis. *Int. Urol. Nephrol.* **2018**, *50*, 2081–2090. [CrossRef]
27. Omari, A.M.; Omari, L.S.; Dagash, H.H.; Sweileh, W.M.; Natour, N.; Zyoud, S.H. Assessment of nutritional status in the maintenance of haemodialysis patients: A cross-sectional study from Palestine. *BMC Nephrol.* **2019**, *20*, 92. [CrossRef]
28. Noack, B.; Genco, R.J.; Trevisan, M.; Grossi, S.; Zambon, J.J.; De Nardin, E. Periodontal infections contribute to elevated systemic C-reactive protein level. *J. Periodontol.* **2001**, *72*, 1221–1227. [CrossRef]
29. D'Aiuto, F.; Nibali, L.; Parkar, M.; Suvan, J.; Tonetti, M.S. Short-term effects of intensive periodontal therapy on serum inflammatory markers and cholesterol. *J. Dent. Res.* **2005**, *84*, 269–273. [CrossRef]
30. Kadiroglu, A.K.; Kadiroglu, E.T.; Sit, D.; Dag, A.; Yilmaz, M.E. Periodontitis is an important and occult source of inflammation in hemodialysis patients. *Blood. Purif.* **2006**, *24*, 400–404. [CrossRef]
31. Zhao, D.; Zhang, S.; Chen, X.; Liu, W.; Sun, N.; Guo, Y.; Dong, Y.; Mo, A.; Yuan, Q. Evaluation of periodontitis and bone loss in patients undergoing hemodialysis. *J. Periodontol.* **2014**, *85*, 1515–1520. [CrossRef]

32. Franek, E.; Blaschyk, R.; Kolonko, A.; Mazur-Psonka, L.; Łangowska-Adamczyk, H.; Kokot, F.; Wiecek, A. Chronic periodontitis in hemodialysis patients with chronic kidney disease is associated with elevated serum C-reactive protein concentration and greater intima-media thickness of the carotid artery. *J. Nephrol.* **2006**, *19*, 346–351.
33. Kshirsagar, A.V.; Craig, R.G.; Beck, J.D.; Moss, K.; Offenbacher, S.; Kotanko, P.; Yoshino, M.; Levin, N.W.; Yip, J.K.; Almas, K.; et al. Severe periodontitis is associated with low serum albumin among patients on maintenance hemodialysis therapy. *Clin. J. Am. Soc. Nephrol.* **2007**, *2*, 239–244. [CrossRef]
34. Pallos, D.; Leão, M.V.; Togeiro, F.C.; Alegre, L.; Ricardo, L.H.; Perozini, C.; Ruivo, G.F. Salivary markers in patients with chronic renal failure. *Arch. Oral Biol.* **2015**, *60*, 1784–1788. [CrossRef]
35. Chen, L.P.; Chiang, C.K.; Chan, C.P.; Hung, K.Y.; Huang, C.S. Does periodontitis reflect inflammation and malnutrition status in hemodialysis patients? *Am. J. Kidney Dis.* **2006**, *47*, 815–822. [CrossRef]
36. Hou, Y.; Wang, X.; Zhang, C.X.; Wei, Y.D.; Jiang, L.L.; Zhu, X.Y.; Du, Y.J. Risk factors of periodontal disease in maintenance hemodialysis patients. *Medicina (Baltim.)* **2017**, *96*, e7892. [CrossRef]
37. de Souza, C.M.; Braosi, A.P.; Luczyszyn, S.M.; Olandoski, M.; Kotanko, P.; Craig, R.G.; Trevilatto, P.C.; Pecoits-Filho, R. Association among oral health parameters, periodontitis, and its treatment and mortality in patients undergoing hemodialysis. *J. Periodontol.* **2014**, *85*, e169–178. [CrossRef]
38. Siribamrungwong, M.; Puangpanngam, K. Treatment of periodontal diseases reduces chronic systemic inflammation in maintenance hemodialysis patients. *Ren. Fail.* **2012**, *34*, 171–175. [CrossRef]
39. Rahmati, M.A.; Craig, R.G.; Homel, P.; Kaysen, G.A.; Levin, N.W. Serum markers of periodontal disease status and inflammation in hemodialysis patients. *Am. J. Kidney Dis.* **2002**, *40*, 983–989. [CrossRef]
40. Mandic, A.; Cavar, I.; Skoro, I.; Tomic, I.; Ljubic, K.; Coric, S.; Mikulic, I.; Azinovic, I.; Pravdic, D. Body composition and inflammation in hemodialysis patients. *Apher. Dial.* **2017**, *21*, 556–564. [CrossRef]
41. Iwasaki, M.; Taylor, G.W.; Awano, S.; Yoshida, A.; Kataoka, S.; Ansai, T.; Nakamura, H. Periodontal disease and pneumonia mortality in haemodialysis patients: A 7-year cohort study. *J. Clin. Periodontol.* **2018**, *45*, 38–45. [CrossRef]
42. Choi, S.R.; Lee, Y.K.; Cho, A.J.; Park, H.C.; Han, C.H.; Choi, M.J.; Koo, J.R.; Yoon, J.W.; Noh, J.W. Malnutrition, inflammation, progression of vascular calcification and survival: Inter-relationships in hemodialysis patients. *PLoS ONE* **2019**, *14*, e0216415. [CrossRef]
43. Kanda, E.; Kato, A.; Masakane, I.; Kanno, Y. A new nutritional risk index for predicting mortality in hemodialysis patients: Nationwide cohort study. *PLoS ONE* **2019**, *14*, e0214524. [CrossRef]
44. Ruospo, M.; Palmer, S.C.; Wong, G.; Craig, J.C.; Petruzzi, M.; De Benedittis, M.; Ford, P.; Johnson, D.W.; Tonelli, M.; Natale, P.; et al. Periodontitis and early mortality among adults treated with hemodialysis: A multinational propensity-matched cohort study. *BMC Nephrol.* **2017**, *18*, 166. [CrossRef]
45. Matsuura, S.; Shirai, Y.; Kubo, M.; Nayama, C.; Okitsu, M.; Oiwa, Y.; Yasui, S.; Suzuki, Y.; Murata, T.; Ishikawa, E.; et al. Body fat mass is correlated with serum transthyretin levels in maintenance hemodialysis patients. *J. Med. Invest.* **2017**, *64*, 222–227. [CrossRef]
46. Avramovski, P.; Avramovska, M.; Sotiroski, K.; Sikole, A. Acute-phase proteins as promoters of abdominal aortic calcification in chronic dialysis patients. *Saudi. J. Kidney Dis. Transpl.* **2019**, *30*, 376–386. [CrossRef]
47. Kim, M.; Kim, C.S.; Bae, E.H.; Ma, S.K.; Kim, S.W. Risk factors for peptic ulcer disease in patients with end-stage renal disease receiving dialysis. *Kidney Res. Clin. Pr.* **2019**, *38*, 81–89. [CrossRef]
48. Naghsh, N.; Sabet, N.K.; Vahidi, F.; Mogharehabed, A.; Yaghini, J. Relationship between periodontal disease and serum factors in patients undergoing hemodialysis. *Open Dent. J.* **2017**, *11*, 701–709. [CrossRef]
49. Malhotra, R.; Grover, V.; Kapoor, A.; Kapur, R. Alkaline phosphatase as a periodontal disease marker. *Indian J. Dent. Res.* **2010**, *21*, 531–536. [CrossRef]
50. Tanaka, K.; Miyake, Y.; Okubo, H.; Hanioka, T.; Sasaki, S.; Miyatake, N.; Arakawa, M. Calcium intake is associated with decreased prevalence of periodontal disease in young Japanese women. *Nutr. J.* **2014**, *13*, 109. [CrossRef]
51. Frankenthal, S.; Nakhoul, F.; Machtei, E.E.; Green, J.; Ardekian, L.; Laufer, D.; Peled, M. The effect of secondary hyperparathyroidism and hemodialysis therapy on alveolar bone and periodontium. *J. Clin. Periodontol.* **2002**, *29*, 479–483. [CrossRef]
52. Sousa, L.H.; Linhares, E.V.; Alexandre, J.T.; Lisboa, M.R.; Furlaneto, F.; Freitas, R.; Ribeiro, I.; Val, D.; Marques, M.; Chaves, H.V.; et al. Effects of atorvastatin on periodontitis of rats subjected to glucocorticoid-induced osteoporosis. *J. Periodontol.* **2016**, *87*, 1206–1216. [CrossRef]

53. Dağ, A.; Firat, E.T.; Kadiroğlu, A.K.; Kale, E.; Yilmaz, M.E. Significance of elevated gingival crevicular fluid tumor necrosis factor-alpha and interleukin-8 levels in chronic hemodialysis patients with periodontal disease. *J. Periodontal. Res.* **2010**, *45*, 445–450.
54. Rocha, L.A.; Barreto, D.V.; Barreto, F.C.; Dias, C.B.; Moysés, R.; Silva, M.R.; Moura, L.A.; Draibe, S.A.; Jorgetti, V.; Carvalho, A.B.; et al. Serum ferritin level remains a reliable marker of bone marrow iron stores evaluated by histomorphometry in hemodialysis patients. *Clin. J. Am. Soc. Nephrol.* **2009**, *4*, 105–109. [CrossRef]
55. Kell, D.B.; Pretorius, E. Serum ferritin is an important inflammatory disease marker, as it is mainly a leakage product from damaged cells. *Metallomics* **2014**, *6*, 748–773. [CrossRef]
56. Kalantar-Zadeh, K.; Rodriguez, R.A.; Humphreys, M.H. Association between serum ferritin and measures of inflammation, nutrition and iron in haemodialysis patients. *Nephrol. Dial. Transpl.* **2004**, *19*, 141–149. [CrossRef]
57. Ganu, V.J.; Boima, V.; Adjei, D.N.; Yendork, J.S.; Dey, I.D.; Yorke, E.; Mate-Kole, C.C.; Mate-Kole, M.O. Depression and quality of life in patients on long term hemodialysis at a nationalhospital in Ghana: A cross-sectional study. *Ghana Med. J.* **2018**, *52*, 22–28. [CrossRef]
58. Kondo, T.; Sasa, N.; Yamada, H.; Takagi, T.; Iizuka, J.; Kobayashi, H.; Yoshida, K.; Fukuda, H.; Ishihara, H.; Tanabe, K.; et al. Acquired cystic disease-associated renal cell carcinoma is the most common subtype in long-term dialyzed patients: Central pathology results according to the 2016 WHO classification in a multi-institutional study. *Pathol. Int.* **2018**, *68*, 543–549. [CrossRef]
59. El-Gamasy, M.A. Study of some pulmonary function tests in Egyptian children with end-stage renal disease under regular hemodialysis in correlation with dialysis duration. *Saudi. J. Kidney Dis. Transpl.* **2019**, *30*, 119–128. [CrossRef]
60. Matsumoto, Y.; Mori, Y.; Kageyama, S.; Arihara, K.; Sato, H.; Nagata, K.; Shimada, Y.; Nojima, Y.; Iguchi, K.; Sugiyama, T. Changes in QTc interval in long-term hemodialysis patients. *PLoS ONE* **2019**, *14*, e0209297. [CrossRef]
61. Parkar, S.M.; Ajithkrishnan, C.G. Periodontal status in patients undergoing hemodialysis. *Indian J. Nephrol.* **2012**, *22*, 246–250. [CrossRef]
62. Sekiguchi, R.T.; Pannuti, C.M.; Silva, H.T., Jr.; Medina-Pestana, J.O.; Romito, G.A. Decrease in oral health may be associated with length of time since beginning dialysis. *Spec. Care Dent.* **2012**, *32*, 6–10. [CrossRef]
63. Castillo, A.; Mesa, F.; Liébana, J.; García-Martinez, O.; Ruiz, S.; García-Valdecasas, J.; O'Valle, F. Periodontal and oral microbiological status of an adult population undergoing haemodialysis: A cross-sectional study. *Oral Dis.* **2007**, *13*, 198–205. [CrossRef]
64. Tonetti, M.S.; Freiburghaus, K.; Lang, N.P.; Bickel, M. Detection of interleukin-8 and matrix metalloproteinases transcripts in healthy and diseased gingival biopsies by RNA/PCR. *J. Periodontal. Res.* **1993**, *28*, 511–513. [CrossRef]
65. Afacan, B.; Öztürk, V.Ö.; Paşalı, Ç.; Bozkurt, E.; Köse, T.; Emingil, G. Gingival crevicular fluid and salivary HIF-1α, VEGF, and TNF-α levels in periodontal health and disease. *J. Periodontol.* **2018**, in press. [CrossRef]
66. Sedý, J.; Horká, E.; Foltán, R.; Spacková, J.; Dusková, J. Mechanism of increased mortality in hemodialysed patients with periodontitis. *Med. Hypotheses* **2010**, *74*, 374–376. [CrossRef]
67. Craig, R.G. Interactions between chronic renal disease and periodontal disease. *Oral Dis.* **2008**, *14*, 1–7. [CrossRef]
68. Bayraktar, G.; Kurtulus, I.; Kazancioglu, R.; Bayramgurler, I.; Cintan, S.; Bural, C.; Bozfakioglu, S.; Issever, H.; Yildiz, A. Oral health and inflammation in patients with end-stage renal failure. *Perit. Dial. Int.* **2009**, *29*, 472–479.
69. Malekmakan, L.; Haghpanah, S.; Pakfetrat, M.; Ebrahimic, Z.; Hasanlic, E. Oral health status in Iranian hemodialysis patients. *Indian J. Nephrol.* **2011**, *21*, 235–238.
70. Palmer, S.C.; Ruospo, M.; Wong, G.; Craig, J.C.; Petruzzi, M.; De Benedittis, M.; Ford, P.; Johnson, D.W.; Tonelli, M.; Natale, P.; et al. ORAL-D Study Investigators. Dental health and mortality in people with end-stage kidney disease treated with hemodialysis: A multinational cohort study. *Am. J. Kidney Dis.* **2015**, *66*, 666–676. [CrossRef]
71. Lagdive, S.S.; Marawar, P.P.; Byakod, G.; Lagdive, S.B. Evaluation and comparison of interleukin-8 (IL-8) level in gingival crevicular fluid in health and severity of periodontal disease: A clinico-biochemical study. *Indian J. Dent. Res.* **2013**, *24*, 188–192. [CrossRef]

72. Branco-de-Almeida, L.S.; Cruz-Almeida, Y.; Gonzalez-Marrero, Y.; Huang, H.; Aukhil, I.; Harrison, P.; Wallet, S.M.; Shaddox, L.M. Local and plasma biomarker profiles in localized aggressive periodontitis. *JDR Clin. Trans. Res.* **2017**, *2*, 258–268. [CrossRef]
73. Chatzopoulos, G.S.; Mansky, K.C.; Lunos, S.; Costalonga, M.; Wolff, L.F. Sclerostin and WNT-5a gingival protein levels in chronic periodontitis and health. *J. Periodontal. Res.* **2019**, in press. [CrossRef]
74. Zekeridou, A.; Mombelli, A.; Cancela, J.; Courvoisier, D.; Giannopoulou, C. Systemic inflammatory burden and local inflammation in periodontitis: What is the link between inflammatory biomarkers in serum and gingival crevicular fluid? *Clin. Exp. Dent. Res.* **2019**, *5*, 128–135. [CrossRef]
75. Palmer, S.C.; Ruospo, M.; Wong, G.; Craig, J.C.; Petruzzi, M.; De Benedittis, M.; Ford, P.; Johnson, D.W.; Tonelli, M.; Natale, P.; et al. Patterns of oral disease in adults with chronic kidney disease treated with hemodialysis. *Nephrol. Dial. Transpl.* **2016**, *31*, 1647–1653. [CrossRef]
76. Chen, L.P.; Hsu, S.P.; Peng, Y.S.; Chiang, C.K.; Hung, K.Y. Periodontal disease is associated with metabolic syndrome in hemodialysis patients. *Nephrol. Dial. Transpl.* **2011**, *26*, 4068–4073. [CrossRef]
77. Tavakoli, M.; Izadi, M.; Yaghini, J.; Rastegari, A.; Abed, A.M. A survey on the effects of metabolic syndrome on the periodontal indices of hemodialysis patients. *Dent. Res. J. (Isfahan)* **2016**, *13*, 333–337.
78. Huang, S.T.; Lin, C.L.; Yu, T.M.; Wu, M.J.; Kao, C.H. Intensive periodontal treatment reduces risk of infection-related hospitalization in hemodialysis population: A nationwide population-based cohort study. *Medicina (Baltim.)* **2015**, *94*, e1436. [CrossRef]
79. Casanova, L.; Hughes, F.J.; Preshaw, P.M. Diabetes and periodontal disease: A two-way relationship. *Br. Dent. J.* **2014**, *217*, 433–437. [CrossRef]
80. Gayathri, S.; Elizabeth, K.; Sadasivan, A.; Arunima, P.R.; Jaya Kumar, K. Effect of initial periodontal therapy on serum nitric oxide levels in chronic periodontitis patients with or without type 2 diabetes mellitus. *J. Contemp. Dent. Pract.* **2019**, *20*, 197–203. [CrossRef]
81. Teratani, G.; Awano, S.; Soh, I.; Yoshida, A.; Kinoshita, N.; Hamasaki, T.; Takata, Y.; Sonoki, K.; Nakamura, H.; Ansai, T. Oral health in patients on haemodialysis for diabetic nephropathy and chronic glomerulonephritis. *Clin. Oral Investig.* **2013**, *17*, 483–489. [CrossRef]
82. Chambrone, L.; Chambrone, D.; Lima, L.A.; Chambrone, L.A. Predictors of tooth loss during long-term periodontal maintenance: A systematic review of observational studies. *J. Clin. Periodontol.* **2010**, *37*, 675–684. [CrossRef]
83. Psaltopoulou, T.; Ilias, I.; Alevizaki, M. The role of diet and lifestyle in primary, secondary, and tertiary diabetes prevention: A review of meta-analyses. *Rev. Diabet. Stud.* **2010**, *7*, 26–35. [CrossRef]
84. Schmalz, G.; Schiffers, N.; Schwabe, S.; Vasko, R.; Müller, G.A.; Haak, R.; Mausberg, R.F.; Ziebolz, D. Dental and periodontal health, and microbiological and salivary conditions in patients with or without diabetes undergoing haemodialysis. *Int. Dent. J.* **2017**, *67*, 186–193. [CrossRef]
85. Chuang, S.F.; Sung, J.M.; Kuo, S.C.; Huang, J.J.; Lee, S.Y. Oral and dental manifestations in diabetic and nondiabetic uremic patients receiving hemodialysis. *Oral Surg. Oral Med. Oral Pathol. Oral Radiol. Endod.* **2005**, *99*, 689–695. [CrossRef]
86. Murali, P.; Narasimhan, M.; Periasamy, S.; Harikrishnan, T.C. A comparison of oral and dental manifestations in diabetic and non-diabetic uremic patients receiving hemodialysis. *J. Oral Maxillofac. Pathol.* **2012**, *16*, 374–379. [CrossRef]
87. Swapna, L.A.; Reddy, R.S.; Ramesh, T.; Reddy, R.L.; Vijayalaxmi, N.; Karmakar, P.; Pradeep, K. Oral health status in haemodialysis patients. *J. Clin. Diagn. Res.* **2013**, *7*, 2047–2050. [CrossRef]
88. Pilot, T.; Miyazaki, H. Global results: 15 years of CPITN epidemiology. *Int. Dent. J.* **1994**, *44*, 553–560.
89. Sung, J.M.; Kuo, S.C.; Guo, H.R.; Chuang, S.F.; Lee, S.Y.; Huang, J.J. The role of oral dryness in interdialytic weight gain by diabetic and non-diabetic haemodialysis patients. *Nephrol. Dial. Transpl.* **2006**, *21*, 2521–2528. [CrossRef]
90. Bayraktar, G.; Kurtulus, I.; Kazancioglu, R.; Bayramgurler, I.; Cintan, S.; Bural, C.; Bozfakioglu, S.; Besler, M.; Trablus, S.; Issever, H.; et al. Evaluation of periodontal parameters in patients undergoing peritoneal dialysis or hemodialysis. *Oral Dis.* **2008**, *14*, 185–189. [CrossRef]
91. Vissink, A.; Panders, A.K.; Gravenmade, E.J.; Vermey, A. The causes and consequences of hyposalivation. *Ear Nose Throat J.* **1988**, *67*, 166–168, 173–176.
92. Sakallioğlu, E.E.; Lütfioğlu, M.; Ozkaya, O.; Aliyev, E.; Açikgöz, G.; Firatli, E. Fluid dynamics of gingiva and gingival health in children with end stage renal failure. *Arch. Oral Biol.* **2007**, *52*, 1194–1199. [CrossRef]

93. Yoshioka, M.; Shirayama, Y.; Imoto, I.; Hinode, D.; Yanagisawa, S.; Takeuchi, Y. Current status of collaborative relationships between dialysis facilities and dental facilities in Japan: Results of a nationwide survey. *BMC Nephrol.* **2015**, *16*, 17. [CrossRef]
94. Yoshioka, M.; Shirayama, Y.; Imoto, I.; Hinode, D.; Yanagisawa, S.; Takeuchi, Y.; Bando, T.; Yokota, N. Factors associated with regular dental visits among hemodialysis patients. *World J. Nephrol.* **2016**, *5*, 455–460. [CrossRef]
95. Ohyama, K.; Yoshimi, H.; Aibara, N.; Nakamura, Y.; Miyata, Y.; Sakai, H.; Fujita, F.; Imaizumi, Y.; Chauhan, A.K.; Kishikawa, N.; et al. Immune complexome analysis reveals the specific and frequent presence of immune complex antigens in lung cancer patients: A pilot study. *Int. J. Cancer.* **2017**, *140*, 370–380. [CrossRef]
96. Aibara, N.; Kamohara, C.; Chauhan, A.K.; Kishikawa, N.; Miyata, Y.; Nakashima, M.; Kuroda, N.; Ohyama, K. Selective, sensitive and comprehensive detection of immune complex antigens by immune complexome analysis with papain-digestion and elution. *J. Immunol. Methods* **2018**, *461*, 85–90. [CrossRef]

12

Pathological Characteristics of Periodontal Disease in Patients with Chronic Kidney Disease and Kidney Transplantation

Mineaki Kitamura [1,2], Yasushi Mochizuki [2,3], Yasuyoshi Miyata [3,*], Yoko Obata [1], Kensuke Mitsunari [3], Tomohiro Matsuo [3], Kojiro Ohba, Hiroshi Mukae [4], Atsutoshi Yoshimura [5], Tomoya Nishino [1] and Hideki Sakai [2,3]

1 Department of Nephrology, Nagasaki University Hospital, Nagasaki 852-8501, Japan
2 Division of Blood Purification, Nagasaki University Hospital, Nagasaki 852-8501, Japan
3 Department of Urology, Nagasaki University Graduate School of Biomedical Sciences, Nagasaki 852-8501, Japan
4 Department of Respiratory Medicine, Unit of Basic Medical Sciences, Nagasaki University Graduate School of Biomedical Sciences, Nagasaki 852-8501, Japan
5 Department of Periodontology and Endodontology, Nagasaki University Graduate School of Biomedical Sciences, Nagasaki 852-8501, Japan
* Correspondence: yasu-myt@nagasaki-u.ac.jp

Abstract: Chronic kidney disease (CKD) is recognized as an irreversible reduction of functional nephrons and leads to an increased risk of various pathological conditions, including cardiovascular disease and neurological disorders, such as coronary artery calcification, hypertension, and stroke. In addition, CKD patients have impaired immunity against bacteria and viruses. Conversely, kidney transplantation (KT) is performed for patients with end-stage renal disease as a renal replacement therapy. Although kidney function is almost normalized by KT, immunosuppressive therapy is essential to maintain kidney allograft function and to prevent rejection. However, these patients are more susceptible to infection due to the immunosuppressive therapy required to maintain kidney allograft function. Thus, both CKD and KT present disadvantages in terms of suppression of immune function. Periodontal disease is defined as a chronic infection and inflammation of oral and periodontal tissues. Periodontal disease is characterized by the destruction of connective tissues of the periodontium and alveolar bone, which may lead to not only local symptoms but also systemic diseases, such as cardiovascular diseases, diabetes, liver disease, chronic obstructive pulmonary disease, and several types of cancer. In addition, the prevalence and severity of periodontal disease are significantly associated with mortality. Many researchers pay special attention to the pathological roles and clinical impact of periodontal disease in patients with CKD or KT. In this review, we provide information regarding important modulators of periodontal disease to better understand the relationship between periodontal disease and CKD and/or KT. Furthermore; we evaluate the impact of periodontal disease on various pathological conditions in patients with CKD and KT. Moreover, pathogens of periodontal disease common to CKD and KT are also discussed. Finally, we examine the importance of periodontal care in these patients. Thus, this review provides a comprehensive overview of the pathological roles and clinical significance of periodontal disease in patients with CKD and KT.

Keywords: periodontal disease; chronic kidney disease; kidney transplantation; immunosuppressive therapy

1. Introduction

Chronic kidney disease (CKD) is defined as either the presence of kidney damage, such as proteinuria and hematuria, or decreased kidney function (estimated glomerular filtration rate (eGFR) < 60 mL/min/1.73 m^2 for >3 months) [1]. CKD is a crucial health issue, as it has a negative impact on prognosis and quality of life (QoL) due to the increasing risk of various pathological conditions including hypertension, diabetes, smoking, aging, autoimmune diseases, systemic inflammation, urinary tract infections, urinary stones, lower urinary tract obstruction, recovery from acute kidney injury, low birth weight, and drug toxicity [2–5]. Conversely, several risk factors of CKD, such as hypertension, diabetes, smoking, and aging have also been identified [1]. Thus, early recognition of CKD and the prevention of CKD progression are highly desirable. Furthermore, growing research has shown that periodontal disease and CKD are positively correlated, although periodontal disease is an important risk factor for CKD as it has the potential to be modified and treated. Several cohort studies have investigated the relationship between CKD and periodontal disease [6–8]. Systematic reviews have also reported that periodontal disease is associated with CKD [9–11]. Moreover, the severity of periodontal disease is correlated with a decline in kidney function [12]. Although periodontal disease is a mixed infection, gram-negative bacilli play a major role. *Porphyromonas gingivalis* is implicated in periodontal disease, and elevated levels of immunoglobulin G (IgG) antibodies against *P. gingivalis* were shown to positively correlate with the onset and progression of CKD [13]. Despite speculations that CKD is closely associated with the occurrence and progression of periodontal disease, detailed pathological characteristics at the molecular level and the clinical significance of periodontal disease in CKD patients are not fully understood and still remain unknown.

Renal replacement therapy is performed to maintain QoL and life in patients with end-stage renal disease (ESRD). As renal replacement therapy, peritoneal dialysis, hemodialysis, and kidney transplantation (KT) are usually selected according to the patient's wishes; his/her clinical condition, the original disease, and/or the presence of transplant organ donor sources. In general, KT has some advantages in the improvement of life expectancy and QoL compared with dialytic therapies [14,15]. In fact, in contrast to peritoneal dialysis and hemodialysis, limitation of amount of drinking water and excessive dietary restriction are necessary the patients received KT when transplanted renal graft achieves normal function [16]. In addition, concentrations of uremic toxins in patients with KT are remarkably lower than those dialysis patients even though technology of dialysis is improving [17]. Such advantages are important to prevent the periodontal disease because oral health is improved by increased drinking of water and normalization of salivary properties [18,19]. Conversely, we also should note that kidney function in KT patients is usually equal to that of CKD patients because there may be still a functional contralateral kidney. Although the differences in renal function are limited between CKD and KT patients, KT should be considered an immunosuppressive status due to the immunosuppressive therapy required in these patients, and this immunoreactivity plays an important role in periodontal disease [20].

In this review, at first, we summarize information regarding the pathogenesis of periodontal disease to provide a better understanding of the specific pathological mechanisms of periodontal disease in CKD and KT patients. Briefly, we pay special attention to common pathological conditions in patients with periodontal diseases and in patients with CKD or KT. Based on this information, we then introduce the impact of periodontal disease on various other diseases and on the pathological status of CKD patients. Moreover, this review also reveals the clinical significance of periodontal disease in patients with KT. Specifically, we discuss the influence of immunosuppressive drugs used to treat oral pathological conditions including gingival overgrowth in patients with KT. Furthermore, we compare the periodontal pathogens implicated in CKD and KT patients. Finally, the impact of periodontal therapy on outcome of kidney function in these patients is discussed, and we comment on the importance of periodic oral care and appropriate periodontal treatment. Thus, this review provides comprehensive and cross-sectional information on the pathological roles of periodontal disease in CKD and KT, while we emphasize that a better understanding of pathogens, pathological roles, and the impact of immunosuppressive therapy is essential to maintain the QoL, avoid complications, and improve survival in these patients.

2. Modulators of Periodontal Disease

It is necessary to exacerbate inflammation in distant tissues for local inflammation of the teeth to injure distant organs. There are several mechanisms through which periodontal bacteria affect multiple organs, such as systemic bacteremia, cytokine release and inflammation, swallowing to the gastrointestinal tract, and direct exposure through alveolar bone destruction. The first two mechanisms are common pathways for multiple organ failure. Bacteremia caused by bacteria invades the blood stream through the periodontitis lesion and an influx of inflammation mediators, such as interleukin (IL)-6 and tumor necrosis factor (TNF)-α, produced in the lesion can be introduced into the systemic circulation. Importantly, the pathological significance of such processes in patients with CKD is different from that of healthy individuals. For example, case fatality rates at 30 and 90 days in ESRD patients with bloodstream infections was 15% and 25%, respectively; however, the rate in control patients was 0% [21]. In addition, a uremic environment due to CKD was reported to modulate the levels of various cytokines and inflammation-related molecules, including toll-like receptor in immune cells, leading to increased inflammation [22]. Furthermore, other investigators have paid special attention to the relationships between CKD and oxidative stress, endothelial dysfunction, and adhesion molecules [23–25]. However, these factors that may be modulated by CKD play important roles in inflammation under various physiological and pathological conditions [23,26–28]. Based on these considerations, we review previous reports describing the pathological significance of bacteremia, cytokines and inflammation-related molecules, oxidative stress, and endothelial dysfunction in periodontal disease.

2.1. Bacteremia

How do periodontal bacteria move via the blood stream and damage multiple organs? First, gingival ulceration in the periodontal pocket enables bacteria to enter the systemic circulation [29]. Recirculating leukocytes engulf and destroy foreign antigens in the immune response; however, some periodontal disease bacteria, such as *P. gingivalis* and *Actinobacillus actinomycetemcomitans*, can survive intracellularly, and may exploit macrophages and/or dendritic cells as vehicles, much like a Trojan horse, which causes silent systemic inflammation [29]. Although it remains unknown as to whether periodontal bacteria proliferate on blood vessel walls, components of periodontitis bacteria have been detected in arteriosclerotic lesions [30]. Thus, bacteremia is an important step in the progression to systematic inflammation in patients with periodontal diseases. In fact, blood bacteria levels were higher in patients with periodontitis than in those with gingivitis ($p < 0.0001$), and its level was positively associated with worse periodontal parameters [31].

2.2. Cytokines and Inflammation-Related Molecules

The biological activity observed in periodontal lesions has suggested that various cytokines are involved in the pathogenesis of periodontal disease [32]. Numerous cytokines are known to be associated with periodontal disease, and cytokines are categorized by their function. Representative inflammatory cytokines include IL-1, IL-6, IL-8, and TNF-α. These inflammatory cytokines enhance vascular permeability, which may enhance bacteremia and stimulate fibroblasts and inflammatory cells, which in turn induce other cytokines. They also enhance the expression of endothelial adhesion molecules, such as intercellular adhesion molecule (ICAM)-1 and vascular cell adhesion molecule (VCAM)-1, E-selectin, and chemokines such as monocyte chemoattractant protein (MCP)-1 and IL-8 [33]. In addition, inflammatory cytokines regulate bone resorption and inhibit bone formation, which are associated with the local expansion of periodontal lesions through alveolar bone loss [32] and systemically with CKD-mineral bone disorder (CKD-MBD). Fibroblast growth factor (FGF)-23, which has been suggested to have a central role in CKD-MBD and in the regulation of serum phosphorus levels, has been associated with higher inflammatory cytokine levels [34]. Moreover, inflammatory cytokines cause an expansion of the mesangial matrix or induce interstitial fibrosis [35]. If bacteremia does not cause direct damage through in situ inflammatory cytokine production in the targeted organ, increased inflammatory cytokines in local periodontal lesions cause systematic inflammation via the blood stream. Other important cytokines are growth factors, such as FGF, platelet-derived growth factor (PDGF), and transforming growth factor-β (TGF-β). Connective tissue growth factor (CTGF), which normally maintains tissue homeostasis, can induce fibrosis during the inflammatory response. Renal fibrosis has a negative impact on renal prognosis, especially in patients with CKD. Considering these findings, cytokines in periodontal diseases increase vascular permeability, enhance the expression of adhesion molecules, and cause up-regulation of TGF-β. These responses may be associated with proteinuria via glomerular permeability, renal thrombosis, and renal fibrosis, respectively, and result in a deterioration of renal function [35,36].

Periodontal disease, which is associated with systemic disorders, is associated with gram-negative organisms such as *P. gingivalis*, rather than gram-positive organisms. Generally, gram-positive cocci and rods are primarily detected in subgingival plaques of healthy people. However, in plaques formed in the gingival pocket of chronic periodontitis patients, gram-negative anaerobic bacilli increase resulting in the transition to bacterial flora, which cause the formation of more complex pathogenic plaques [37]. Lipopolysaccharides (LPS) derived from the periodontal pathogens will be delivered systemically in blood vessels to other organs. An increase in inflammation through Toll-like receptor 2 and/or 4 in the innate immune system will be observed in these organs [29]. The interaction between LPS and toll-like receptors is quite complicated: The toll-like receptor-mediated pathogenic action of LPS in the immune system differs depending on the derived pathogens and the toll-like receptors [38]. For example, LPS derived from *P. gingivalis* has been associated with inducing urinary protein via Toll-like receptor 2 of the renal glomerular vascular endothelial cells and the progression of kidney diseases via Toll-like receptor 4 signaling in a diabetic animal model [39]. Nonetheless, it should be noted that the downstream signaling of Toll-like receptors has crucial roles in inflammation [32].

2.3. Oxidative Stress

Reactive oxygen species (ROS) are an important primary defense factor in periodontal disease [40]. ROS are produced by inflammatory cells such as polymorphonuclear leukocytes and vascular smooth muscle cells, and nicotine adenine dinucleotide phosphate oxidase is a major source of ROS generation. However, although the main target of ROS is nuclear DNA, excessive ROS production will generate lipid peroxide through homeostasis of oxidative balance in tissues, and lipid peroxide in local periodontal lesions is associated with periodontal diseases [41]. Moreover, ROS are associated with oxidative stress and long-lasting systemic oxidative stress, which is thought to cause multi-organ failure [42]. Reactive nitrogen intermediates are also important in oxidative stress. For example, peroxynitrite, which is produced by nitric oxide and superoxide anion causes endothelial damage [43]. There are several oxidative stress markers such as malondialdehyde (MDA), 8-hydroxydeoxyguanosine (8-OHdG), and 4-hydroxy-2-nonenal (4-HNE). It is plausible that oxidative stress has a significant impact on local periodontal lesions, and the effects of oxidative stress on the systemic inflammation have been shown by several research groups. For example, tissue 8-OHdG levels increased in multiple organs, such as the liver, heart, kidneys, and brain in a periodontal inflammation model [41]. Furthermore, in saliva, MDA and 8-OHdG levels are thought to be associated with oxidative periodontal lesions, and 4-HNE levels in the saliva may reflect systemic inflammation [44]. Conversely, there has been a report indicating that nuclear factor erythroid 2-related factor (NrF2), which is a key regulator of antioxidants, plays an important role in protecting against tissue destruction in periodontitis [45]. Thus, the balance between oxidative stress and antioxidants is speculated to be associated with occurrence, severity, and progression of periodontal disease.

2.4. Inflammatory Reaction and Endothelial Dysfunction

One of the most important mechanisms in systemic organ dysfunction in periodontal disease is due to endothelial dysfunction, which is associated with platelet aggregation, foam-cell formation, and development of atheroma [46]. In CKD, proteinuria is one of the most important surrogate markers of kidney prognosis and reflects endothelial dysfunction [34]. As stated above, inflammatory cytokines originating from bacteremia or paracrine from distal periodontal lesions will cause vascular permeability and vascular wall injury [32]. In addition to inflammatory cytokines, endothelial adhesion molecules, such as ICAM-1 and VCAM-1, play an important role in vascular injury via the activation of endothelial cells and smooth muscle cell proliferation [47]. Endothelial injury will cause arterial stenosis, resulting in hypertension [47].

In addition to the above observations, an animal model showed that ridocaine inhibited endothelial dysfunction of the systematic artery in rats with periodontal inflammation and decreased ROS was associated with such a mechanism [48]. Furthermore, investigation in patients with chronic periodontitis demonstrated that endothelial dysfunction of the branchial artery occurred with greater frequency in patients with periodontitis than in those without periodontitis [46]. Interestingly, this study and other investigators showed that together with various cytokines and inflammation-related molecules, oxidative stress regulated the relationship between periodontitis and endothelial dysfunction [49,50].

2.5. Matrix Metalloproteinases and Transglutaminases

When discussing the pathological mechanisms and development of periodontal disease, information regarding gingival remodeling and healing steps is important. In addition, an understanding of the protective system of oral tissues from microbial challenge in periodontal disease is also essential. From this standpoint, there is an interesting study that focused on the pathological roles of matrix metalloproteinase (MMP) and transglutaminases in patients with chronic periodontitis [51]. In short, when MMP-2 and -9 and transglutaminase-1–3 were analyzed in 22 patients with chronic periodontitis and healthy controls, transglutaminase-1 and 3 mRNA levels in chronic periodontitis patients were lower than those in healthy controls [51]. Finally, this study showed that different transglutaminases might regulate gingival remodeling/healing and adaptive processes in patients with chronic periodontitis. Conversely, it has also been reported that transglutaminase-2 may play an important role in vascular calcification in CKD [52]. Thus, the pathological roles of transglutaminases in CKD are not fully understood.

3. Periodontal Disease and Chronic Kidney Disease

3.1. Impact on Periodontal Disease from other Pathological Conditions

As discussed above, there is evidence suggesting that there is a direct relationship between the inflammation of periodontal disease and CKD, and renal function may decline for various reasons. CKD may evolve from any chronic renal disorder etiology, and typically includes diabetes, hypertension, and chronic nephritis [1,4]. In contrast, periodontal diseases can cause dysfunction of various organs, such as the heart, liver, and kidney. Therefore, the reduction in renal function due to the burden of other diseases as a result of periodontal disease should be considered.

3.1.1. Diabetes

The most important complication of periodontal disease is diabetes, and the risk of diabetes mellitus is increased by periodontal disease, suggesting that this association is bidirectional. In fact, the prevalence of diabetes is higher in patients with periodontal disease than in those without periodontitis [53]. Furthermore, the Hisayama study in Japan showed that patients who developed glucose intolerance were more likely to have periodontal disease than the group that did not develop glucose intolerance [54]. Diabetic nephropathy with overt proteinuria occurs as a result of long-term diabetes, but diabetes patients with periodontal disease have a higher risk of cardiovascular disease compared with patients without periodontal disease [55]. Therefore, diabetic nephropathy caused by periodontal disease shortens the clinical course of ESRD [56]. With regard to the molecular mechanisms involved, the inflammatory cytokines IL-1 and IL-6, TNF-α; fibrotic growth factors TGF-β and CTGF; and oxidative stress have all been implicated in the original pathogenesis of diabetic nephropathy [57]. There is a close relationship between diabetes and periodontal disease and glycemic control is crucial, not only for kidney function, but also periodontal disease. Leukocyte function is poorly controlled in diabetic patients and this may worsen and exacerbate periodontal disease [58]. The effects of periodontal disease on diabetic nephropathy vary depended upon the patients' condition. Thus, diabetic patients with periodontal disease should be treated intensively both for glycemic control and periodontal diseases.

3.1.2. Hypertension

Hypertension is one of the most important risk factors of premature cardiovascular disease, including CKD. A systematic review has shown the relationship between periodontal disease and hypertension [59]. As stated above, inflammation in response to bacteremia or inflammatory mediators from periodontal lesions plays a role in hypertension. Possible pathophysiological mechanisms in periodontal disease and high blood pressure are endothelial dysfunction, reduction of nitric oxide bioavailability, oxidative stress, renin-angiotensin-aldosterone system activation, arterial stiffness, and atherosclerosis [47]. Conversely, cross-sectional clinical studies have shown that risk factors for CKD in patients with periodontal disease include diabetes [60,61] and hypertension [60].

3.1.3. Liver Diseases

Periodontal disease is considered to be associated with different forms of liver disease, one of which is nonalcoholic fatty liver disease (s). The correlation between IgG antibody titers against periodontal pathogens has been shown to be increased in non-alcoholic fatty liver disease (NAFLD) patients [62]. Similar to injuries in other organs, the mechanisms involved in periodontal diseases and NAFLD are described as follows: LPS derived from periodontopathic bacteria are transferred to the blood and act directly on the liver, or LPS-derived inflammatory cytokines act indirectly on the liver [63]. NAFLD can affect multiple extrahepatic organs, such as the cardiovascular system, and increases the risk of developing CKD, with insulin resistance being an important mediating factor [64].

3.1.4. Others

In recent years, nutritional status in kidney disease has attracted increasing attention and patients with CKD are facing protein energy wasting (PEW) complications [59]. Since proinflammatory cytokines affect the brain and cause anorexia, persistent inflammation is associated with PEW [65]. CKD is a very complicated disease, and the etiologies of inflammation observed in patients with CKD are multifactorial. Although any form of inflammation can cause PEW, periodontal disease is a potential etiology for persistent inflammation [66]. Periodontal pathogens that are swallowed and reach the intestine cause changes in the intestinal microbiota, resulting in a situation resembling metabolic bacteremia such as that found in obesity. Although the direct effect of periodontal pathogens on the gut microbiota is controversial, oral microbiota could also alter the gut microbiota [67]. Recent studies have revealed that not only diabetes and obesity but also CKD is closely associated with the intestinal flora [68]. Dysbiosis of the gut microbiota is believed to be associated with periodontal disease, and administration of *P. gingivalis* was shown to alter the gut microbiota and affect multiple organs in an animal model [69]. Thus, CKD should be considered a multifactorial disease; it is extremely difficult to identify specific etiological factors, but it should be taken into consideration that periodontal disease indirectly causes renal dysfunction.

A scheme illustrating the complex mechanisms involved in periodontal disease and CKD is shown in Figure 1.

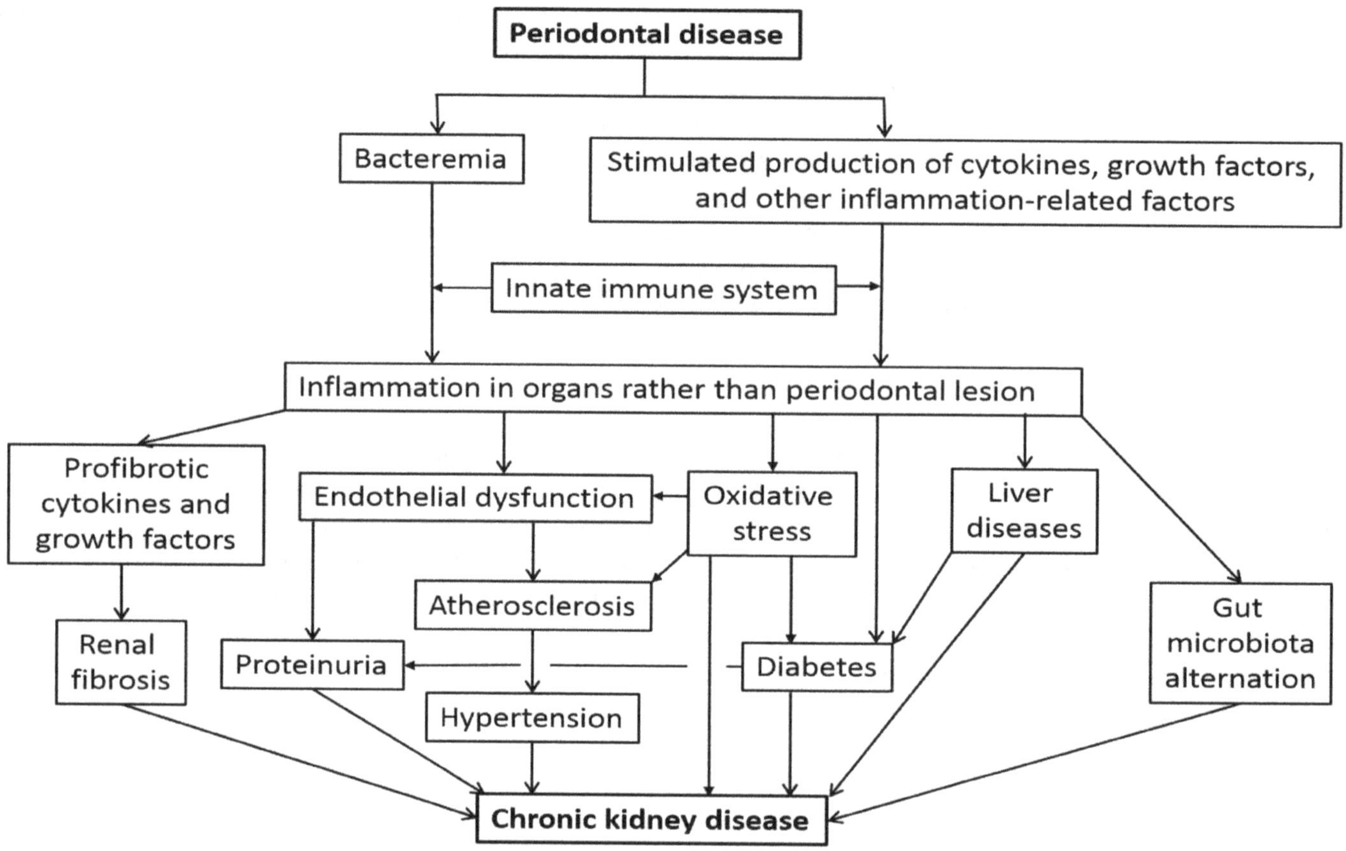

Figure 1. Impact of periodontal disease in the pathogenesis in chronic kidney disease.

3.2. Periodontal Therapy and CKD Patients with Periodontal Disease

There is a bidirectional relationship between periodontal disease and CKD, and between periodontal disease and diabetes [70]. The results of this study still remain unclear, although if CKD proceeds and renal function deteriorates, lymphocyte function and monocyte/macrophage function will be impaired and the immune system will aggregate; consequently, the risk of infection will increase compared to the healthy population [4]. When it comes to CKD-MBD, hyperphosphatemia increases phosphate levels in saliva, which is associated with a higher risk of inflammation of the periodontium. Furthermore, higher levels of phosphorus itself are linked to systemic inflammation [71]. This will enhance the association of periodontal disease and CKD. Although periodontal disease is a crucial risk factor for the onset of kidney disease and progression of renal failure, it is a treatable and modifiable risk factor. eGFR might improve in patients with CKD, however patients with ESRD cannot improve their eGFR.

The treatment of periodontal disease attenuates systemic inflammation and improves surrogate markers of endothelial function [72]. Through the reduction of inflammatory cytokines, renal function was shown to improve after treatment of periodontal disease [73]. A systematic review also showed a favorable effect of periodontal treatment on eGFR [74]. Other reports have indicated that treatment for periodontal disease decreases asymmetric dimethylarginine [75] and 4-hydroxy-2-nonenal, surrogate markers of systemic inflammation [44] and endothelial function [9], respectively.

In a discussion on periodontal therapy in patients with CKD, we must also take into consideration the influence of immunosuppressive agents. In short, a variety of CKD, such as lupus nephritis and IgA nephropathy, is commonly treated with immunosuppressive agents [76,77]. Undoubtedly, the immune response is closely associated with infection control in almost organs and tissues including oral and periodontal tissues. Therefore, in CKD patients treated with immunosuppressive agents, a treatment strategy for periodontal disease must be planned according to its severity, renal function, and response to anti-bacterial agents. In addition, in some patients, decreasing exposure to immunosuppressive agents should also be discussed. Unfortunately, however, there is little information regarding appropriate dosage in these patients. We emphasize the importance of further studies on appropriate dosage and types of immunosuppressive agents to be used in CKD patients with severe periodontal disease, especially in non-responders to anti-bacterial agents.

4. Periodontal Disease and Kidney Transplantation

As mentioned above, KT is one of the major renal replacement approaches to maintain QoL in patients with ESRD, and KT might be the choice of renal replacement therapy to achieve normalized kidney function, which undeniably leads to both social and physical advantages for the patient [14,15]. However, immunosuppressive therapy is essential for maintenance of kidney allograft function to prevent rejection and renal dysfunction, although it may be the cause of several infectious diseases including periodontitis. In addition, there is a general agreement that immunosuppressive conditions sometimes lead to the progression of local infections to general bacteremia. In Japan a total of 1742 KT including 1544 from living donors (LD) and 198 from deceased donors (DD) were performed in the proportion of patients with ABO blood type, incompatible with KT and requiring desensitization for antibody removal before KT, was as large as 27.7% of KT from LD, while the dialysis period before KT was as long as 15.1 years from DD in a Japanese survey [78]. ABO incompatibility and exposure of long-term dialysis therapy lead to susceptibility to immunosuppression, which leads to the risk of developing infectious diseases including periodontal disease. It is important to understand the underlying biological mechanisms of periodontal disease and the immunological status of KT recipients. Moreover, it is important to identify an approach to treat periodontal diseases for the management of KT.

4.1. The Screening of Periodontal Disease Before and After KT

Screening for infectious diseases is important in the preparation of KT. It is well-known that poor oral health is common among CKD patients [79]. KT candidates are considered to have a high prevalence of periodontal disease due to the status of end-stage of renal insufficiency, which is called stage-five CKD. There has been a recent increase in the number of preemptive kidney transplantation (PEKT) procedures, which are defined as transplant before initiation of maintenance dialysis therapy, for the avoidance of complication by dialysis therapy [80]. PEKT is often performed at the progression of renal deterioration in the pre-dialysis stage. Moreover, the progressed renal insufficiency may occasionally fall into a severe immunocompromised state. Oral infections should be treated completely before exposure to immunosuppression for KT candidates, since recent potent immunosuppressive therapy regimens might lead to unexpected onset of infection including periodontitis. Oral health has been reported to be better during the KT period than at the pre-dialysis stage, and it thus it is important to treat oral infectious foci at the pre-dialysis stage in order to prevent adverse outcomes after KT [81]. However, lower salivary flow rates and higher numbers of drugs at the KT stage might influence the clinical outcome [81]. Patients with diabetic nephropathy associate with worse periodontal health and higher oral inflammatory conditions at the pre-dialysis stage to the same degree as the pre-transplant stage [82]. Due to the high prevalence of cardiovascular disease and requirements of extracorporeal circulation for hemodialysis, anti-coagulant therapy is used in many KT candidates. The surgical treatment of oral diseases in this condition may lead to active bleeding and cause general bacteremia or fatal sepsis. Preconditioning and necessary treatment are important for the KT recipient before and after exposure to immunosuppressive therapy. Finally, it should be considered that appropriate timing of treatment must be provided to KT recipients depending on the patient's general status, CKD stage, and original cause of renal insufficiency [81,82].

4.2. Periodontal Condition and Clinical Outcome

Several investigators have examined the effects of periodontal conditions in relation to clinical outcome following KT. The studies reported a higher [83,84], similar [85], or lower [86] incidence of periodontitis in transplant recipients than in healthy controls. A limitation to the study results is that these differ depending on the definition of occurrence of periodontitis used. Ioannidou et al. [87] reported that none of the continuous periodontal variables were significantly associated with deterioration of allograft function due to the presence of strict criteria such as HLA-matching or history of acute rejection. A systematic review described the associations between periodontal status and clinical outcomes in KT recipients. A patient's periodontal status might be associated with a larger left ventricular mass, greater carotid thickness, graft rejection, lower graft survival, and higher mortality rate in early KT periods among KT recipients [88]. These studies suggest that periodontal status may affect clinical outcomes of patient survival and graft survival due to the occurrence of cardiovascular disease and abnormal immunological responses with essential immunosuppressive therapy [86–88].

4.3. *Influence of Immunosuppressive Drugs*

Recently, potent strong immunosuppressive therapy is becoming more commonly used to prevent acute rejection, which has improved outcomes of KT in the modern era [89]. A protocol using everolimus (ERL) is often performed in addition to a standard protocol consisting of mycophenolate mofetil (MMF), tacrolimus (Tac), and corticosteroid (CS), which has allowed further improvements in treatment outcomes of KT [90,91]. However, protocols using multiple agents can lead to a condition of excessive immunosuppression, which may worsen oral status. There are currently different immunosuppressive agents available and it is clinically important to understand differences in each drug relative to the possible occurrence of periodontal disease. Calcineurin inhibitors (CNI) such as Cyclosporin A (CsA) and Tac have played a central role in immunosuppressive therapy of KT since the 1980s. CsA is characterized by a major side effect of gingival overgrowth (GO), which may lead to occasionally worsening of oral health. CsA-induced gingival enlargement has been reported to vary from 7–80% in different transplant centers [92]. Conversely, the use of ERL frequently results in adverse events of stomatitis and compromised status, and so it may be important to properly manage the oral environment during treatment [93]. However, few reports have examined the risk of developing periodontitis and other oral diseases in patients using ERL. Pereira-Lopes et al. compared the oral health status of KT recipients receiving Tac or ERL as immunosuppressants. The study showed that KT recipients receiving the ERL protocol presented reduced periodontal inflammation in comparison with patients receiving Tac [94]. In the study, patients receiving ERL were older and they experienced more limited periodontal inflammation. There might be a bias in the patient selection in the study. ERL is used for CNI minimization or corticosteroid elimination due to protection from CNI nephrotoxicity or various side effects of steroid therapy, which might affect long-term graft survival or patient survival [95–97]. Tac has similar adverse effects as CsA because both drugs share the same pharmacological mechanism of calcineurin inhibition. Several investigators have examined the occurrence of GO with the use of Tac, which has been less frequent than the use of CsA [98,99]. In a clinical study comparing exposure to CsA and Tac, it was reported that GO occurred later in the group using Tac, with the severity of GO in the Tac group being lower than that in the CA group [100]. Another study including a post-hoc analysis revealed that the prevalence of GO was 60.0% for CsA, 28.9% for Tac, and 15.6% for sirolimus, which was used as an mTOR inhibitor for the same purpose of ERL [101]. Tac may be an alternative agent to CsA in attempting to avoid adverse effects of GO [102,103]. Tac seems advantageous with regard to periodontal effects when using CNI as a standard immunosuppression protocol.

4.4. *Immunosuppressant-Induced Gingival Overgrowth and Periodontal Condition*

Gingival enlargement is commonly observed as a side effect of several different types of drugs, including anticonvulsants, calcium channel blockers, and immunosuppressants [92]. As previously mentioned, GO is common adverse effect of CsA usage, which may lead to the worsening of periodontal conditions in KT recipients. A multitude of factors may affect clinical and histopathological manifestations of immunosuppressant-induced GO. Several investigators have examined the causes of CsA-induced GO, which might associate with periodontal disease. The results of several studies examining specific factors found in the gingival crevicular fluid (GCF) were indicative of CsA-induced GO. Increased LL-37 peptide levels in the GCF is observed at the CsA-induced GO positive site with neutrophil infiltration and extended inflammation. LL-37 is an antimicrobial peptide and an important defense molecule of the host immune response [104]. Gürkan et al. [105] examined the association of many types of cytokine families with CsA-induced GO by the examination of the GCF. TGF-β_1, whose levels are associated with clinical periodontal parameters, might be an exclusive mediator of CsA- or Tac-induced GO. Increased IL-6 and oncostain M under CsA usage have been reported to be involved in regulating the severity of inflammation and presence of GO, but cytokines of the IL-6 family might not be directly involved in the biological mechanisms associated with CsA-induced GO [106]. A study examining transgultaminase (TGM)-2, which had been shown to play a role in fibrosis by extracellular matrix accumulation, showed that TGM-2 might contribute to CsA-induced GO by modifying the GCF and plasma levels of oxidative stress markers [107].

The investigation of molecules contained in the GCF may provide researchers with a variety of insights associated with medication-induced GO. Conversely, several study groups have attempted to elucidate the mechanism of GO by investigating gene polymorphisms. IL-10 gene polymorphism might be associated with CsA-induced GO in KT recipients. A special genotype and allele might indicate an association with susceptibility to GO [108]. Alpha-2 integrin gene polymorphisms were not associated with CsA-induced GO but were associated with CsA-independent GO in KT recipients [109]. Interestingly, the length of the CAG repeat of the androgen receptor gene might link to CsA-induced GO via the analysis of polymorphisms [110]. Thus, many studies have been attempted to elucidate the mechanisms involved in drug-induced GO [104–110], but the biological mechanism of the gingival tissue response involved in immunosuppressant-induced GO is still not fully understood. Since gingival enlargement is directly associated with QoL, it is necessary to elucidate the causes of drug-induced GO by further scientific research and the challenge is to modify present immunosuppressive therapy regimens to avoid GO.

4.5. Inflammatory Markers of Periodontitis in KT

Inflammation may be associated with the deterioration of solid-organ function in transplantation recipients. Systemic inflammation occasionally originates from periodontal inflammation. There is clinical evidence that periodontal inflammation is linked to the occurrence of different systemic diseases including ESRD [111]. Moreover, the chronic inflammation of kidney allograft is often modulated by alloimmune-dependent mechanisms. The main cause of inflammation in solid-organ transplantation is dependent on human leukocyte antigen (HLA) mismatches or panel reactive antibody (PRA) scores, which may lead to acute humoral rejection [112,113]. Several inflammatory markers such as IL-6 and C-reactive protein (CRP) may be predictors of renal allograft survival associated with alloimmune-dependent acute rejection [114,115]. Moreover, specific cells associated with periodontal disease may produce significantly higher levels of IL-6, and serum CRP was reported to be elevated in patients with periodontal inflammation [116]. Shaqman et al. [117] compared periodontal disease and systemic inflammatory status of transplant recipients and age-matched controls, which led to the conclusion of the absence of any significant predictors of systemic inflammation in the population. In another study Blach et al. [118] examined several inflammatory markers such as TNF-α, IL-6, and high-sensitive CRP (hs-CRP) in KT recipients. The study demonstrated that severe chronic periodontitis was associated with increased serum hs-CRP, but not with any significant elevation of TNF- α or CRP. Elevated hs-CRP levels appeared to influence mortality after KT [118]; thus, it is important to monitor the levels of inflammatory markers such as hs-CRP, which may lead to the early detection and early treatment of periodontal disease. Furthermore, it would be more useful if an inflammatory marker specific to KT recipients undergoing immunosuppressive therapy were identified in real world studies.

5. Periodontal Pathogens in Chronic Kidney Disease and Kidney Transplantation

Several investigators have reported an increased frequency of periodontal pathogens in CKD and KT patients. There is general agreement that periodontal disease occurred by mixed infection, but not by a single pathogen alone [119,120]. With regard to CKD, Bastos et al. [121] reported that the frequencies of *P. gingivalis* and *Candida albicans* in pre-dialysis CKD patients showed a higher trend than the control group (94.7 versus 72.2% and 52.0% versus 26.3%, respectively); however, such difference did not reach statistical significance ($p = 0.078$ and $p = 0.079$, respectively). Conversely, the frequencies of *P. gingivalis* and *Treponema denticola* (*T. denticola*) were significantly associated with clinical detectable levels ($p = 0.008$ and $p = 0.013$, respectively) in CKD patients with periodontitis [121]. Conversely, other investigators have shown that *T. denticola*, *Tanerella forsythia* (*T. forsythia*), and *Parvimonas micra* (*P. micra*) were significantly associated with periodontal disease in patients with CKD [122]. In addition, the authors also found that *T. forsythia* was independently associated with periodontal disease in a multivariate analysis model including other significant pathogens, age, and estimated glomerular filtration rate ($p = 0.008$) [122].

Regarding KT patients, the frequency of *Streptococcus constellatus* in plaque samples form subjects with alveolar bone loss (36.4%) was significantly higher ($p = 0.019$) than that in samples without alveolar bone loss (3.7%) [83]. Conversely, a report also indicated that total counts of micro-organisms were increased between day 0 and day 90 after renal transplantation and between day 30 and day 90 after surgery [123]. In addition, the same study also showed that the frequency of β-hemolytic Streptococcus on day 90 after surgery (28.6%) was significantly lower ($p = 0.031$) than that on day 30 (44.4%) in KT patients with GO, but not in patients without GO [123]. Thus, in KT patients, quantitative and qualitative changes of microorganisms in the subgingival plaque might occur 90 days after surgery, and GO had an effect on expression of these microorganisms [117]. Unfortunately, there is limited information on the pathological significance of pathogens in patients with KT.

Conversely, a recent study evaluated the relationships between immunosuppressive agents and periodontal pathogenic bacteria in patients following solid organ transplantation [124]. Although it should be noted that the study population included three different types of organs (kidney, liver, and lung), the study demonstrated that changes in the levels of periodontal pathogenic bacteria dependent on immunosuppressive agents. In short, the prevalence of *P. micra*, was associated with immunosuppression exclusively with glucocorticoids; however, *P. gingivalis* was associated with combined immunosuppression of glucocorticoids, MMF, and Tac [124]. A summary is shown in Table 1.

Table 1. Pathological significance and levels of pathogens according to kidney status.

Pathogens	Status	Pathological Significance and Level of Pathogens	Ref.
β-hemolytic Streptococcus	KT	Associated with gingival overgrowth after transplantation	[123]
Capnocytophaga spec	KT	Lower compared to HD	[120]
Enterococcus faecalis	CKD	Higher compared to control	[125]
Fusobacterium nucleatum	KT	Lower in immunosuppression with glucocorticoid and mycophenolate	[124]
	CRF	Correlation with periodontal disease in multi-variate analysis model	[122]
Parvimonas micra	KT	Lower compared to HD	[122]
	SOT	Higher in immunosuppression with glucocorticoid	[124]
Porphyromonasgingivalis	CRF	Positively associated with clinical attachment level	[122]
	SOT	Lower immunosuppression with glucocorticoid, mycophenolate, and tacrolimus	[124]
Prevotella nigrescens	CRF	Higher compared to control	[125]
Streptococcus constellatus	KT	Lower in subjects with peritoneal destruction	[83]
Tanerella forsythia	CKD	Correlation with periodontal disease in a multi-variate analysis model	[122]
	SOT	Lower in immunosuppression with glucocorticoid and mycophenolate	[124]
Treponema denticola	CRF	Positively associated with clinical attachment level	[121]
	CKD	Associated with periodontal disease	[122]

CKD—chronic kidney disease, KT—kidney transplantation, SOT—solid organ transplantation, and ref—reference.

6. Care of Periodontal Conditions in Chronic Kidney Disease and Kidney Transplantation

Many investigators pay special attention to the prevalence and severity of periodontal disease. In addition, the importance of periodontal treatment has been reported in CKD and KT patients because they may exhibit periodontal conditions worse than that of the healthy general population [124,125]. Currently, several pilot studies support this opinion in these patient groups [75,126]. Unfortunately, CRF or KT patients do not have much interest in screening and/or treatment of periodontal disease. Although we have no data in CRF and KT, there is a report that approximately 70% of hemodialysis facilities have no associated dental clinic [127]. There is an opinion that immunosuppressive therapy is not associated with the necessity of dental and periodontal treatment in patients with transplantation [124]. However, there is no general consensus for KT patients. Conversely, other investigators have suggested the importance of appropriate oral health in KT patients because oral hygiene status was closely associated with the development and degree of GO [128]. Finally, we also emphasize that periodic oral care and appropriate periodontal treatment with dentists are important to maintain QoL, inhibit the complications, and prolong the survival periods in CKD and KT patients. In recent years, the usefulness of various treatment strategies for improvement of oral health has been analyzed [129,130]. In addition, there is the opinion that clinical conditions, such as lipidemia in obesity, affect preventive and treatment strategies of chronic periodontitis [131]. Based on these facts, further detailed studies with larger study populations, longer observation periods, and analyses including broader periodontal disease-related factors are necessary to be able to reach definitive conclusions.

7. Conclusions

In this review, we introduced the pathological significance of periodontal diseases in patients with CKD. Specifically, we showed the increased risks of various pathological conditions, such as diabetes, hypertension, atherosclerosis, liver diseases, and gut microbiota alternation in these patients. Furthermore, in addition to the pathological roles of periodontal diseases in KT patients, we focused on the influence of immunosuppressive drugs on oral health, such as periodontitis, periodontal inflammation, and gingival enlargement. Moreover, the pathological significance and levels of pathogens were compared between patients with CKD and those with KT. Finally, we emphasized the importance of care of oral and periodontal condition to maintain the QoL, prevent complications, and improve survival in patients with CKD and KT. Conversely, a discussion regarding comprehensive preventive strategies of oral health, information on genetic polymorphisms and DNA methylation of oral diseases-related molecules is essential [132]. Based on such information, we suggest that further detailed prospective studies with larger populations and analyses at the molecular level should be performed to clarify the importance of oral health in these patients.

Acknowledgments: We would like to thank Editage (www.editage.jp) for English language editing.

References

1. National Kidney Foundation. K/DOQI clinical practice guidelines for chronic kidney disease: Evaluation, classification, and stratification. *Am. J. Kidney Dis.* **2002**, *39* (Suppl. 1), S1–S266.
2. Ishigami, J.; Grams, M.E.; Chang, A.R.; Carrero, J.J.; Coresh, J.; Matsushita, K. CKD and Risk for Hospitalization with Infection: The Atherosclerosis Risk in Communities (ARIC) Study. *Am. J. Kidney Dis.* **2017**, *69*, 752–761. [CrossRef] [PubMed]
3. Chen, D.P.; Davis, B.R.; Simpson, L.M.; Cushman, W.C.; Cutler, J.A.; Dobre, M.; Ford, C.E.; Louis, G.T.; Muntner, P.; Oparil, S.; et al. Association between chronic kidney disease and cancer mortality: A report from the ALLHAT. *Clin. Nephrol.* **2017**, *87*, 11–20. [CrossRef] [PubMed]
4. Webster, A.C.; Nagler, E.V.; Morton, R.L.; Masson, P. Chronic Kidney Disease. *Lancet* **2017**, *389*, 1238–1252. [CrossRef]

5. Jabbari, B.; Vaziri, N.D. The nature, consequences, and management of neurological disorders in chronic kidney disease. *Hemodial. Int.* **2018**, *22*, 150–160. [CrossRef] [PubMed]
6. Grubbs, V.; Vittinghoff, E.; Taylor, G.; Kritz-Silverstein, D.; Powe, N.; Bibbins-Domingo, K.; Ishani, A.; Cummings, S.R. Osteoporotic Fractures in Men (MrOS) Study Research Group. The association of periodontal disease with kidney function decline: A longitudinal retrospective analysis of the MrOS dental study. *Nephrol. Dial. Transplant.* **2016**, *31*, 466–472. [CrossRef]
7. Ricardo, A.C.; Athavale, A.; Chen, J.; Hampole, H.; Garside, D.; Marucha, P.; Lash, J.P. Periodontal disease, chronic kidney disease and mortality: Results from the third National Health and Nutrition Examination Survey. *BMC Nephrol.* **2015**, *16*, 97. [CrossRef]
8. Sharma, P.; Dietrich, T.; Ferro, C.J.; Cockwell, P.; Chapple, I.L. Association between periodontitis and mortality in stages 3-5 chronic kidney disease: NHANES III and linked mortality study. *J. Clin. Periodontol.* **2016**, *43*, 104–113. [CrossRef] [PubMed]
9. Deschamps-Lenhardt, S.; Martin-Cabezas, R.; Hannedouche, T.; Huck, O. Association between periodontitis and chronic kidney disease: Systematic review and meta-analysis. *Oral Dis.* **2019**, *25*, 385–402. [CrossRef]
10. Kapellas, K.; Singh, A.; Bertotti, M.; Nascimento, G.G.; Jamieson, L.M. Perio-CKD collaboration. Periodontal and chronic kidney disease association: A systematic review and meta-analysis. *Nephrology* **2019**, *24*, 202–212. [CrossRef]
11. Zhang, J.; Jiang, H.; Sun, M.; Chen, J. Association between periodontal disease and mortality in people with CKD: A meta-analysis of cohort studies. *BMC Nephrol.* **2017**, *18*, 269. [CrossRef] [PubMed]
12. Grubbs, V.; Vittinghoff, E.; Beck, J.D.; Kshirsagar, A.V.; Wang, W.; Griswold, M.E.; Powe, N.R.; Correa, A.; Young, B. Association Between Periodontal Disease and Kidney Function Decline in African Americans: The Jackson Heart Study. *J. Periodontol.* **2015**, *86*, 1126–1132. [CrossRef] [PubMed]
13. Kshirsagar, A.V.; Offenbacher, S.; Moss, K.L.; Barros, S.P.; Beck, J.D. Antibodies to periodontal organisms are associated with decreased kidney function. The Dental Atherosclerosis Risk in Communities study. *Blood Purif.* **2007**, *25*, 125–132. [CrossRef] [PubMed]
14. Wang, J.H.; Skeans, M.A.; Israni, A.K. Current Status of Kidney Transplant Outcomes: Dying to Survive. *Adv. Chronic Kidney Dis.* **2016**, *23*, 281–286. [CrossRef] [PubMed]
15. Ju, A.; Chow, B.Y.; Ralph, A.F.; Howell, M.; Josephson, M.A.; Ahn, C.; Butt, Z.; Dobbels, F.; Fowler, K.; Jowsey-Gregoire, S.; et al. Patient-reported outcome measures for life participation in kidney transplantation: A systematic review. *Am. J. Transplant.* **2019**, in press. [CrossRef]
16. Nagaoka, Y.; Onda, R.; Sakamoto, K.; Izawa, Y.; Kono, H.; Nakagawa, K.; Shinoda, K.; Morita, S.; Kanno, Y. Dietary intake in Japanese patients with kidney transplantation. *Clin. Exp. Nephrol.* **2016**, *20*, 972–981. [CrossRef]
17. Liabeuf, S.; Cheddani, L.; Massy, Z.A. Uremic Toxins and Clinical Outcomes: The Impact of Kidney Transplantation. *Toxins* **2018**, *10*, 229. [CrossRef]
18. Björnsson, M.J.; Velschow, S.; Stoltze, K.; Havemose-Poulsen, A.; Schou, S.; Holmstrup, P. The influence of diet consistence, drinking water and bedding on periodontal disease in Sprague-Dawley rats. *J. Periodontal Res.* **2003**, *38*, 543–550. [CrossRef]
19. Podzimek, S.; Vondrackova, L.; Duskova, J.; Janatova, T.; Broukal, Z. Salivary Markers for Periodontal and General Diseases. *Dis. Markers* **2016**, *2016*. [CrossRef]
20. Park, C.S.; Lee, J.Y.; Kim, S.J.; Choi, J.I. Identification of immunological parameters associated with the alveolar bone level in periodontal patients. *J. Periodontal Implant Sci.* **2010**, *40*, 61–68. [CrossRef]
21. Dagasso, G.; Conley, J.; Parfitt, E.; Pasquill, K.; Steele, L.; Laupland, K. Risk factors associated with bloodstream infections in end-stage renal disease patients: A population-based study. *Infect. Dis.* **2018**, *50*, 831–836. [CrossRef] [PubMed]
22. Grabulosa, C.C.; Manfredi, S.R.; Canziani, M.E.; Quinto, B.M.R.; Barbosa, R.B.; Rebello, J.F.; Batista, M.C.; Cendoroglo, M.; Dalboni, M.A. Chronic kidney disease induces inflammation by increasing Toll-like receptor-4, cytokine and cathelicidin expression in neutrophils and monocytes. *Exp. Cell Res.* **2018**, *365*, 157–162. [CrossRef] [PubMed]
23. Feng, Y.M.; Thijs, L.; Zhang, Z.Y.; Yang, W.Y.; Huang, Q.F.; Wei, F.F.; Kuznetsova, T.; Jennings, A.M.; Delles, C.; Lennox, R.; et al. Glomerular function in relation to circulating adhesion molecules and inflammation markers in a general population. *Nephrol. Dial. Transplant.* **2018**, *33*, 426–435. [CrossRef] [PubMed]

24. Krata, N.; Zagożdżon, R.; Foroncewicz, B.; Mucha, K. Oxidative Stress in Kidney Diseases: The Cause or the Consequence? *Arch. Immunol. Ther. Exp.* **2018**, *66*, 211–220. [CrossRef] [PubMed]
25. Khukhlina, O.S.; Antoniv, A.A.; Mandryk, O.Y.; Smandych, V.S.; Matushchak, M.R. The role of endothelial dysfunction in the progression mechanisms of non-alcoholic steatohepatitis in patients with obesity and chronic kidney disease. *Wiad. Lek.* **2019**, *72*, 523–526. [PubMed]
26. Yang, X.; Chang, Y.; Wei, W. Endothelial Dysfunction and Inflammation: Immunity in Rheumatoid Arthritis. *Mediat. Inflamm.* **2016**, *2016*, 6813016. [CrossRef]
27. Molteni, M.; Gemma, S.; Rossetti, C. The Role of Toll-Like Receptor 4 in Infectious and Noninfectious Inflammation. *Mediat. Inflamm.* **2016**, *2016*, 6978936. [CrossRef] [PubMed]
28. Nasef, N.A.; Mehta, S.; Ferguson, L.R. Susceptibility to chronic inflammation: An update. *Arch. Toxicol.* **2017**, *91*, 1131–1141. [CrossRef]
29. Hajishengallis, G. Periodontitis: From microbial immune subversion to systemic inflammation. *Nat. Rev. Immunol.* **2015**, *15*, 30–44. [CrossRef]
30. Tsuchida, S.; Satoh, M.; Takiwaki, M.; Nomura, F. Ubiquitination in Periodontal Disease: A Review. *Int. J. Mol. Sci.* **2017**, *18*, 1476. [CrossRef]
31. Balejo, R.D.P.; Cortelli, J.R.; Costa, F.O.; Cyrino, R.M.; Aquino, D.R.; Cogo-Müller, K.; Miranda, T.B.; Moura, S.P.; Cortelli, S.C. Effects of chlorhexidine preprocedural rinse on bacteremia in periodontal patients: A randomized clinical trial. *J. Appl. Oral Sci.* **2017**, *25*, 586–595. [CrossRef]
32. Okada, H.; Murakami, S. Cytokine expression in periodontal health and disease. *Crit. Rev. Oral Biol. Med.* **1998**, *9*, 248–266. [CrossRef] [PubMed]
33. Gimbrone, M.A., Jr.; García-Cardeña, G. Endothelial Cell Dysfunction and the Pathobiology of Atherosclerosis. *Circ. Res.* **2016**, *118*, 620–636. [CrossRef] [PubMed]
34. Munoz Mendoza, J.; Isakova, T.; Ricardo, A.C.; Xie, H.; Navaneethan, S.D.; Anderson, A.H.; Bazzano, L.A.; Xie, D.; Kretzler, M.; Nessel, L.; et al. Fibroblast growth factor 23 and Inflammation in CKD. *Clin. J. Am. Soc. Nephrol.* **2012**, *7*, 1155–1162. [CrossRef] [PubMed]
35. Gewin, L.; Zent, R.; Pozzi, A. Progression of chronic kidney disease: Too much cellular talk causes damage. *Kidney Int.* **2017**, *91*, 552–560. [CrossRef] [PubMed]
36. Paisley, K.E.; Beaman, M.; Tooke, J.E.; Mohamed-Ali, V.; Lowe, G.D.; Shore, A.C. Endothelial dysfunction and inflammation in asymptomatic proteinuria. *Kidney Int.* **2003**, *63*, 624–633. [CrossRef] [PubMed]
37. Larsen, T.; Fiehn, N.E. Dental biofilm infections—An update. *APMIS.* **2017**, *125*, 376–384. [CrossRef]
38. Pulendran, B.; Kumar, P.; Cutler, C.W.; Mohamadzadeh, M.; Van Dyke, T.; Banchereau, J. Lipopolysaccharides from distinct pathogens induce different classes of immune responses in vivo. *J. Immunol.* **2001**, *167*, 5067–5076. [CrossRef]
39. Kajiwara, K.; Takata, S.; To, T.T.; Takara, K.; Hatakeyama, Y.; Tamaoki, S.; Darveau, R.P.; Ishikawa, H.; Sawa, Y. The promotion of nephropathy by Porphyromonas gingivalis lipopolysaccharide via toll-like receptors. *Diabetol. Metab. Syndr.* **2017**, *9*, 73. [CrossRef]
40. Kanzaki, H.; Wada, S.; Narimiya, T.; Yamaguchi, Y.; Katsumata, Y.; Itohiya, K.; Fukaya, S.; Miyamoto, Y.; Nakamura, Y. Pathways that Regulate ROS Scavenging Enzymes, and Their Role in Defense Against Tissue Destruction in Periodontitis. *Front. Physiol.* **2017**, *8*, 51. [CrossRef]
41. Tomofuji, T.; Ekuni, D.; Irie, K.; Azuma, T.; Tamaki, N.; Maruyama, T.; Yamamoto, T.; Watanabe, T.; Morita, M. Relationships between periodontal inflammation, lipid peroxide and oxidative damage of multiple organs in rats. *Biomed. Res.* **2011**, *32*, 343–349. [CrossRef] [PubMed]
42. D'Aiuto, F.; Nibali, L.; Parkar, M.; Patel, K.; Suvan, J.; Donos, N. Oxidative stress, systemic inflammation, and severe periodontitis. *J. Dent. Res.* **2010**, *89*, 1241–1246. [CrossRef]
43. Jha, N.; Ryu, J.J.; Choi, E.H.; Kaushik, N.K. Generation and Role of Reactive Oxygen and Nitrogen Species Induced by Plasma, Lasers, Chemical Agents, and Other Systems in Dentistry. *Oxid. Med. Cell. Longev.* **2017**, *2017*, 7542540. [CrossRef] [PubMed]
44. Önder, C.; Kurgan, Ş.; Altıngöz, S.M.; Bağış, N.; Uyanık, M.; Serdar, M.A.; Kantarcı, A.; Günhan, M. Impact of non-surgical periodontal therapy on saliva and serum levels of markers of oxidative stress. *Clin. Oral Investig.* **2017**, *21*, 1961–1969. [CrossRef] [PubMed]
45. Chiu, A.V.; Saigh, M.A.; McCulloch, C.A.; Glogauer, M. The Role of NrF2 in the Regulation of Periodontal Health and Disease. *J. Dent. Res.* **2017**, *96*, 975–983. [CrossRef] [PubMed]

46. Bartova, J.; Sommerova, P.; Lyuya-Mi, Y.; Mysak, J.; Prochazkova, J.; Duskova, J.; Janatova, T.; Podzimek, S. Periodontitis as a risk factor of atherosclerosis. *J. Immunol. Res.* **2014**, *2014*, 636893. [CrossRef] [PubMed]
47. Macedo Paizan, M.L.; Vilela-Martin, J.F. Is there an association between periodontitis and hypertension? *Curr. Cardiol. Rev.* **2014**, *10*, 355–361. [CrossRef]
48. Saito, T.; Yamamoto, Y.; Feng, G.G.; Kazaoka, Y.; Fujiwara, Y.; Kinoshita, H. Lidocaine Prevents Oxidative Stress-Induced Endothelial Dysfunction of the Systemic Artery in Rats with Intermittent Periodontal Inflammation. *Anesth. Analg.* **2017**, *124*, 2054–2062. [CrossRef]
49. Moura, M.F.; Navarro, T.P.; Silva, T.A.; Cota, L.O.M.; Soares Dutra Oliveira, A.M.; Costa, F.O. Periodontitis and Endothelial Dysfunction: Periodontal Clinical Parameters and Levels of Salivary Markers Interleukin-1β, Tumor Necrosis Factor-α, Matrix Metalloproteinase-2, Tissue Inhibitor of Metalloproteinases-2 Complex, and Nitric Oxide. *J. Periodontol.* **2017**, *88*, 778–787. [CrossRef]
50. Scicchitano, P.; Cortese, F.; Gesualdo, M.; De Palo, M.; Massari, F.; Giordano, P.; Ciccone, M.M. The role of endothelial dysfunction and oxidative stress in cerebrovascular diseases. *Free Radic. Res.* **2019**, *20*, 1–471. [CrossRef]
51. Currò, M.; Matarese, G.; Isola, G.; Caccamo, D.; Ventura, V.P.; Cornelius, C.; Lentini, M.; Cordasco, G.; Ientile, R. Differential expression of transglutaminase genes in patients with chronic periodontitis. *Oral Dis.* **2014**, *20*, 616–623. [CrossRef]
52. Chen, N.X.; O'Neill, K.; Chen, X.; Kiattisunthorn, K.; Gattone, V.H.; Moe, S.M. Transglutaminase 2 accelerates vascular calcification in chronic kidney disease. *Am. J. Nephrol.* **2013**, *37*, 191–198. [CrossRef] [PubMed]
53. Ziukaite, L.; Slot, D.E.; Van der Weijden, F.A. Prevalence of diabetes mellitus in people clinically diagnosed with periodontitis: A systematic review and meta-analysis of epidemiologic studies. *J. Clin. Periodontol.* **2018**, *45*, 650–662. [CrossRef] [PubMed]
54. Saito, T.; Shimazaki, Y.; Kiyohara, Y.; Kato, I.; Kubo, M.; Iida, M.; Koga, T. The severity of periodontal disease is associated with the development of glucose intolerance in non-diabetics: The Hisayama study. *J. Dent. Res.* **2004**, *83*, 485–490. [CrossRef] [PubMed]
55. Liccardo, D.; Cannavo, A.; Spagnuolo, G.; Ferrara, N.; Cittadini, A.; Rengo, C.; Rengo, G. Periodontal Disease: A Risk Factor for Diabetes and Cardiovascular Disease. *Int. J. Mol. Sci.* **2019**, *20*, 1414. [CrossRef] [PubMed]
56. Shultis, W.A.; Weil, E.J.; Looker, H.C.; Curtis, J.M.; Shlossman, M.; Genco, R.J.; Knowler, W.C.; Nelson, R.G. Effect of periodontitis on overt nephropathy and end-stage renal disease in type 2 diabetes. *Diabetes Care* **2007**, *30*, 306–311. [CrossRef] [PubMed]
57. Elmarakby, A.A.; Sullivan, J.C. Relationship between oxidative stress and inflammatory cytokines in diabetic nephropathy. *Cardiovasc. Ther.* **2012**, *30*, 49–59. [CrossRef] [PubMed]
58. Mauri-Obradors, E.; Estrugo-Devesa, A.; Jané-Salas, E.; Viñas, M.; López-López, J. Oral manifestations of Diabetes Mellitus. A systematic review. *Med. Oral Patol. Oral Cir. Bucal* **2017**, *22*, e586–e594. [CrossRef] [PubMed]
59. Martin-Cabezas, R.; Seelam, N.; Petit, C.; Agossa, K.; Gaertner, S.; Tenenbaum, H.; Davideau, J.L.; Huck, O. Association between periodontitis and arterial hypertension: A systematic review and meta-analysis. *Am. Heart J.* **2016**, *180*, 98–112. [CrossRef]
60. Han, S.S.; Shin, N.; Lee, S.M.; Lee, H.; Kim, D.K.; Kim, Y.S. Correlation between periodontitis and chronic kidney disease in Korean adults. *Kidney Res. Clin. Pract.* **2013**, *32*, 164–170. [CrossRef]
61. Liu, K.; Liu, Q.; Chen, W.; Liang, M.; Luo, W.; Wu, X.; Ruan, Y.; Wang, J.; Xu, R.; Zhan, X.; et al. Prevalence and risk factors of CKD in Chinese patients with periodontal disease. *PLoS ONE* **2013**, *8*, e70767. [CrossRef] [PubMed]
62. Komazaki, R.; Katagiri, S.; Takahashi, H.; Maekawa, S.; Shiba, T.; Takeuchi, Y.; Kitajima, Y.; Ohtsu, A.; Udagawa, S.; Sasaki, N.; et al. Periodontal pathogenic bacteria, Aggregatibacter actinomycetemcomitans affect non-alcoholic fatty liver disease by altering gut microbiota and glucose metabolism. *Sci. Rep.* **2017**, *7*, 13950. [CrossRef] [PubMed]
63. Tomofuji, T.; Ekuni, D.; Yamanaka, R.; Kusano, H.; Azuma, T.; Sanbe, T.; Tamaki, N.; Yamamoto, T.; Watanabe, T.; Miyauchi, M.; et al. Chronic administration of lipopolysaccharide and proteases induces periodontal inflammation and hepatic steatosis in rats. *J. Periodontol.* **2007**, *78*, 1999–2006. [CrossRef] [PubMed]
64. Targher, G.; Byrne, C.D. Non-alcoholic fatty liver disease: An emerging driving force in chronic kidney disease. *Nat. Rev. Nephrol.* **2017**, *13*, 297–310. [CrossRef] [PubMed]

65. Lodebo, B.T.; Shah, A.; Kopple, J.D. Is it Important to Prevent and Treat Protein-Energy Wasting in Chronic Kidney Disease and Chronic Dialysis Patients? *J. Ren. Nutr.* **2018**, *28*, 369–379. [CrossRef]
66. Machowska, A.; Carrero, J.J.; Lindholm, B.; Stenvinkel, P. Therapeutics targeting persistent inflammation in chronic kidney disease. *Transl. Res.* **2016**, *167*, 204–213. [CrossRef]
67. Atarashi, K.; Suda, W.; Luo, C.; Kawaguchi, T.; Motoo, I.; Narushima, S.; Kiguchi, Y.; Yasuma, K.; Watanabe, E.; Tanoue, T.; et al. Ectopic colonization of oral bacteria in the intestine drives T(H)1 cell induction and inflammation. *Science* **2017**, *358*, 359–365. [CrossRef]
68. Tang, W.H.; Kitai, T.; Hazen, S.L. Gut Microbiota in Cardiovascular Health and Disease. *Circ. Res.* **2017**, *120*, 1183–1196. [CrossRef]
69. Nakajima, M.; Arimatsu, K.; Kato, T.; Matsuda, Y.; Minagawa, T.; Takahashi, N.; Ohno, H.; Yamazaki, K. Oral Administration of P. gingivalis Induces Dysbiosis of Gut Microbiota and Impaired Barrier Function Leading to Dissemination of Enterobacteria to the Liver. *PLoS ONE* **2015**, *10*, e0134234. [CrossRef]
70. Fisher, M.A.; Taylor, G.W.; West, B.T.; McCarthy, E.T. Bidirectional relationship between chronic kidney and periodontal disease: A study using structural equation modeling. *Kidney Int.* **2011**, *79*, 347–355. [CrossRef]
71. Brown, R.B. Dysregulated Phosphate Metabolism, Periodontal Disease, and Cancer: Possible Global Health Implications. *Dent. J.* **2019**, *7*, 18. [CrossRef] [PubMed]
72. Tonetti, M.S.; D'Aiuto, F.; Nibali, L.; Donald, A.; Storry, C.; Parkar, M.; Suvan, J.; Hingorani, A.D.; Vallance, P.; Deanfield, J. Treatment of periodontitis and endothelial function. *N. Engl. J. Med.* **2007**, *356*, 911–920. [CrossRef] [PubMed]
73. Fang, F.; Wu, B.; Qu, Q.; Gao, J.; Yan, W.; Huang, X.; Ma, D.; Yue, J.; Chen, T.; Liu, F.; et al. The clinical response and systemic effects of non-surgical periodontal therapy in end-stage renal disease patients: A 6-month randomized controlled clinical trial. *J. Clin. Periodontol.* **2015**, *42*, 537–546. [CrossRef] [PubMed]
74. Chambrone, L.; Foz, A.M.; Guglielmetti, M.R.; Pannuti, C.M.; Artese, H.P.; Feres, M.; Romito, G.A. Periodontitis and chronic kidney disease: A systematic review of the association of diseases and the effect of periodontal treatment on estimated glomerular filtration rate. *J. Clin. Periodontol.* **2013**, *40*, 443–456. [CrossRef] [PubMed]
75. Almeida, S.; Figueredo, C.M.; Lemos, C.; Bregman, R.; Fischer, R.G. Periodontal treatment in patients with chronic kidney disease: A pilot study. *J. Periodontal Res.* **2017**, *52*, 262–267. [CrossRef] [PubMed]
76. Park, D.J.; Kang, J.H.; Lee, J.W.; Lee, K.E.; Kim, T.J.; Park, Y.W.; Lee, J.S.; Choi, Y.D.; Lee, S.S. Risk factors to predict the development of chronic kidney disease in patients with lupus nephritis. *Lupus* **2017**, *26*, 1139–1148. [CrossRef] [PubMed]
77. Tomino, Y. How to treat patients with chronic kidney disease: With special focus on IgA nephropathy. *Nephrology* **2018**, *23*, 76–79. [CrossRef] [PubMed]
78. Japanese Society for Clinical Renal Transplantation; The Japan Society for Transplantation. Annual progress report from the Japanese renal transplant registry: Number of renal transplantations in 2017 and a follow-up survey. *Ishoku* **2018**, *53*, 89–108.
79. Ruospo, M.; Palmer, S.C.; Craig, J.C.; Gentile, G.; Johnson, D.W.; Ford, P.J.; Tonelli, M.; Petruzzi, M.; De Benedittis, M.; Strippoli, G.F. Prevalence and severity of oral disease in adults with chronic kidney disease: A systematic review of observational studies. *Nephrol. Dial. Transplant.* **2014**, *29*, 364–375. [CrossRef]
80. Okumi, M.; Sato, Y.; Unagami, K.; Hirai, T.; Ishida, H.; Tanabe, K.; Japan Academic Consortium of Kidney Transplantation (JACK). Preemptive kidney transplantation: A propensity score matched cohort study. *Clin. Exp. Nephrol.* **2017**, *21*, 1105–1112. [CrossRef]
81. Nylund, K.M.; Meurman, J.H.; Heikkinen, A.M.; Furuholm, J.O.; Ortiz, F.; Ruokonen, H.M. Oral health in patients with renal disease: A longitudinal study from predialysis to kidney transplantation. *Clin. Oral. Investig.* **2018**, *22*, 339–347. [CrossRef] [PubMed]
82. Nylund, K.; Meurman, J.H.; Heikkinen, A.M.; Honkanen, E.; Vesterinen, M.; Ruokonen, H. Oral health in predialysis patients with emphasis on periodontal disease. *Quintessence Int.* **2015**, *46*, 899–907. [PubMed]
83. Leung, W.K.; Yau, J.Y.; Jin, L.J.; Chan, A.W.; Chu, F.C.; Tsang, C.S.; Chan, T.M. Subgingival microbiota of renal transplant recipients. *Oral Microbiol. Immunol.* **2003**, *18*, 37–44. [CrossRef] [PubMed]
84. Lessem, J.; Drisko, C.; Greenwell, H.; Persson, R.; Newman, H.; Smart, G.; Hopkins, L.; Parameshwar, J.; Fishbein, D.; Partridge, C.; et al. Are cardiac transplant patients more likely to have periodontitis? A case record study. *J. Int. Acad. Periodontol.* **2002**, *4*, 95–100. [PubMed]

85. Oshrain, H.I.; Telsey, B.; Mandel, I.D. A longitudinal study of periodontal disease in patients with reduced immunocapacity. *J. Periodontol.* **1983**, *54*, 151–154. [CrossRef] [PubMed]
86. Rahman, M.M.; Caglayan, F.; Rahman, B. Periodontal health parameters in patients with chronic renal failure and renal transplants receiving immunosuppressive therapy. *J. Nihon Univ. Sch. Dent.* **1992**, *34*, 265–272.
87. Ioannidou, E.; Shaqman, M.; Burleson, J.; Dongari-Bagtzoglou, A. Periodontitis case definition affects the association with renal function in kidney transplant recipients. *Oral Dis.* **2010**, *16*, 636–642. [CrossRef] [PubMed]
88. Nunes-Dos-Santos, D.L.; Gomes, S.V.; Rodrigues, V.P.; Pereira, A.L.A. Periodontal status and clinical outcomes in kidney transplant recipients: A systematic review. *Oral Dis.* **2019**, in press. [CrossRef]
89. Bamoulid, J.; Staeck, O.; Halleck, F.; Khadzhynov, D.; Brakemeier, S.; Dürr, M.; Budde, K. The need for minimization strategies: Current problems of immunosuppression. *Transpl. Int.* **2015**, *28*, 891–900. [CrossRef]
90. Karam, S.; Wali, R.K. Current State of Immunosuppression: Past, Present, and Future. *Crit. Rev. Eukaryot. Gene Expr.* **2015**, *25*, 113–134. [CrossRef]
91. Ventura-Aguiar, P.; Campistol, J.M.; Diekmann, F. Safety of mTOR inhibitors in adult solid organ transplantation. *Expert Opin. Drug Saf.* **2016**, *15*, 303–319. [CrossRef] [PubMed]
92. Dongari-Bagtzoglou, A. Research, Science and Therapy Committee, American Academy of Periodontology. Drug-associated gingival enlargement. *J. Periodontol.* **2004**, *75*, 1424–1431.
93. Ji, Y.D.; Aboalela, A.; Villa, A. Everolimus-associated stomatitis in a patient who had renal transplant. *BMJ Case Rep.* **2016**, *2016*, 2016217513. [CrossRef] [PubMed]
94. Pereira-Lopes, O.; Sampaio-Maia, B.; Sampaio, S.; Vieira-Marques, P.; Monteiro-da-Silva, F.; Braga, A.C.; Felino, A.; Pestana, M. Periodontal inflammation in renal transplant recipients receiving everolimus or tacrolimus—Preliminary results. *Oral Dis.* **2013**, *19*, 666–672. [CrossRef] [PubMed]
95. Diekmann, F. Immunosuppressive minimization with mTOR inhibitors and belatacept. *Transpl. Int.* **2015**, *28*, 921–927. [CrossRef] [PubMed]
96. Sommerer, C.; Budde, K.; Zeier, M.; Wüthrich, R.P.; Reinke, P.; Eisenberger, U.; Mühlfeld, A.; Arns, W.; Stahl, R.; Heller, K.; et al. Early conversion from cyclosporine to everolimus following living-donor kidney transplantation: Outcomes at 5 years posttransplant in the randomized ZEUS trial. *Clin. Nephrol.* **2016**, *85*, 215–225. [CrossRef] [PubMed]
97. Sommerer, C.; Duerr, M.; Witzke, O.; Lehner, F.; Arns, W.; Kliem, V.; Ackermann, D.; Guba, M.; Jacobi, J.; Hauser, I.A.; et al. Five-year outcomes in kidney transplant patients randomized to everolimus with cyclosporine withdrawal or low-exposure cyclosporine versus standard therapy. *Am. J. Transplant.* **2018**, *18*, 2965–2976. [CrossRef] [PubMed]
98. Ellis, J.S.; Seymour, R.A.; Taylor, J.J.; Thomason, J.M. Prevalence of gingival overgrowth in transplant patients immunosuppressed with tacrolimus. *J. Clin. Periodontol.* **2004**, *31*, 126–131. [CrossRef] [PubMed]
99. Sekiguchi, R.T.; Paixão, C.G.; Saraiva, L.; Romito, G.A.; Pannuti, C.M.; Lotufo, R.F. Incidence of tacrolimus-induced gingival overgrowth in the absence of calcium channel blockers: A short-term study. *J. Clin. Periodontol.* **2007**, *34*, 545–550. [CrossRef] [PubMed]
100. Paixão, C.G.; Sekiguchi, R.T.; Saraiva, L.; Pannuti, C.M.; Silva, H.T.; Medina-Pestana, J.; Romito, G.A. Gingival overgrowth among patients medicated with cyclosporin A and tacrolimus undergoing renal transplantation: A prospective study. *J. Periodontol.* **2011**, *82*, 251–258. [CrossRef] [PubMed]
101. Cota, L.O.; Aquino, D.R.; Franco, G.C.; Cortelli, J.R.; Cortelli, S.C.; Costa, F.O. Gingival overgrowth in subjects under immunosuppressive regimens based on cyclosporine, tacrolimus, or sirolimus. *J. Clin. Periodontol.* **2010**, *37*, 894–902. [CrossRef] [PubMed]
102. Greenberg, K.V.; Armitage, G.C.; Shiboski, C.H. Gingival enlargement among renal transplant recipients in the era of new-generation immunosuppressants. *J. Periodontol.* **2008**, *79*, 453–460. [CrossRef] [PubMed]
103. Párraga-Linares, L.; Almendros-Marqués, N.; Berini-Aytés, L.; Gay-Escoda, C. Effectiveness of substituting cyclosporin A with tacrolimus in reducing gingival overgrowth in renal transplant patients. *Med. Oral Patol. Oral Cir. Bucal* **2009**, *14*, e429–e433.
104. Türkoğlu, O.; Gürkan, A.; Emingil, G.; Afacan, B.; Töz, H.; Kütükçüler, N.; Atilla, G. Are antimicrobial peptides related to cyclosporine A-induced gingival overgrowth? *Arch. Oral Biol.* **2015**, *60*, 508–515. [CrossRef] [PubMed]

105. Gürkan, A.; Afacan, B.; Emingil, G.; Töz, H.; Başkesen, A.; Atilla, G. Gingival crevicular fluid transforming growth factor-beta1 in cyclosporine and tacrolimus treated renal transplant patients without gingival overgrowth. *Arch. Oral Biol.* **2008**, *53*, 723–728. [CrossRef]
106. Gürkan, A.; Becerik, S.; Öztürk, V.Ö.; Atmaca, H.; Atilla, G.; Emingil, G. Interleukin-6 Family of Cytokines in Crevicular Fluid of Renal Transplant Recipients with and Without Cyclosporine A-Induced Gingival Overgrowth. *J. Periodontol.* **2015**, *86*, 1069–1077. [CrossRef] [PubMed]
107. Becerik, S.; Celec, P.; Gürkan, A.; Öztürk, V.Ö.; Kamodyova, N.; Atilla, G.; Emingil, G. Gingival Crevicular Fluid and Plasma Levels of Transglutaminase-2 and Oxidative Stress Markers in Cyclosporin A-Induced Gingival Overgrowth. *J. Periodontol.* **2016**, *87*, 1508–1516. [CrossRef]
108. Luo, Y.; Gong, Y.; Yu, Y. Interleukin-10 gene promoter polymorphisms are associated with cyclosporin A-induced gingival overgrowth in renal transplant patients. *Arch. Oral Biol.* **2013**, *58*, 1199–1207. [CrossRef]
109. Gürkan, A.; Emingil, G.; Afacan, B.; Berdeli, A.; Atilla, G. Alpha 2 integrin gene (ITGA2) polymorphism in renal transplant recipients with and without drug inducedgingival overgrowth. *Arch. Oral Biol.* **2014**, *59*, 283–288. [CrossRef]
110. Al Sayed, A.A.; Al Sulaiman, M.H.; Mishriky, A.; Anil, S. The role of androgen receptor gene in cyclosporine induced gingival overgrowth. *J. Periodontal Res.* **2014**, *49*, 609–614. [CrossRef]
111. Kshirsagar, A.V.; Craig, R.G.; Moss, K.L.; Beck, J.D.; Offenbacher, S.; Kotanko, P.; Klemmer, P.J.; Yoshino, M.; Levin, N.W.; Yip, J.K.; et al. Periodontal disease adversely affects the survival of patients with end-stage renal disease. *Kidney Int.* **2009**, *75*, 746–751. [CrossRef] [PubMed]
112. Ramzy, D.; Rao, V.; Brahm, J.; Miriuka, S.; Delgado, D.; Ross, H.J. Cardiac allograft vasculopathy: A review. *Can. J. Surg.* **2005**, *48*, 319–327. [PubMed]
113. Yates, P.J.; Nicholson, M.L. The aetiology and pathogenesis of chronic allograft nephropathy. *Transpl. Immunol.* **2006**, *16*, 148–157. [CrossRef] [PubMed]
114. Hartono, C.; Dadhania, D.; Suthanthiran, M. Noninvasive diagnosis of acute rejection of solid organ transplants. *Front. Biosci.* **2004**, *9*, 145–153. [CrossRef] [PubMed]
115. van Ree, R.M.; Oterdoom, L.H.; de Vries, A.P.; Gansevoort, R.T.; van der Heide, J.J.; van Son, W.J.; Ploeg, R.J.; de Jong, P.E.; Gans, R.O.; Bakker, S.J. Elevated levels of C-reactive protein independently predict accelerated deterioration of graft function in renal transplant recipients. *Nephrol. Dial. Transplant.* **2007**, *22*, 246–253. [CrossRef] [PubMed]
116. Paraskevas, S.; Huizinga, J.D.; Loos, B.G. A systematic review and meta-analyses on C-reactive protein in relation to periodontitis. *J. Clin. Periodontol.* **2008**, *35*, 277–290. [CrossRef] [PubMed]
117. Shaqman, M.; Ioannidou, E.; Burleson, J.; Hull, D.; Dongari-Bagtzoglou, A. Periodontitis and inflammatory markers in transplant recipients. *J. Periodontol.* **2010**, *81*, 666–672. [CrossRef]
118. Blach, A.; Franek, E.; Witula, A.; Kolonko, A.; Chudek, J.; Drugacz, J.; Wiecek, A. The influence of chronic periodontitis on serum TNF-alpha, IL-6 and hs-CRP concentrations, and function of graft and survival of kidney transplant recipients. *Clin. Transplant.* **2009**, *23*, 213–219. [CrossRef]
119. Alves, L.A.; Souza, R.C.; da Silva, T.M.; Watanabe, A.; Dias, M.; Mendes, M.A.; Ciamponi, A.L. Identification of microorganisms in biofluids of individuals with periodontitis and chronic kidney disease using matrix-assisted laser desorption/ionization time-of-flight mass spectrometry. *Rapid Commun. Mass Spectrom.* **2016**, *30*, 1228–1232. [CrossRef]
120. Schmalz, G.; Kauffels, A.; Kollmar, O.; Slotta, J.E.; Vasko, R.; Müller, G.A.; Haak, R.; Ziebolz, D. Oral behavior, dental, periodontal and microbiological findings in patients undergoing hemodialysis and after kidney transplantation. *BMC Oral Health* **2016**, *16*, 72. [CrossRef]
121. Bastos, J.A.; Diniz, C.G.; Bastos, M.G.; Vilela, E.M.; Silva, V.L.; Chaoubah, A.; Souza-Costa, D.C.; Andrade, L.C. Identification of periodontal pathogens and severity of periodontitis in patients with and without chronic kidney disease. *Arch. Oral Biol.* **2011**, *56*, 804–811. [CrossRef] [PubMed]
122. Ismail, F.B.; Ismail, G.; Dumitriu, A.S.; Baston, C.; Berbecar, V.; Jurubita, R.; Andronesi, A.; Dumitriu, H.T.; Sinescu, I. Identification of subgingival periodontal pathogens and association with the severity of periodontitis in patients with chronic kidney diseases: A cross-sectional study. *Biomed. Res. Int.* **2015**, *2015*, 370314. [CrossRef] [PubMed]
123. Saraiva, L.; Lotufo, R.F.; Pustiglioni, A.N.; Silva, H.T., Jr.; Imbronito, A.V. Evaluation of subgingival bacterial plaque changes and effects on periodontal tissues in patients with renal transplants under immunosuppressive therapy. *Oral Surg. Oral Med. Oral Pathol. Oral Radiol. Endodontol.* **2006**, *101*, 457–462. [CrossRef] [PubMed]

124. Schmalz, G.; Berisha, L.; Wendorff, H.; Widmer, F.; Marcinkowski, A.; Teschler, H.; Sommerwerck, U.; Haak, R.; Kollmar, O.; Ziebolz, D. Association of time under immunosuppression and different immunosuppressive medication on periodontal parameters and selected bacteria of patients after solid organ transplantation. *Med. Oral Patol. Oral Cir. Bucal* **2018**, *23*, e326–e334. [CrossRef] [PubMed]
125. Artese, H.P.; de Sousa, C.O.; Torres, M.C.; Silva-Boghossian, C.M.; Colombo, A.P. Effect of non-surgical periodontal treatment on the subgingival microbiota of patients with chronic kidney disease. *Braz. Oral Res.* **2012**, *26*, 366–372. [CrossRef]
126. Grubbs, V.; Garcia, F.; Jue, B.L.; Vittinghoff, E.; Ryder, M.; Lovett, D.; Carrillo, J.; Offenbacher, S.; Ganz, P.; Bibbins-Domingo, K.; et al. The Kidney and Periodontal Disease (KAPD) study: A pilot randomized controlled trial testing the effect of non-surgical periodontal therapy on chronic kidney disease. *Contemp. Clin. Trials* **2017**, *53*, 143–150. [CrossRef]
127. Yoshioka, M.; Shirayama, Y.; Imoto, I.; Hinode, D.; Yanagisawa, S.; Takeuchi, Y. Current status of collaborative relationships between dialysis facilities and dental facilities in Japan: Results of a nationwide survey. *BMC Nephrol.* **2015**, *16*, 17. [CrossRef]
128. Pejcic, A.; Djordjevic, V.; Kojovic, D.; Zivkovic, V.; Minic, I.; Mirkovic, D.; Stojanovic, M. Effect of periodontal treatment in renal transplant recipients. *Med. Princ. Pract.* **2014**, *23*, 149–153. [CrossRef]
129. Isola, G.; Matarese, M.; Ramaglia, L.; Iorio-Siciliano, V.; Cordasco, G.; Matarese, G. Efficacy of a drug composed of herbal extracts on postoperative discomfort after surgical removal of impacted mandibular third molar: A randomized, triple-blind, controlled clinical trial. *Clin. Oral Investig.* **2019**, *23*, 2443–2453. [CrossRef]
130. Matarese, G.; Ramaglia, L.; Fiorillo, L.; Cervino, G.; Lauritano, F.; Isola, G. Implantology and Periodontal Disease: The Panacea to Problem Solving? *Open Dent. J.* **2017**, *11*, 460–465. [CrossRef]
131. Cury, E.Z.; Santos, V.R.; Maciel, S.D.S.; Gonçalves, T.E.D.; Zimmermann, G.S.; Mota, R.M.S.; Figueiredo, L.C.; Duarte, P.M. Lipid parameters in obese and normal weight patients with or without chronic periodontitis. *Clin. Oral Investig.* **2018**, *22*, 161–167. [CrossRef] [PubMed]
132. Ferlazzo, N.; Currò, M.; Zinellu, A.; Caccamo, D.; Isola, G.; Ventura, V.; Carru, C.; Matarese, G.; Ientile, R. Influence of MTHFR Genetic Background on p16 and MGMT Methylation in Oral Squamous Cell Cancer. *Int. J. Mol. Sci.* **2017**, *18*, 724. [CrossRef] [PubMed]

Changes in Metabolic Profiles of Human Oral Cells by Benzylidene Ascorbates and Eugenol

Hiroshi Sakagami [1,*], Masahiro Sugimoto [2,3,4], Yumiko Kanda [5], Yukio Murakami [6], Osamu Amano [7], Junko Saitoh [8] and Atsuko Kochi [8]

1 Meikai University Research Institute of Odontology (M-RIO), 1-1 Keyakidai, Sakado, Saitama 350-0283, Japan
2 Institute for Advanced Biosciences, Keio University, Tsuruoka 997-0052, Japan; msugi@sfc.keio.ac.jp
3 Health Promotion and Preemptive Medicine, Research and Development Center for Minimally Invasive Therapies, Tokyo Medical University, Shinjuku, Tokyo 160-0022, Japan
4 Research and Development Center for Precision Medicine, University of Tsukuba, Tukuba, Ibaraki 305-8550, Japan
5 Department of Microscope, Meikai University School of Dentistry, 1-1 Keyakidai, Sakado, Saitama 350-0283, Japan; k-yumiko@dent.meikai.ac.jp
6 Division of Oral Diagnosis and General Dentistry, Meikai University School of Dentistry, 1-1 Keyakidai, Sakado, Saitama 350-0283, Japan; ymura@dent.meikai.ac.jp
7 Division of Anatomy, Meikai University School of Dentistry, 1-1 Keyakidai, Sakado, Saitama 350-0283, Japan; oamano@dent.meikai.ac.jp
8 Ichijokai Hospital, 4-26-1 Kitakokubu, Ichikawa, Chiba 272-0836, Japan; junchan@kve.biglobe.ne.jp (J.S.); ichi-1@ya2.so-net.ne.jp (A.K.)
* Correspondence: sakagami@dent.meikai.ac.jp

Abstract: Background: Sodium-5,6-benzylidene-L-ascorbate (SBA), and its component units, benzaldehyde (BA) and sodium ascorbate (SA), are known to exert antitumor activity, while eugenol exerts anti-inflammatory activity. To narrow down their intracellular targets, metabolomic analysis was performed. **Methods:** Viable cell number was determined by the 3-(4,5-dimethylthiazol-2-yl)-2,5-diphenyltetrazolium bromide (MTT) method. Fine cell structures were observed under transmission electron microscope. Cellular metabolites were extracted with methanol and subjected to capillary electrophoresis-mass spectrometry (CE-MS) for quantification of intracellular metabolites. **Results:** SBA was cleaved into BA and SA under acidic condition. Among these three compounds, BA showed the highest-tumor specificity in vitro against human oral squamous cell carcinoma (OSCC) cell line. BA did not induce the vacuolization in HSC-2 OSCC cells, and its cytotoxicity was not inhibited by catalase, in contrast to SBA and SA. Only BA suppressed the tricarboxylic acid (TCA) cycle at early stage of cytotoxicity induction. Eugenol more rapidly induced the vacuolization and suppressed the TCA cycle in three human normal oral cells (gingival fibroblast, periodontal ligament fibroblast, pulp cell). Neither BA nor eugenol affected the ATP utilization, further supporting that they do not induce apoptosis. **Conclusions:** The present study demonstrated for the first time that both BA and eugenol suppressed the TCA cycle in tumor cells and normal cells, respectively. It is crucial to design methodology that enhances the antitumor potential of BA and reduces the cytotoxicity of eugenol to allow for safe clinical application.

Keywords: metabolomics; oral cell; benzaldehyde; eugenol; inflammation; cytotoxicity

---

1. Introduction

Benzaldehyde (BA) is an antitumor principle of the volatile fraction of figs [1]. Several BA derivatives have been prepared for clinical application. Oral administration of β-cyclodextrin benzaldehyde inclusion compound [2] and intravenous administration of 4,6-benzylidene-α-D-glucose [3] or sodium-5,6-benzylidene-L-ascorbate (SBA) [4,5] to patients with advanced, inoperable carcinoma induced remarkable necrotic changes of the tumor, although they showed weak or no antitumor activity against implanted tumors in mice. SBA had no apparent host immunopotentiation activity such as stimulation of cytokine action or production; activation of monocyte or polymorphonuclear cells; or modulation of poly (ADP-ribose) glycohydrolase activity, suggesting the antitumor activity of SBA might be produced by direct action of authentic SBA or its metabolized form(s) [5]. Using a newly established high-performance liquid chromatography (HPLC) separation technique [6], we demonstrated that under acidic condition the acetal linkage in SBA is hydrolyzed, producing benzaldehyde (BA) and sodium ascorbate (SA) [7] (Figure 1A). However, BA level was not changed during incubation for 48 h in culture medium [7].

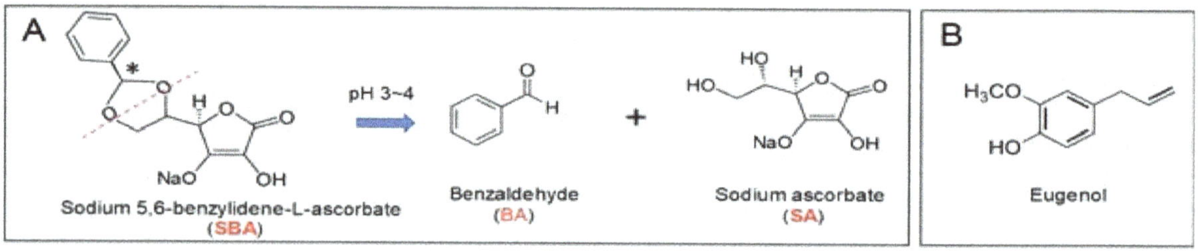

Figure 1. Chemical structure of sodium 5,6-benzylidene-L-ascorbate (SBA) and its hydrolyzed products (benzaldehyde (BA), sodium ascorbate (SA)) (**A**) and eugenol (**B**). SBA has two diastereomers (*S* and *R* configurations at stereogenic center indicated by asterisk in A) present at 31% and 69% (determined by chromato-integrator), respectively [6,7].

In vitro study with human oral squamous cell carcinoma (OSCC) cell lines (HSC-2, HSC-3, and HSC-4) and human normal oral cells (gingival fibroblast (HGF), periodontal ligament fibroblast (HPLF), and pulp cell (HPC)) demonstrated that tumor-specificity of BA (TS = 8.8) was four times higher than that of SBA (TS = 2.0), and that neither compounds induced apoptosis (internucleosomal DNA fragmentation, caspase-3, caspase-8, and caspase-9 activation) in OSCC cell line (HSC-2) [8,9], in contrast to HL-60 human promyelocytic leukemic cells [10]. SBA and SA showed common biological properties such as apoptosis induction of HL-60 cells [10], cytotoxicity augmentation with cupper ions, radical generation, and prooxidant action (oxidation potential, hydrogen peroxide production, and methionine oxidation) but showed different properties such as a propensity to react with iron and cysteine analog and catalase sensitivity [11–15] (Table 1). However, to our knowledge, comparative metabolomic study of SBA or SA with BA has not been reported.

Table 1. Biological activities of SBA and its cleaved products, BA and SA.

Biological Activities	SBA	SA	BA	Ref.
Antitumor activity (in vivo)	Yes	No	Yes	[5]
Tumor-specificity (TS = CC_{50} (normal)/CC_{50} (tumor))	2	2.5	8.8	[8,9]
Apoptosis-induction in HSC-2 cells	No	N.D.	No	[8,9]
Apoptosis-induction in HL-60 cells	Yes	Yes	No	[10]
Cytotoxicity by addition of copper	Increase	Increase	N.D.	[11,12]
Cytotoxicity by addition of iron, cysteine analog, catalase	Not clear	Decrease	N.D.	[11–13]
Radical generation	Yes	Yes	N.D.	[11,12]
Oxidation potential, H_2O_2 production, methionine oxidation	Yes	Yes	N.D.	[11–15]

N.D., not determined.

In dentistry, zinc oxide-eugenol formulations have been used for many years as bases, liners, cements, and temporary restorative materials [16], and were previously considered as the preferred material for root canal fillings [17]. However, zinc oxide-eugenol released cytotoxic concentrations of eugenol (Figure 1B) [18], and induced chronic inflammation, without healing the pulp, nor forming the dentin bridge up to 12 weeks postoperatively [19]. However, due to the lack of randomized clinical trials, long-term follow-up studies, and proper coronal sealing, whether eugenol is the best root canal filling material for endodontically treated deciduous teeth is still questionable [20,21]. Eugenol induced very rapid and irreversible cell death [22,23] in both human OSCC cell lines (HSC-2, HSC-4, Ca9-22) and normal oral cells (HGF, HPLF, and HCP) to comparable extents [23]. Eugenol induced apoptotic cell death in human promyelocytic leukemia [24], colon cancer [25], and breast cancer cells [26], but not in human normal oral cells and OSCC cell lines [23].

Apoptosis and non-apoptosis are two alternative forms of cell death, with well-defined morphological and biochemical differences [27]. One crucial physiological difference between apoptotic and non-apoptotic cells is the intracellular ATP level. Since apoptosis is an energy-dependent process, a decrease in ATP to below critical levels may impede the execution of apoptosis and promote necrosis [28,29]. This was supported by our findings that sodium fluoride (NaF), which induced apoptosis in HSC-2 cells [30,31], increased the ATP utilization (assessed by AMP/ATP ratio) [32], whereas eugenol, which induced non-apoptosis [19], did not significantly change the ATP utilization in OSCC cells [33]. However, to our knowledge, the effect of eugenol on cellular metabolites of human normal oral cells has not been investigated.

In the present study, we investigated which metabolic pathways are mostly affected by short treatment with SBA-related compounds and eugenol. To accomplish this, we first determined the minimum exposure time required for the irreversible cell death induction, and then performed the metabolomic analysis. The present study demonstrated for the first time that BA shows several properties distinct from those of SBA and SA, and that both BA and eugenol targeted the tricarboxylic acid (TCA) cycle at early stage of cell death induction.

2. Materials and Methods

2.1. Materials

The following chemicals and materials were obtained from the indicated companies: Dulbecco's modified Eagle's medium (DMEM) from Gibco BRL, Grand Island, NY, USA; fetal bovine serum (FBS), benzaldehyde (MW = 106) (purity: >98%), sodium ascorbate (MW = 198), eugenol (MW = 164) (purity: >98%), NaF, D-mannitol, 20% glutaraldehyde solution, dimethylsulfoxide (DMSO) from Wako Pure Chemical, Osaka, Japan; doxorubicin, catalase (EC1.11.1.6, from bovine liver, 41,000 unit/mg protein) from Sigma-Aldrich Inc., St. Louis, MO, USA; mitomycin C from Merck KGaA, Darmstadt, Germany; 5-fluorouracil (5-FU) from Kyowa, Tokyo, Japan; methotrexate from Nacalai Tesque, Inc., Kyoto, Japan; docetaxel from Toronto Research Chemicals, New York, NY, USA; gefitinib from LC Laboratories®, PKC Pharmaceuticals, Inc., Woburn, MA, USA; SBA (MW = 286) from ChemiScience, Tokyo, Japan; culture plastic dishes and plates (96-well) from Becton Dickinson Labware, Franklin Lakes, NJ, USA. Eugenol was dissolved in DMSO at 400 mM before use, and diluted with medium. As a control, cells treated with 0.5% DMSO were used.

2.2. Cytotoxic Assay

Human OSCC cell line (HSC-2), purchased from Riken Cell Bank (Ibaragi, Japan), and human oral normal cells (HGF, HPLF, and HPC), established from the first premolar tooth extracted from the lower jaw of a 12-year-old girl [34], were cultured in DMEM supplemented with 10% heat-inactivated FBS. Cells were inoculated at 2×10^3 cells per each well of 96-microwell plate. After 48 h, cells were treated with SBA, BA, or SA, as described below. The viable cell number was then determined by MTT method as described previously [8,9,23].

2.3. Fine Cell Structure

HSC-2 cells (2×10^5 cells) were inoculated into 8.4-cm (inner diameter) dish. After 48 h, cells were incubated with 0, 1.25, 2.5, 5, or 10 mM SBA, BA, or SA for 3 h, 3 h, or 30 min, respectively.

Near confluent HPC (19 population doubling level (PDL)), HPLF (15 PDL), and HGF (20 PDL) cells were incubated with 2 mM eugenol for 0, 20, or 40 min (HPLF, HGF) or 0, 30, or 60 min (HPC). Aliquots of the cells were washed three times with 5 mL of cold phosphate-buffered saline without calcium and magnesium (PBS (−)) and then fixed for 1 h with 2% glutaraldehyde in 0.1 M cacodylate buffer (pH 7.4) at 4 °C. The cells were scraped with a rubber policemen, pelleted by centrifugation, post-fixed for 90 min with 1% osmium tetraoxide-0.1 M cacodylate buffer (pH 7.4), dehydrated, and embedded in Araldite M (CIBA-GEIGY Swiss; NISSHIN EN Co., Ltd., Tokyo, Japan). Thin sections were stained with uranyl acetate and lead citrate and were then observed under a JEM-1210 transmission electron microscope, Japan Electron Optics Laboratory (JEOL, Co., Ltd., Tokyo, Japan) (magnification: ×3000 or ×5000) at an accelerating voltage of 100 kV [8,9,35].

2.4. Processing for Metabolomic Analysis

The cells (2~5 × 10^5) were inoculated on a 8.4-cm (inner diameter) dish and grown to near confluency. After replacing medium with fresh culture medium, cells were treated for each sample. Experiments were performed twice. The following conditions of incubation time and concentrations were used.

Exp. I: HSC-2 cells were treated for 60 min with 0, 0.625, 1.25, 2.5, 5, or 10 mM SBA for 90 min with 0, 1.25, 2.5, 5, 10, or 20 mM BA or for 30 min with 0, 0.625, 1.25, 2.5, 5, or 10 mM SA. Aliquots of the cells were trypsinized for counting the viable cell number with hemocytometer after staining with trypan blue. The cell numbers recovered from the dishes ranged between 2.65~3.03 × 10^6 cells (SBA), 1.55~1.84 × 10^6 cells (BA), and 2.75~3.10 × 10^6 cells (SA) at the time of cell harvest, respectively.

Exp. II: HSC-2 cells were treated for 70 min without (control), or with 4 or 8 mM SBA, or with 8 or 16 mM BA. HGF (19 PDL), HPLF (15 PDL), and HPC (17 PDL) cells were treated with 2 mM eugenol for 0, 20, 40, 60, or 80 min (HGF, HPLF) or for 0, 30, 60, 80, or 100 min (HPC). The cell numbers recovered from the dishes at the time of cell harvest ranged between 3.83~4.22 × 10^6 cells (HSC-2), 0.195~ 0.322 × 10^6 cells (HGF), 0.280~0.495 × 10^6 cells (HPLF), and 0.640~0.873 × 10^6 cells (HPC), respectively.

Aliquots of cells were washed twice with 10 mL of ice-cold 5% D-mannitol and then immersed for 10 min with 1 mL methanol containing internal standard (25 μmol/L each of methionine sulfone, 2-[*N*-morpholino]-ethanesulfonic acid and D-camphor-10-sulfonic acid). The supernatant (methanol extract) was collected. To 400 μL of the dissolved samples, 400 μL of chloroform and 200 μL of Milli-Q water were added and the mixture was centrifuged at 10,000× *g* for 3 min at 4 °C. The aqueous layer was filtered to remove large molecules by centrifugation through a 5-kDa cut-off filter (Millipore, Billerica, MA) at 9100× *g* for 2.0 h at 4 °C. Three hundred and twenty microliters of the filtrate was concentrated by freeze drying and dissolved in 50 μL of Milli-Q water containing reference compounds (200 μM each of 3-aminopyrrolidine and trimesate) immediately before capillary electrophoresis (CE)-time-of-flight (TOF)-mass spectrometry (MS) analysis [33,35,36].

2.5. CE-MS Analysis

The instrumentation and measurement conditions used for CE-TOF-MS were described previously [37,38] with slight modification [36].

For cationic metabolite analysis using CE-TOF-MS, a sample was prepared in fused silica capillaries filled with 1 mol/L formic acid as the reference electrolyte [32]. The capillary was flushed with formic acid. Sample solutions (3 nL) were injected at 50 mbar for 5 s and a voltage of 30 kV was applied. The capillary temperature was maintained at 20 °C and the temperature of the sample tray was kept below 5 °C. The sheath liquid was delivered at 10 μL/min. Electrospray ionization (ESI)-TOF-MS was conducted in the positive ion mode. The capillary voltage was set at 4 kV and the flow rate of nitrogen gas (heater temperature = 300 °C) was set at 7 psig. In TOF-MS, the fragmentor, skimmer, and OCT RF voltages were 75, 50, and 125 V, respectively. Automatic recalibration of each acquired spectrum was performed using reference standards. Mass spectra were acquired at a rate of 1.5 cycles/s over a m/z range of 50–1000.

For anionic metabolite analysis using CE-TOF-MS, a commercially available COSMO (+) capillary, chemically coated with a cationic polymer, was used for separation. Ammonium acetate solution (50 mmol/L; pH 8.5) was used as the electrolyte for separation. Before the first use, the new capillary was flushed successively with the running electrolyte (pH 8.5), 50 mmol/L acetic acid (pH 3.4), and then the electrolyte again for 10 min each. Before each injection, the capillary was equilibrated for 2 min by flushing with 50 mM acetic acid (pH 3.4) and then with the running electrolyte for 5 min [32]. A sample solution (30 nL) was injected at 50 mbar for 30 s, and a voltage of −30 kV was applied. The capillary temperature was maintained at 20 °C and the sample tray was cooled below 5 °C. An Agilent 1100 series pump equipped with a 1:100 splitter was used to deliver 10 μL/min of 5 mM ammonium acetate in 50% (v/v) methanol/water, containing 0.1 μM Hexakis, to the CE interface. Here, it was used as a sheath liquid surrounding the CE capillary to provide a stable electrical connection between the tip of the capillary and the grounded electrospray needle. ESI-TOF-MS was conducted in the negative ionization mode at a capillary voltage of 3.5 kV. For TOF-MS, the fragmentor, skimmer, and OCT RF voltages were set at 100, 50, and 200 V, respectively. The flow rate of the drying nitrogen gas (heater temperature = 300 °C) was maintained at 7 psig. Automatic recalibration of each acquired spectrum was performed using reference standards ([13C isotopic ion of deprotonated acetic acid dimer (2 CH3COOH–H)]$^-$, m/z 120.03841), and ([Hexakis + deprotonated acetic acid (M + CH3COOH–H)]$^-$, m/z 680.03554). Exact mass data were acquired at a rate of 1.5 spectra/s over a m/z range of 50–1000.

Cation analysis was performed using an Agilent CE capillary electrophoresis system, an Agilent G6220A LC/MSD TOF system, an Agilent 1100 series isocratic HPLC pump, a G1603A Agilent CEMS adapter kit, and a G1607A Agilent CE-ESI-MS sprayer kit [35]. Anion analysis was performed using an Agilent CE capillary electrophoresis system, an Agilent G6220A LC/MSD TOF system, an Agilent 1200 series isocratic HPLC pump, a G1603A Agilent CE-MS adapter kit, and a G7100A Agilent CE-electrospray ionization (ESI) source-MS sprayer kit [35].

2.6. Statistical Analysis

Data are expressed as the mean ± standard deviation (S.D.). Raw data of metabolomics analysis were analyzed using our proprietary software, MasterHands [39,40]. Concentrations were calculated using external standards based on relative area (i.e., the area divided by the area of the internal standards). Overall metabolomic profiles were accessed by principal component (PC) analysis (PCA). XLstat (Ver. 2014.1.04, Addinsoft, Paris, France) GraphPad Prism (Version 5.04, GraphPad Software, San Diego, CA, USA), and MeV (Version 4.9.0, http://mev.tm4.org/, Center for Cancer Computational Biology, Dana-Farber Cancer Institute, Boston, MA, USA) were used for PCA and other statistical tests. Differences were considered significant at $p < 0.05$.

3. Results

3.1. Distinct Biological Properties of BA from SBA and SA

3.1.1. Catalase Sensitivity

The addition of catalase (3000 unit/mL) reduced the cytotoxicity of SBA and SA up to >6.4-fold and >24.6-fold, respectively, confirming our previous finding [13]. On the other hand, the cytotoxicity of BA was not affected by the addition of catalase (Figure 2). This suggests that extracellularly released hydrogen peroxide may not be involved in BA-induced cytotoxicity.

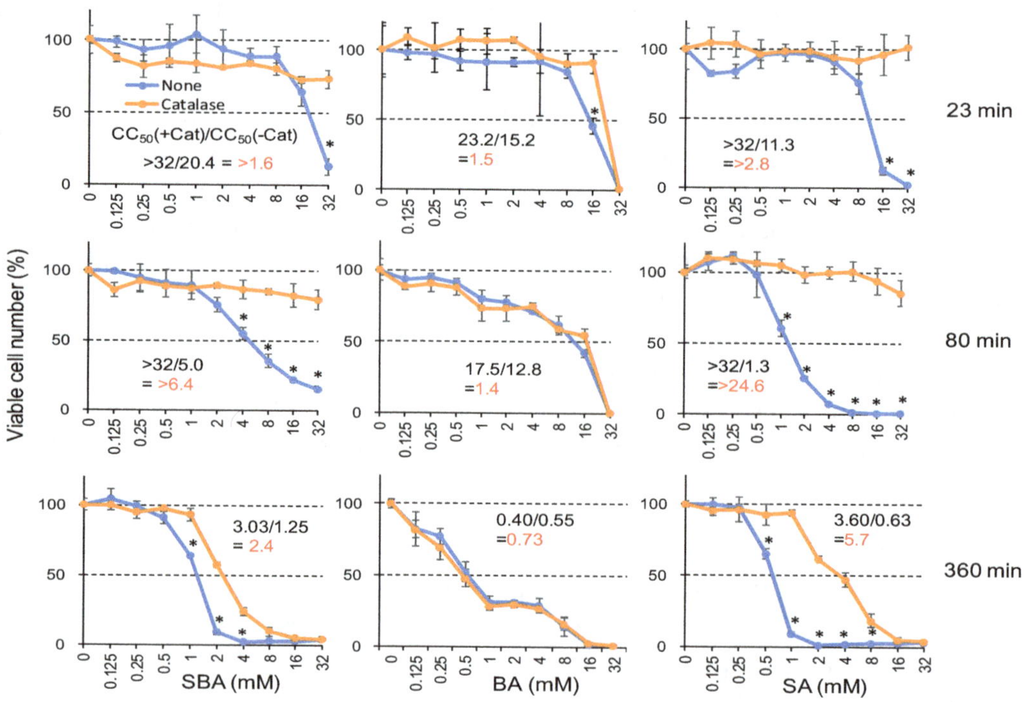

Figure 2. Involvement of extracellularly released hydrogen peroxide in the cytotoxicity induced by SA and SBA, but not BA. HSC-2 cells were incubated for 23, 80, or 360 min with the indicated concentrations of each compound in the presence or absence of catalase (3000 units/mL), and then replaced with fresh medium and incubated for a total of 48 h. Viable cell number was determined by MTT method, and expressed as % of control (drug-free, catalase-free). Each value represents mean ± S.D. of triplicate assays. * Significant difference from control $p < 0.05$.

3.1.2. Minimum Exposure Time Required for Irreversible Cell Death Induction

In order to detect the initial event that leads to irreversible cell death, we first determined the minimum exposure time. HSC-2 cells were incubated for various times, and then medium was replaced with drug-free medium and cells were incubated for up to 48 h. Viable cell number was reduced dose- and time-dependently after treatment with any drugs tested. Cytotoxic action of SA was the fastest, reaching the plateau phase of viable cell number reduction after only 2 h. Cytotoxic action of SBA was slightly slower, requiring 3~6 h to reach the bottom. Cytotoxic action of BA was much slower, requiring 8 h to reach the bottom (Figure 3).

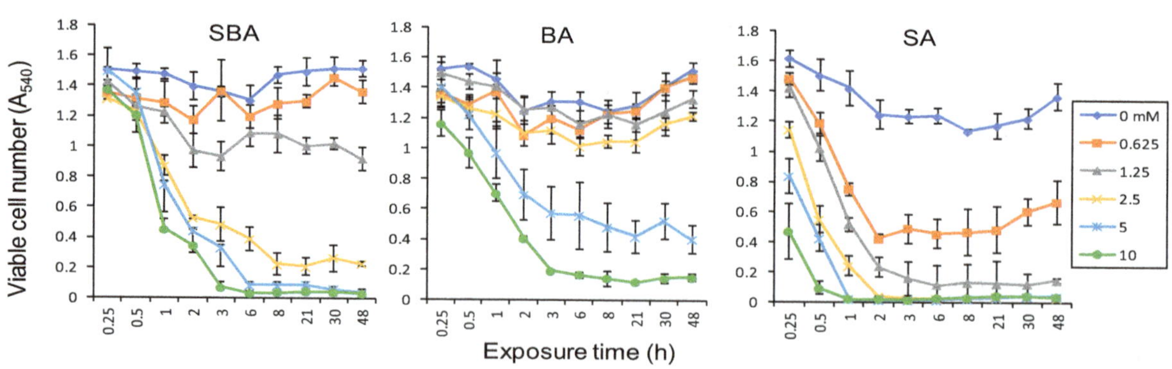

Figure 3. Minimum exposure time required for cytotoxicity induction by SBA, BA, and SA. HSC-2 cells were incubated for the indicated times without (control) or with 0, 0.625, 1.25, 2.5, 5, or 10 mM for each compound, and replaced with fresh drug-free medium. Cells were incubated for a total of 48 h and viable cell number was determined by MTT methods. Each value represents the mean ± S.D. of triplicate assays.

3.1.3. Induction of Mitochondrial Vacuolization

When HSC-2 cells were treated for 3 h with SBA and SA at 2.5 mM or higher concentrations, mitochondrial vacuolization and multivesicular bodies appeared (indicated by red box). On the other hand, BA did not induce such morphological changes (Figure 4).

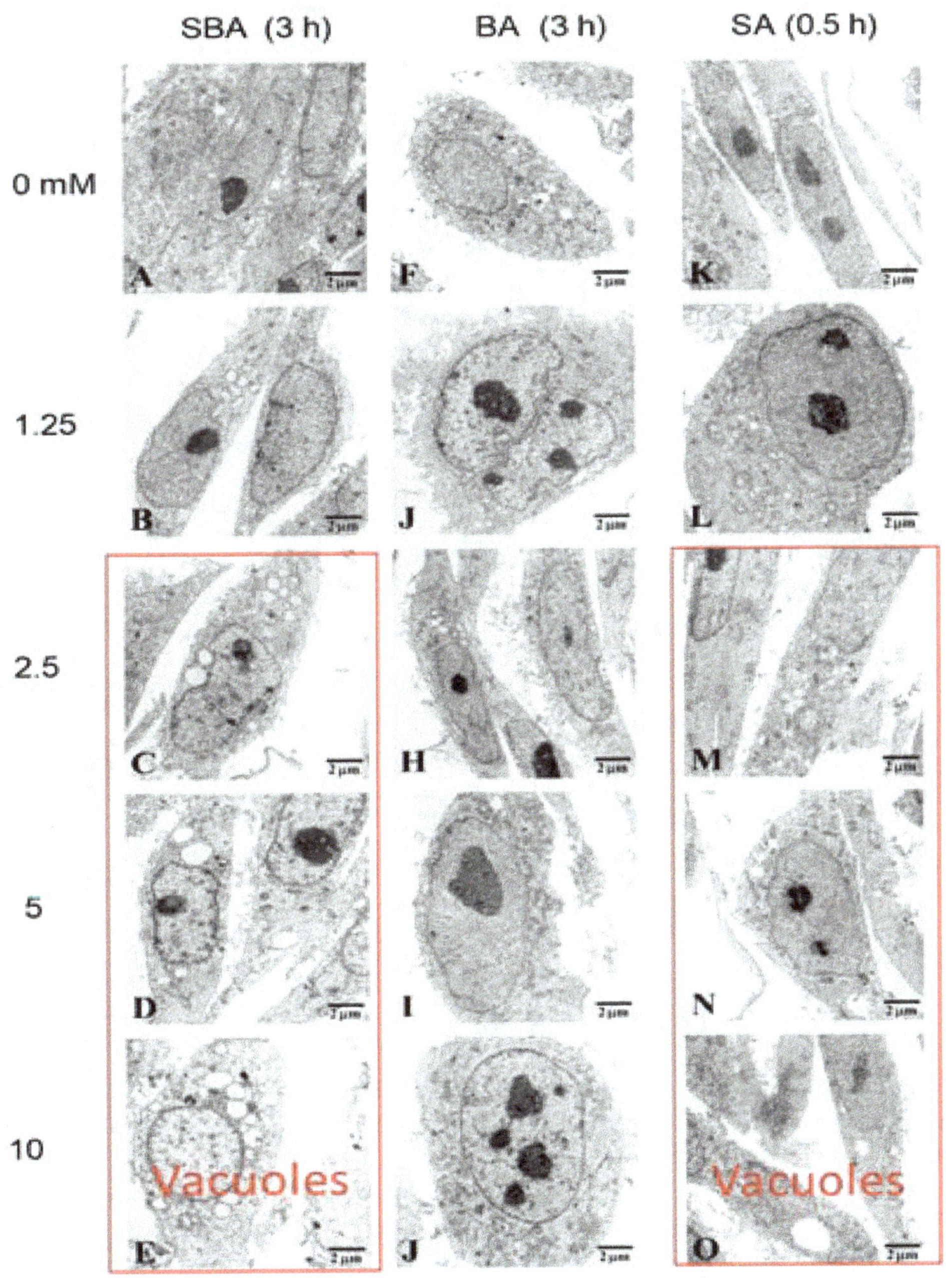

Figure 4. TEM analysis of fine cell structure of HSC-2 cells treated by the indicated concentrations of SBA (**A–E**), benzaldehyde (**F–J**), and sodium ascorbate (**K–O**). Images magnified at ×5000.

3.1.4. Effect on TCA Cycle Metabolites

In order to detect early metabolic changes, HSC-2 cells were incubated for only 60, 90, and 30 min with increasing concentrations of SBA, BA, or SA, respectively, and subjected to metabolomic analysis. We found dramatic changes in the TCA cycle after treatment of BA (Figure 5).

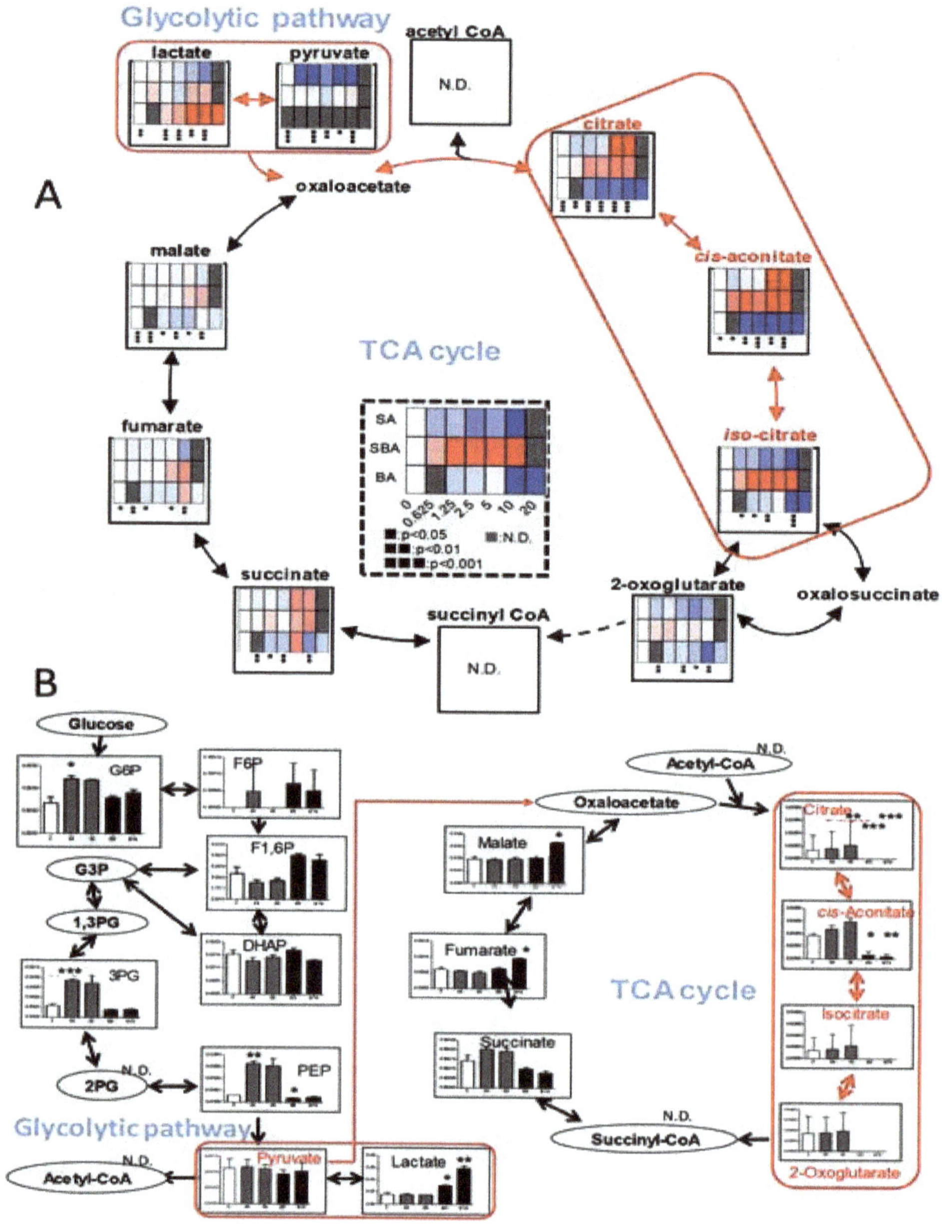

Figure 5. BA, but not SAB nor SA, inhibits the tricarboxylic acid (TCA) cycle. (**A**). Dose-response of SBA (60 min), BA (90 min), SA (30 min). HSC-2 cells were treated as Exp. I in Materials and Methods. Averaged values of quantified metabolites (amol/cell) were calculated by triplicate. To visualize the data in heat maps, each of the values were divided by those of 0 mM, i.e. fold changes were visualized and colored. Blue, white, and red were assigned for the fold changes of 0, 1, and 2, respectively. For the treatments of 0.626 mM, Student's t-tests were used, and for those of 20 mM, no statistical test was conducted. Not detected (N.D.) was colored in gray. One-way ANOVAs were conducted and black boxes were assigned below each heat map. (**B**). Dose-response of SBA and BA. HSC-2 cells were treated as Exp. II in Materials and Methods..Horizontal axis from left to right: C, S4, S8, B8, and B16 represent control, 4 and 8 mM SBA, 8 and 16 mM BA, respectively. Treatment time: 70 min. Control and each group were analyzed using Welch's test (both tail) and p-values were adjusted by Bonferroni correction. * $p < 0.05$, ** $p < 0.01$, and *** $p < 0.001$. Error bar indicates standard deviation of triplicates.

Within 90 min exposure to BA, intracellular concentrations of citrate, *cis*-aconitate, and *iso*-citrate declined to base-line level in HSC-2 cells, whereas that of succinate, fumarate, and malate maintained almost constant levels, indicating the rapid suppression of TCA cycle progression. In contrast, we could not detect such dramatic changes in other pathways (including pyrimidine metabolism, purine metabolism, glycolysis, pentose phosphate pathway, arginine, proline metabolism and urea cycle, glycine, serine and threonine metabolism, alanine, asparagine and aspartate metabolism, lysine metabolism, beta-alanine biosynthesis and metabolism, methionine and cysteine metabolism, histidine metabolism, tryptophan metabolism, phenylalanine, tyrosine metabolism, valine, leucine and isoleucine metabolism, γ-aminobutyric acid (GABA) biosynthesis and metabolism and glutamine metabolism) (Figure S1, Table S1). We checked the reproducibility of the finding (Table S2). The repeated experiment again showed that citrate, *cis*-aconitate, isocitrate, and 2-oxoglutarate were depleted by 8 or 16 mM BA (Figure 5B).

We next investigated which pathway may be involved in suppressing the TCA cycle. We found that BA increased lactate production, maintaining nearly constant levels of pyruvic acid, suggesting that BA may have reduced the amount of pyruvate that enters the TCA cycle (Figure 5A). We confirmed this finding by repeating the experiment (Figure 5B). BA reduced β-alanine, L-aspartic acid, and adenylosuccinate (Figure 6), which may directly or indirectly reduce the production of citrate.

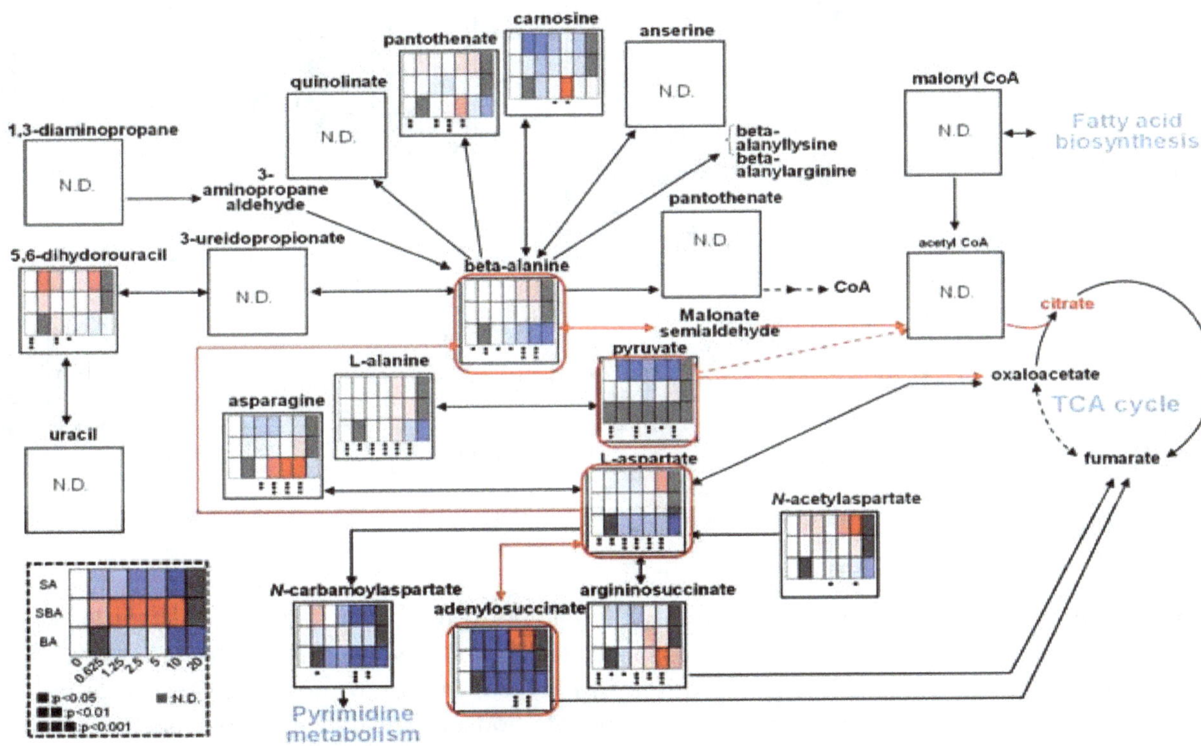

Figure 6. Possible pathway that reduces the supply of citrate by BA. SBA (60 min), BA (90 min), SA (30 min). The procedures used to produce heat maps and statistical analyses were described in Figure 5A.

We next investigated the effect on ATP utilization (Figure 7). BA treatment reproducibly reduced the AMP to less than half of the control level while it maintained a nearly constant ATP level, indicating the reduction of ATP utilization (Figure 7A). SBA treatment slightly elevated ATP but reduced AMP to one-third of the control level, again indicating the reduction of ATP utilization. On the other hand, SA increased the AMP at higher concentration (5 and 10 mM), suggesting the enhancement of ATP utilization (Figure 7A). We checked the reproducibility that both SAB and BA reduced the AMP utilization (Figure 7B). These data suggest that BA may not induce apoptosis in HSC-2 cells, in accord with our previous report [4,5].

We also investigated the changes in redox and amino acids (Figure S1). SBA, BA, and SA increased methionine sulfoxide and oxidized glutathione (GSSG) but reduced Glutathione (GSH) only slightly at higher concentration, suggesting that these compounds showed some minor prooxidant action. It was unexpected that BA dose-dependently reduced GABA, while glutamate was not changed significantly. However, the biological significance of this finding is unclear at present. Glutamine level was kept constant except for at the highest concentration of BA, negating the possibility that BA-induced cell death is not mediated by the deletion of glutamine, one of the energy sources for cell survival.

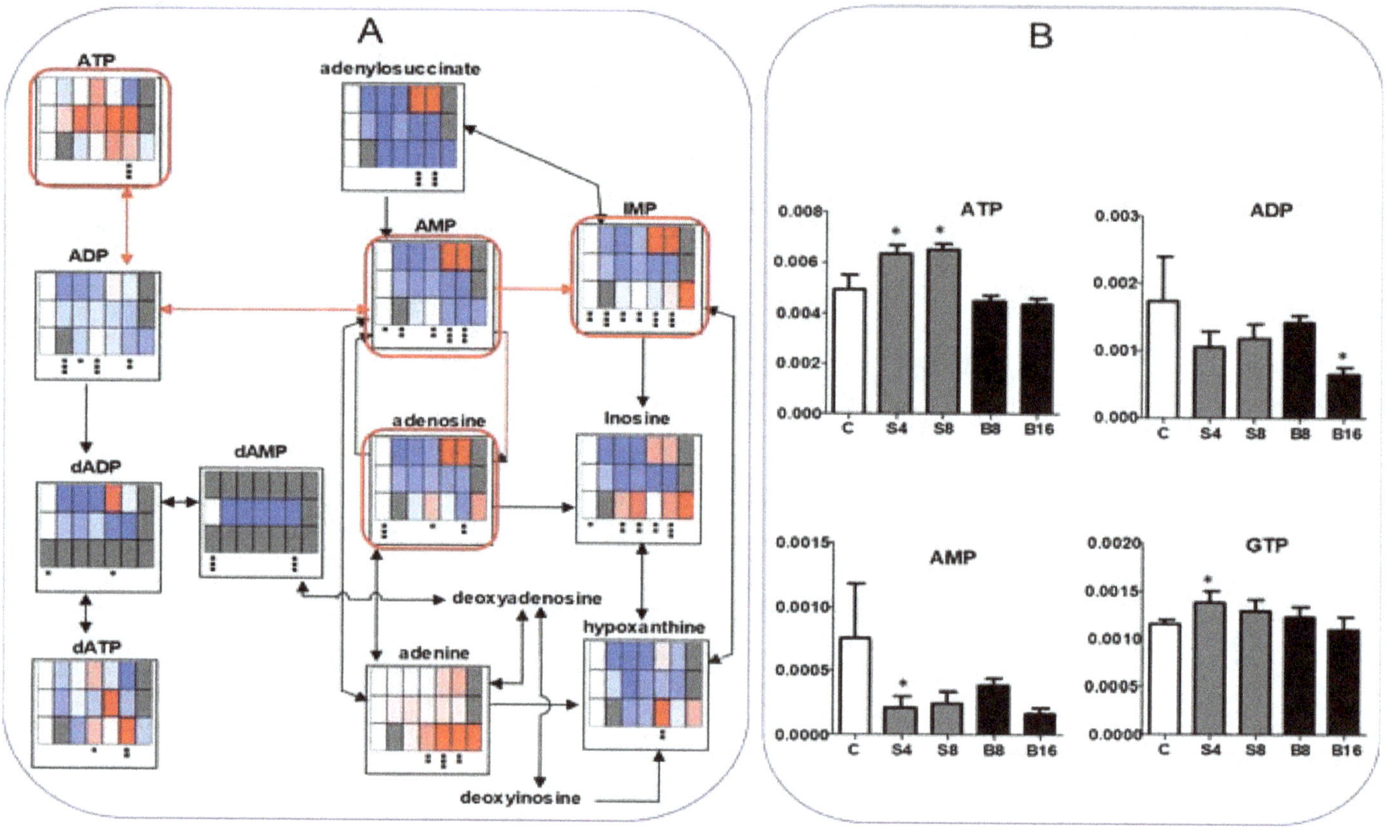

Figure 7. BA as well as SBA, but not, SA, reduce the ATP utilization. (**A**). SBA (60 min), BA (90 min), SA (30 min). HSC-2 cells were treated as Exp. I in Materials and Methods. (**B**). Horizontal axis from left to right: C, S4, S8, B8, and B16 represent control, 4 and 8 mM SBA, 8 and 16 mM BA, respectively. HSC-2 cells were treated as Exp. II in Materials and Methods. Vertical axis, μmol/cell. Each value represents mean ± S.D. ($n = 3$). The procedures used to produce heat maps and statistical analyses were described in the legend of Figure 5. * $p < 0.05$.

Overall metabolomic profiles were accessed by principal component (PC) analysis (PCA) (Figure 8). Plots of SA, SBA, and BA were separated into non-overlapped clusters with each other. Along with the first PC, SBA was clustered at slightly higher values (−2~5) than SA (−8~−4), and BA was clustered at much higher values (2~23) with the exception of two plots. Along with the second PC, SA (−2~13) and SBA (2~6) distributed into an overlapped region, whereas BA distributed at much lower values (0~−17). This indicates that the changes in the intracellular metabolites induced by SBA are more close to those induced by SA, as compared with those induced by BA.

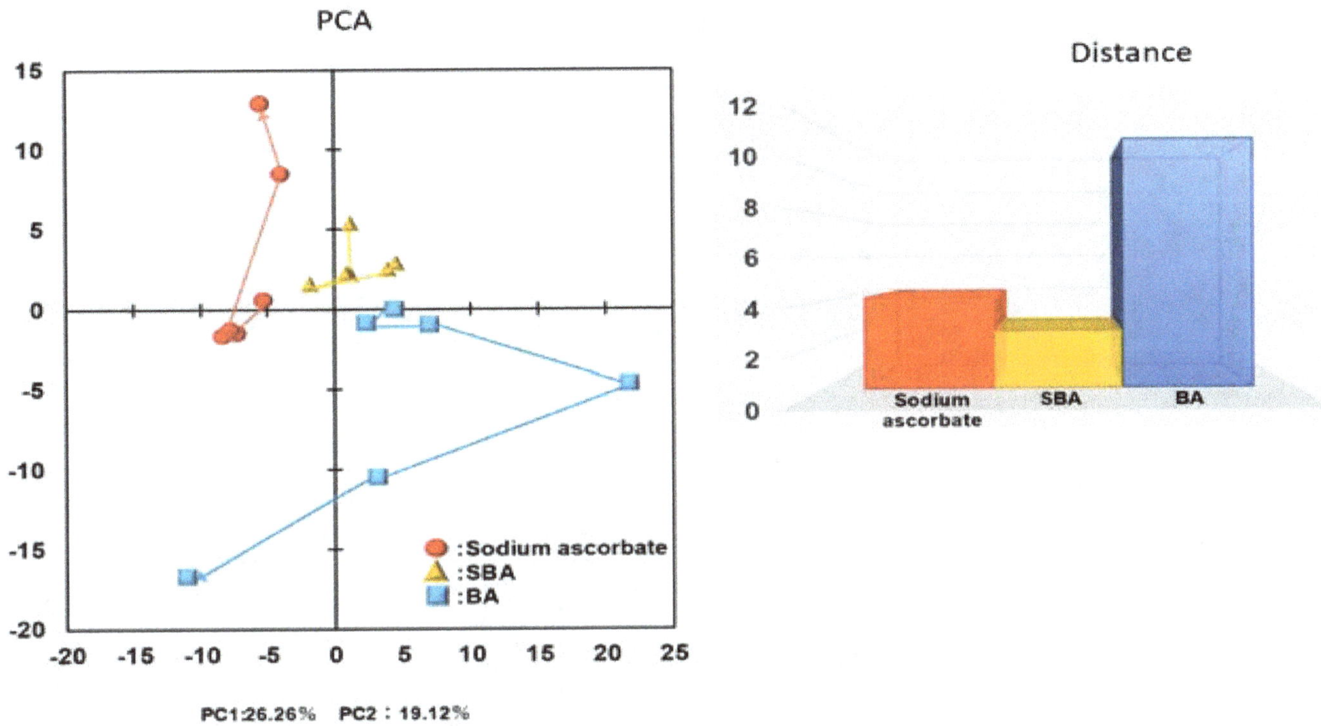

Figure 8. Principal component analysis (PCA) analysis of closeness between SBA related compounds.

3.2. *Changes of Metabolic Profiles in Normal Oral Cells Induced by Eugenol*

3.2.1. Eugenol Induced Rapid Collapse in Mitochondria

We have previously reported that four dental compounds, hydroquinone, benzoquinone, eugenol, and phtharal, induced irreversible cell death in human oral squamous cell carcinoma (OSCC) cell lines (HSC-2, HSC-4, Ca9-22) and normal human oral cells (HGF, HPLF, HPC) and skin keratinocytes within 4 h, without induction of apoptotic markers. The 50% cytotoxic concentration (CC_{50}) of eugenol was about 0.70~0.82 mM for tumor cells, and 0.75~0.79 mM for normal cells, yielding very low tumor-specificity (TS = 0.4–1.3), as compared with anticancer drugs (5-FU, melphalan, peplomycin) (TS = 4.1–9.7) [23]. Based on this finding, three human normal oral cells were exposed to 2 mM eugenol for up to 100 min.

Exposure of human normal oral cells (HPC, HPLF, HPC) to eugenol for only 20~60 min produced changes in mitochondria and endoplasmic reticulum, inducing mitochondrial collapse, vacuolization, and secondary lysosome (Figure 9).

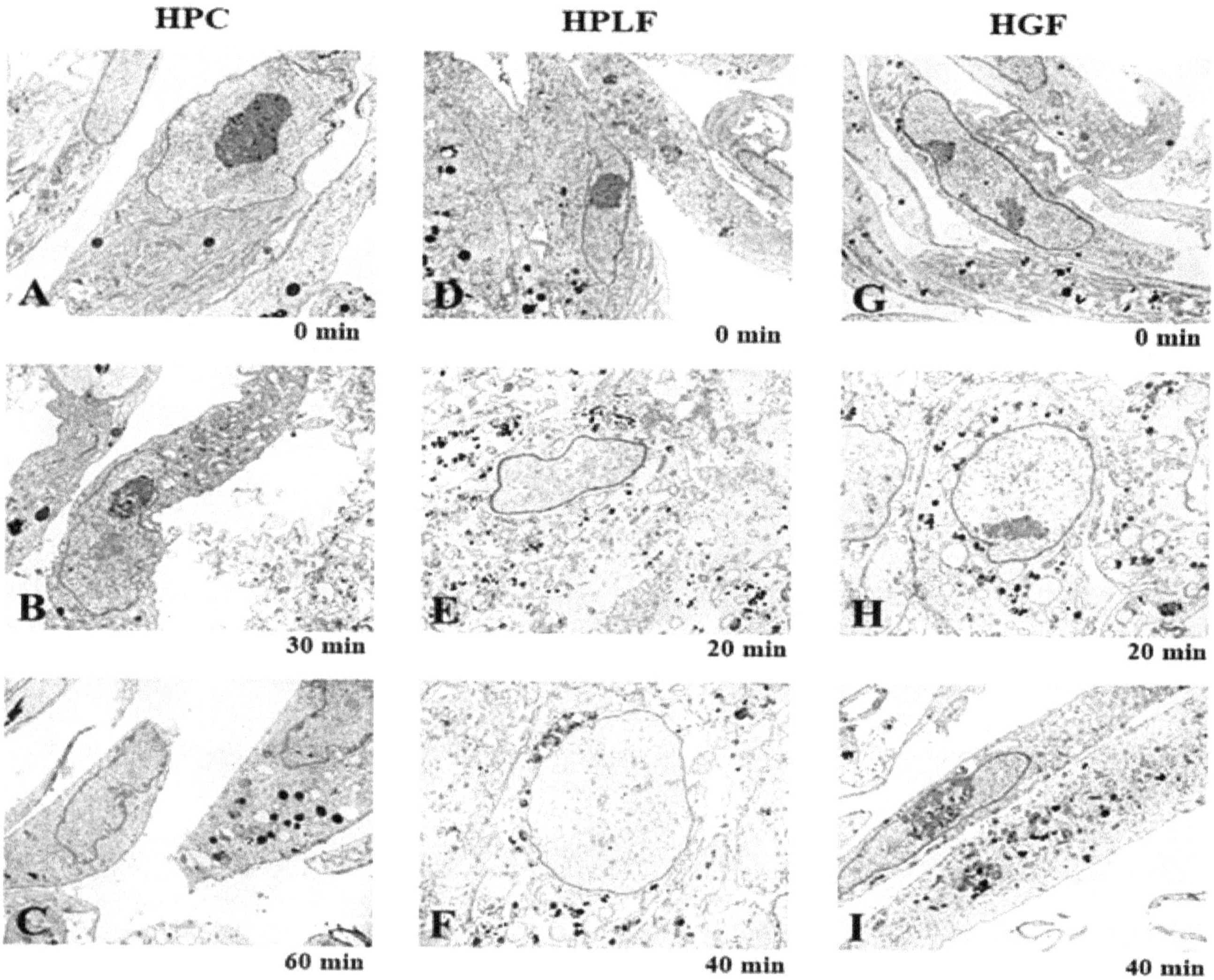

Figure 9. Rapid changes in the mitochondria and endoplasmic reticulum in normal oral cells by eugenol. Human normal oral HCP (**A**–**C**), HPLF (**D**–**F**), and HGF (**G**–**I**) cells were exposed to eugenol (2 mM) for the indicated times, and then subjected to TEM analysis. Images magnified at ×3000.

3.2.2. Eugenol Rapidly Suppressed TCA Cycle

The most dramatic changes to the TCA cycle were observed after treatment with eugenol (Figure 10). Within 20 min exposure to eugenol, intracellular concentrations of citrate, *cis*-aconitate, isocitrate, and 2-oxoglutarate rapidly declined in all three cells, whereas that of succinate, fumarate, and malate maintained almost constant levels over 80~100 min, indicating the rapid suppression of TCA cycle progression. On the other hand, eugenol treatment did not reduce, but rather slightly increased, the intracellular concentration of glycolytic metabolites (G6P, F6P, F1,6P, DHAP, 3PG, PEP, acetyl CoA, pyruvate, lactate) (Figure 10).

Eugenol treatment did not apparently affect the intracellular concentration of ATP in all three cells (Figure 11). Conversion of ATP to ADP was approximately 10%, and that of ADP to AMP was approximately 10% in all cells, indicating the very low incidence of ATP utilization (AMP/ATP = 0.01).

Similarly, eugenol treatment slightly increased the intracellular concentration of 19 amino acids, except for cysteine, which was undetectable in all cells (Table S2).

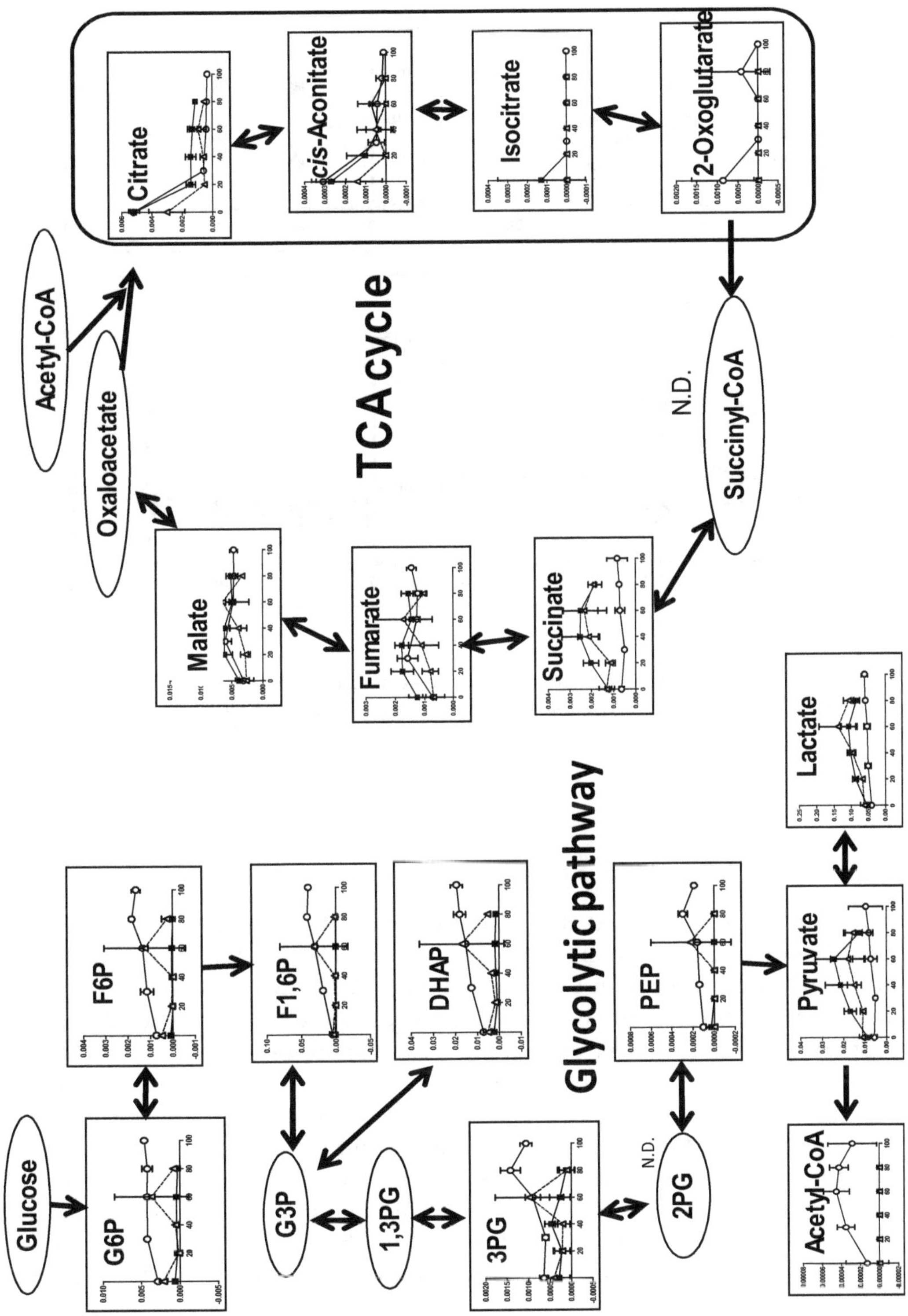

Figure 10. Eugenol suppressed the TCA cycle. HPC (○), HPLF (■), HGF (△). Vertical axis, μmol/cell. Three groups were compared by one-way ANOVA (no post test).

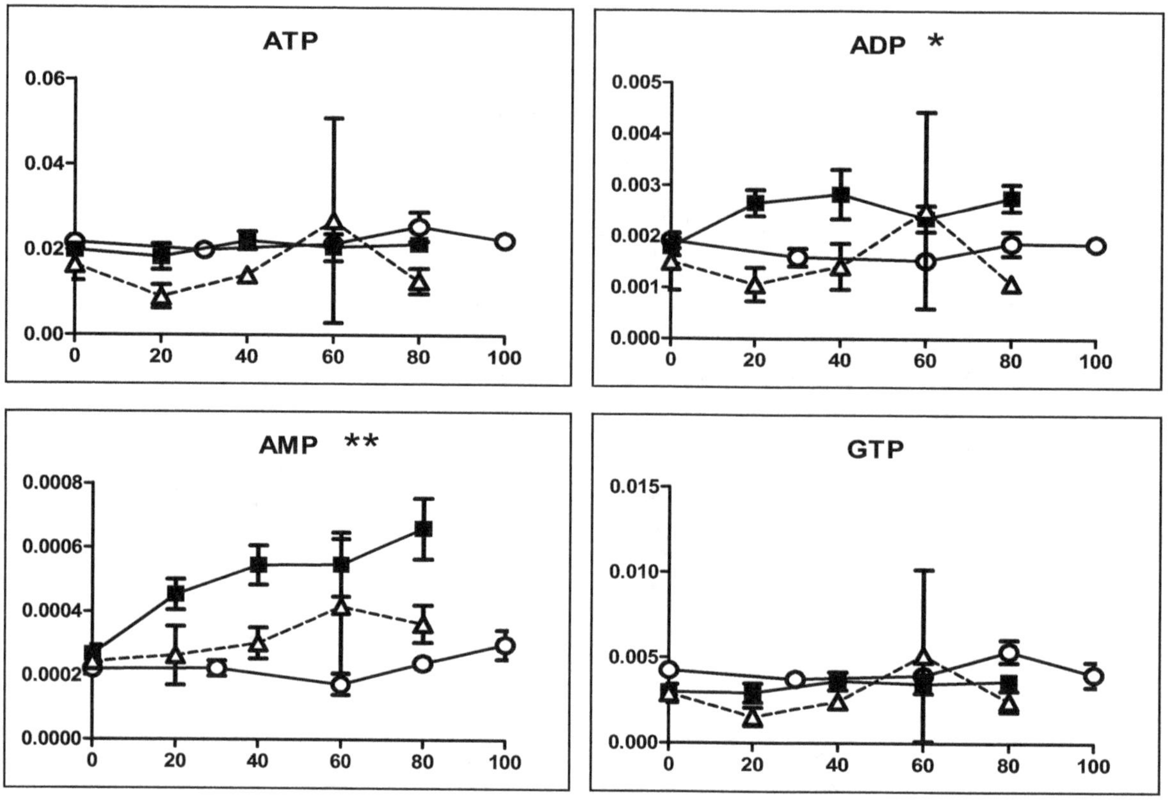

Figure 11. Eugenol generally does not affect the ATP concentrations. HPC (○), HPLF (■), HGF (△). Vertical axis, μmol/cell. Three groups were compared by one-way ANOVA (no post test). * $p < 0.05$, ** $p < 0.01$.

4. Discussion

4.1. Inhibition of TCA Cycle by Benzaldehyde (BA) in Malignant Cells

The present study demonstrated that among three SBA-related compounds (SBA, BA, SA), BA showed the following three distinct properties from others. First, in terms of catalase-sensitivity, the cytotoxicity of BA against human OSCC cell line (HSC-2) was not affected by the addition of catalase, whereas that of SBA and SA was considerably reduced by catalase. This suggests that the release of hydrogen peroxide into the extracellular milieu is important for the cell death induction by SBA and SA, but not so in the cell death induced by BA. Since catalase does not penetrate inside the cells, the possibility that intracellular hydrogen oxide may play a role in the BA-induced cytotoxicity cannot be excluded at present. Second, BA showed an inability to induce vacuolization. Third, BA was shown to inhibit the TCA cycle, possibly due to the poor supply of pyruvate or β-alanine (and their precursors). The reduction of ATP utilization (as assessed by the ratio of AMP/ATP) further supports the non-apoptosis induction by BA [9]. Since BA showed the highest tumor-specificity among three SBA-related compounds, the inhibition of TCA cycle may be the target of anti-cancer therapy.

A closer look at the dose-response of SA revealed its biphasic effect. Lower concentrations (0.625, 1.25, 2.5 mM) of SA increased the intracellular ATP level, while higher concentrations (5, 10 mM) of SA reduced the ATP level. On the other hand, lower concentrations (0.625, 1.25, 2.5 mM) of SA reduced the intracellular concentration of AMP, adenosine, IMP, and inosine, while higher concentrations (5, 10 mM) of SA elevated their concentrations (Figure 7). This further supports the bi-phasic action of SA [12]. We have previously reported that millimolar concentrations of SA (which is a popular reducing agent) produced hydrogen peroxide, reduced intracellular GSH levels, and induced apoptosis in HL-60 human promyelocytic leukemia, in a Ca^{2+}-dependent manner [13].

4.2. Inhibition of TCA Cycle by Eugenol in Non-Malignant Cells

We also found that eugenol (2 mM) induced the rapid suppression of the TCA cycle in all three human normal oral cells (HGF, HPLF, HPC). This was in nice contrast to our previous finding that eugenol slightly elevated the intracellular concentration of isocitrate and did not significantly change that of 2-oxoglutarate [33]. This demonstrated that eugenol reduced the TCA cycle only in normal oral cells, but not in OSCC cells. The present study further confirmed that eugenol induced non-apoptotic cell death, since eugenol did not affect ATP utilization except in HPLF cells (Figure 10). At present, what type of cell death eugenol has induced is yet to be determined. Considering the induction of vacuolization by eugenol, paraptosis (which causes cytoplasmic vacuolization and mitochondria enlargement [41]) may have been induced. Alternatively, considering the pro-inflammatory action of eugenol reported against HGF [42], pyroptosis (called cell inflammatory necrosis), characterized by swelling of the cell, the release of cell contents, and pro-inflammatory cytokines [43] may also be involved. Since natural products can modulate many types of cell death against cancer, such as paraptosis, necroptosis, mitotic catastrophe, and so on [44], further studies are necessary to identify the type of cell death that eugenol induces in normal oral cells. The narrow therapeutic range of eugenol suggests the importance of careful monitoring of its cytotoxicity against oral normal cells during dental treatment.

4.3. Combination Experiments with Anticancer Drugs

We have started the search for anticancer drugs that enhance the cytotoxicity of BA against human OSCC cell line HSC-2 cells. We have previously reported the mean value of CC_{50} of several anticancer drugs against four human OSCC cell lines (Ca9-22, HSC-2, HSC-3, and HSC-4) and their tumor-specificity (TS), which was determined by the ratio of the mean value of CC_{50} against three normal human oral cells (HGF, HPC, and HPC) divided by the mean value of CC_{50} against four OSCC cell lines. The anticancer drugs that we tested for their CC_{50} and TS values are doxorubicin (CC_{50} = 0.09 μM, TS = 70), mitomycin C (CC_{50} = 1.3 μM, TS = 31), methotrexate (CC_{50} < 2.4 μM, TS > 170), 5-FU (CC_{50} = 99 μM, TS > 10), docetaxel (CC_{50} < 0.032 μM, TS > 2708), and gefitinib (CC_{50} = 17 μM, TS = 4) [45]. We found that simultaneous addition of doxorubicin, mitomycin C, methotrexate, 5-FU, docetaxel and gefitinib, and dental medicines such as sodium fluoride and eugenol did not show synergistic augmentation of the cytotoxicity of BA and SBA against HSC-2 cells (Figure 12). Further study is needed to find the optimal condition for enhancing the cytotoxicity of BA against OSCC cells.

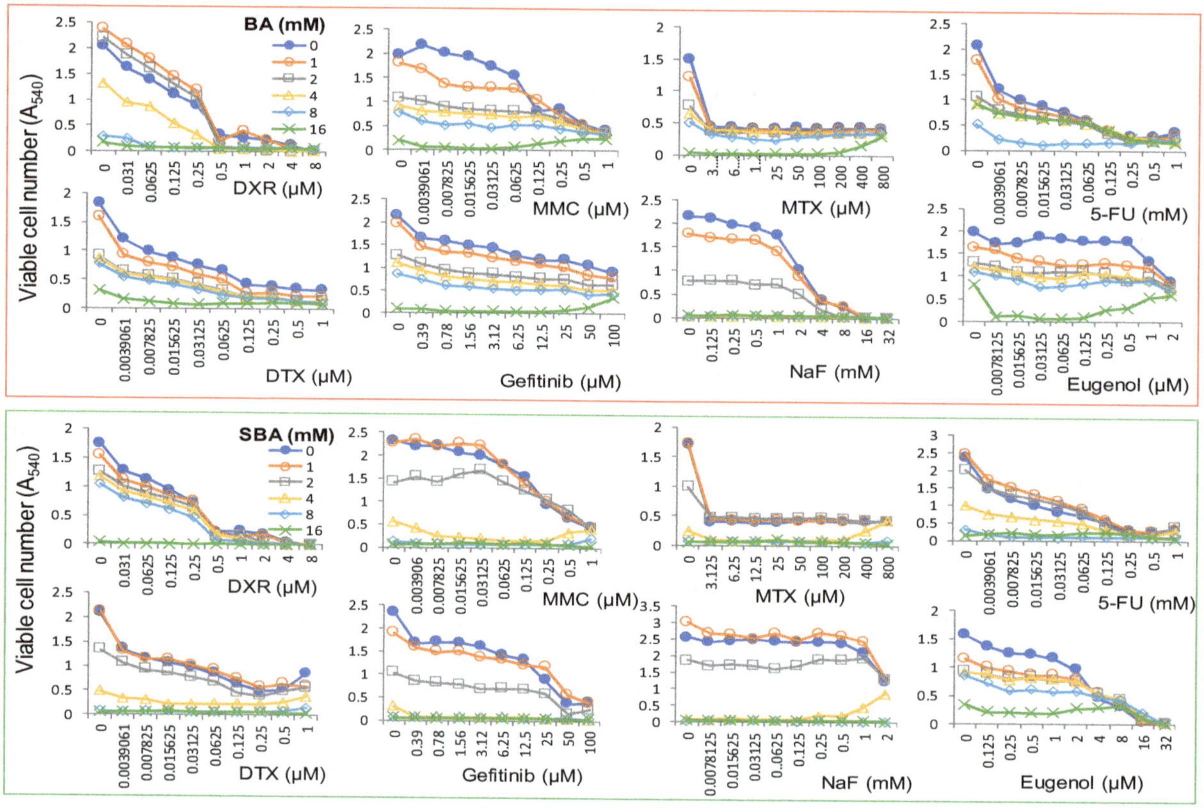

Figure 12. Combination effects of anticancer drugs and dental medicines on the augmentation of the cytotoxicity of BA (upper column) and SBA (lower column). HSC-2 cells were incubated for 48 h with the indicated concentrations of drugs in the presence of 0, 1, 2, 4, 8, or 16 mM BA or SBA, and the viable cell number was determined by MTT methods. Each value represents mean ± S.D. of triplicate assays. DXR, doxorubicin; MMC, mitomycin C; MTX, methotrexate; 5-FU, 5-fluorouracil; DTX, docetaxel; NaF, sodium fluoride.

In conclusion, both BA and eugenol suppressed the TCA cycle at the early stage of non-apoptotic cell death. As compared with eugenol, BA did not induce vacuolization, inhibited growth more slowly, and had higher tumor-specificity. Further studies are needed to design a methodology that enhances the antitumor potential of BA and reduces the cytotoxicity of eugenol in order to allow for safe clinical application. Also, the in vivo metabolic fate of SBA should be monitored for its clinical use.

Supplementary Materials:
Figure S1: Effect of SBA, BA and SA on Pyrimidine metabolism (A), puring metabolism (B), glycolysis (C), TCA cycle (D), pentose phosphate pathway (E), arginine, proline metabolism and urea cycle (F), glycine, serine and threonine metabolism (G), alanine, asparagine and aspartic acid metabolism, β-alanine biosynthesis and metabolism (H), lysine metabolisum (I), methionine and cysteine metabolism (G), histidine metabolism (K), tryptophane metabolism (L), phenylalanine, tyrosine metabolism (M), valine, leucine and isoleucine metabolism (N) and GABA biosynthesis and metabolism, glutamine metabolism (O) in HSC-2 cells. Table S1: Metabolic changes induced by SBA, BA and SA (A). 171 compounds were detected. Each value represents amol/cell, and can be seen by magnifier. Table S2: Metabolic changes induced by SBA, BA in HSC-2 cells (Exp. I), and by eugenol in HGF, HPC and HPLF cells (Exp. II). 188 compounds were detected. Each value represents amol/cell, and can be seen by magnifier.

Author Contributions: H.S. designed the experiment, performed the cytotoxicity assay, and wrote the paper; M.S. designed and analyzed the metabolomic study; Y.K. performed the TEM analysis; Y.M. contributed the eugenol experiment; O.A. interpreted the TEM data; J.S. and A.K. contributed in the set up for the experiment with SBA and BA.

Acknowledgments: The authors acknowledge the intramural support for from Meikai University School of Dentistry.

References

1. Takeuchi, S.; Kochi, M.; Sakaguchi, K.; Nakagawa, K.; Mizutani, T. Benzaldehyde as a carcinostatic principle in figs. *Agric. Biol. Chem.* **1978**, *42*, 1449–1451. [CrossRef]
2. Kochi, M.; Takeuchi, S.; Mizutani, T.; Mochizuki, K.; Matsumoto, Y.; Saito, Y. Antitumor activity of benzaldehyde. *Cancer Treat. Rep.* **1980**, *64*, 21–23.
3. Kochi, M.; Isono, N.; Niwayama, M.; Shirakabe, K. Antitumor activity of a benzaldehyde derivative. *Cancer Treat. Rep.* **1985**, *69*, 533–537. [PubMed]
4. Kochi, M.; Ueda, S.; Hagiwara, T. Antitumor activity of sodium benzylidenascorbate. In *Progress in Cancer Research and Therapy 35: Hormones and Cancer 3*; Bresciani, F., King, R.J.B., Eds.; Raven Press: New York, NY, USA, 1988; pp. 338–343.
5. Sakagami, H.; Asano, K.; Fukuchi, K.; Gomi, K.; Ota, H.; Kazama, K.; Tanuma, S.; Kochi, M. Induction of tumor degeneration by sodium benzylideneascorbate. *Anticancer Res.* **1991**, *11*, 1533–1538. [PubMed]
6. Sakagami, H.; Sakagami, T.; Takeda, M.; Iwaki, K.; Takeda, K. Determination of sodium 5,6-benzylidene-l-ascorbate and related compounds by high-performance liquid chromatography. *J. Chromatogr. Coruña* **1993**, *653*, 37–43. [CrossRef]
7. Sakagami, H.; Sakagami, T.; Yamamura, M.; Takahashi, H.; Shibuya, I.; Takeda, M. Stability of sodium 5,6-benzylidene-L-ascorbate. *Anticancer Res.* **1995**, *15*, 1269–1274. [PubMed]
8. Kishino, K.; Hashimoto, K.; Amano, O.; Kochi, M.; Sakagami, H. Tumor-specific cytotoxicity and type of cell death induced by sodium 5,6-benzylidene-L-ascorbate. *Anticancer Res.* **2008**, *28*, 2577–2584. [PubMed]
9. Ariyoshi-Kishino, K.; Hashimoto, K.; Amano, O.; Kochi, M.; Sakagami, H. Tumor-specific cytotoxicity and type of cell death induced by benzaldehyde. *Anticancer Res.* **2010**, *30*, 5069–5076. [PubMed]
10. Kuribayashi, N.; Sakagami, H.; Sakagami, T.; Niimi, E.; Shiokawa, D.; Ikekita, M.; Takeda, M.; Tanuma, S. Induction of DNA fragmentation in human myelogenous leukemic cell lines by sodium 5,6-benzylidene-L-ascorbate and its related compounds. *Anticancer Res.* **1994**, *14*, 969–976. [PubMed]
11. Sakagami, H.; Satoh, K.; Kochi, M. Comparative study of the antitumor action between sodium 5,6-bnzylidene-L-ascorbate and sodium ascorbate (Minireview). *Anticancer Res.* **1997**, *17*, 4451–4452. [PubMed]
12. Sakagami, H.; Satoh, K.; Hakeda, Y.; Kumegawa, M. Apoptosis-inducing activity of vitamin C and vitamin K. *Cell Mol. Biol.* **2000**, *46*, 129–143. [PubMed]
13. Sakagami, H.; Kuribayashi, N.; Iida, M.; Hagiwara, T.; Takahashi, H.; Yoshida, H.; Shiota, F.; Ohata, H.; Momose, K.; Takeda, M. The requirement for and mobilization of calcium during induction by sodium ascorbate and by hydrogen peroxide of cell death. *Life Sci.* **1996**, *58*, 1131–1138. [CrossRef]
14. Sakagami, H.; Satoh, K.; Kadofuku, T.; Takeda, M. Methionine oxidation and apoptosis induction by ascorbate, gallate and hydrogen peroxide. *Anticancer Res.* **1997**, *17*, 2565–2570. [PubMed]
15. Sakagami, H.; Hosaka, M.; Arakawa, H.; Maeda, M.; Satoh, K.; Ida, Y.; Asano, K.; Hisamitsu, T.; Takimoto, M.; Ota, H.; et al. Role of hydrogen peroxide in antitumor activity induction by sodium 5,6-benzylidene-L-ascorbate. *Anticancer Res.* **1998**, *18*, 2519–2524. [PubMed]
16. Sweet, C. Procedure for treatment of exposed and pulpless deciduous teeth. *J. Am. Dent. Assoc.* **1930**, *17*, 1150–1153.
17. Primosch, R.E. Primary tooth pulp therapy as taught in predoctoral pediatric dental programs in the United States. *Pediatr. Dent.* **1997**, *19*, 118–122. [PubMed]
18. Hume, W. An analysis of the release and the diffusion through dentin of eugenol from zinc oxide-eugenol mixtures. *J. Dent. Res.* **1984**, *63*, 881–884. [CrossRef] [PubMed]
19. Glass, R.; Zander, H. Pulp healing. *J. Dent. Res.* **1949**, *28*, 97–107. [CrossRef] [PubMed]
20. Barja-Fidalgo, F.; Moutinho-Ribeiro, M.; Oliveira, M.A.A.; de Oliveira, B.H. A systematic review of root canal filling materials for deciduous teeth: Is there an alternative for zinc oxide-eugenol? *ISRN Dent.* **2011**, *2011*, 1–7. [CrossRef] [PubMed]

21. Hilton, T.J. Keys to clinical success with pulp capping: A review of the literature. *Oper. Dent.* **2009**, *34*, 615–625. [CrossRef] [PubMed]
22. Hume, W.R. Effect of eugenol on respiration and division in human pulp, mouse fibroblasts, and liver cells in vitro. *J. Dent. Res.* **1984**, *63*, 1262–1265. [CrossRef] [PubMed]
23. Koh, T.; Machino, M.; Murakami, Y.; Umemura, N.; Sakagami, H. Cytotoxicity of dental compounds against human oral squamous cell carcinoma and normal oral cells. *In Vivo* **2013**, *27*, 85–96. [PubMed]
24. Atsumi, T.; Fujisawa, S.; Satoh, K.; Sakagami, H.; Iwakura, I.; Ueha, T.; Sugita, Y.; Yokoe, I. Cytotoxicity and radical intensity of eugenol, isoeugenol or related dimers. *Anticancer Res.* **2000**, *20*, 2519–2524. [PubMed]
25. Jaqanathan, S.K.; Mazumdar, A.; Mondhe, D.; Mandal, M. Apoptotic effect of eugenol in human colon cancer cell lines. *Cell Biol. Int.* **2011**, *35*, 607–615. [CrossRef] [PubMed]
26. Vidhya, N.; Devaraj, S.N. Induction of apoptosis by eugenol in human breast cancer cells. *Indian J. Exp. Biol.* **2011**, *49*, 871–878. [PubMed]
27. Majno, G.; Joris, I. Apoptosis, oncosis, and necrosis. An overview of cell death. *Am. J. Pathol.* **1995**, *146*, 3–15. [PubMed]
28. Halestrap, A.P.; Clarke, S.J.; Javadov, S.A. Mitochondrial permeability transition pore opening during myocardial reperfusion—A target for cardioprotection. *Cardiovasc. Res.* **2004**, *61*, 372–385. [CrossRef]
29. Halestrap, A. Biochemistry: A pore way to die. *Nature* **2005**, *434*, 578–579. [CrossRef] [PubMed]
30. Otsuki, S.; Morshed, S.R.M.; Chowdhury, S.A.; Takayama, F.; Satoh, T.; Hashimoto, K.; Sugiyama, K.; Amano, O.; Yasui, T.; Yokote, Y.; et al. Possible link between glycolysis and apoptosis induced by sodium fluoride. *J. Dent. Res.* **2005**, *84*, 919–923. [CrossRef] [PubMed]
31. Otsuki, S.; Sugiyama, K.; Amano, O.; Yasui, T.; Sakagami, H. Negative regulation of NaF-induced apoptosis by Bad-CAII complex. *Toxicology* **2011**, *287*, 131–136. [CrossRef] [PubMed]
32. Sakagami, H.; Sugimoto, M.; Tanaka, S.; Onuma, H.; Ota, S.; Kaneko, M.; Soga, T.; Tomita, M. Metabolomic profiling of sodium fluoride-induced cytotoxicity in an oral squamous cell carcinoma cell line. *Metabolomics* **2014**, *10*, 270–279. [CrossRef]
33. Koh, T.; Murakami, Y.; Tanaka, S.; Machino, M.; Onuma, H.; Kaneko, M.; Sugimoto, M.; Soga, T.; Tomita, M.; Sakagami, H. Changes of metabolic profiles in an oral squamous cell carcinoma cell line induced by eugenol. *In Vivo* **2013**, *27*, 233–244. [PubMed]
34. Kantoh, K.; Ono, M.; Nakamura, Y.; Nakamura, Y.; Hashimoto, K.; Sakagami, H.; Wakabayashi, H. Hormetic and anti-radiation effects of tropolone-related compounds. *In Vivo* **2010**, *24*, 843–852. [PubMed]
35. Sakagami, H.; Shimada, C.; Kanda, Y.; Amano, O.; Sugimoto, M.; Ota, S.; Soga, T.; Tomita, M.; Sato, A.; Tanuma, S.; et al. Effects of 3-styrylchromones on metabolic profiles and cell death in oral squamous cell carcinoma cells. *Toxocol. Rep.* **2015**, *2*, 1281–1290. [CrossRef] [PubMed]
36. Garcia-Contreras1, R.; Sugimoto, M.; Umemura, N.; Kaneko, M.; Hatakeyama, Y.; Soga, T.; Tomita, M.; Scougall-Vilchis, R.J.; Contreras-Bulnes, R.; Nakajima, H.; et al. Alteration of metabolomic profiles by titanium dioxide nanoparticles in human gingivitis model. *Biomaterials* **2015**, *57*, 33–40. [CrossRef] [PubMed]
37. Soga, T.; Baran, R.; Suematsu, M.; Ueno, Y.; Ikeda, S.; Sakurakawa, T.; Kakazu, Y.; Ishikawa, T.; Robert, T.; Nishioka, T.; et al. Differential metabolomics reveals ophthalmic acid as an oxidative stress biomarker indicating hepatic glutathione consumption. *J. Biol. Chem.* **2006**, *281*, 16768–16776. [CrossRef] [PubMed]
38. Sugimoto, M.; Sakagami, H.; Yokote, Y.; Onuma, H.; Kaneko, M.; Mori, M.; Sakaguchi, Y.; Soga, T.; Tomita, M. Non-targeted metabolite profiling in activated macrophage secretion. *Metabolomics* **2012**, *8*, 624–633. [CrossRef]
39. Sugimoto, M.; Wong, D.T.; Hirayama, A.; Soga, T.; Tomita, M. Capillary electrophoresis mass spectrometry-based saliva metabolomics identified oral, breast and pancreatic cancer-specific profiles. *Metabolomics* **2010**, *6*, 78–95. [CrossRef] [PubMed]
40. Sugimoto, M.; Kawakami, M.; Robert, M.; Soga, T.; Tomita, M. Bioinformatics tools for mass spectroscopy-based metabolomic data processing and analysis. *Curr. Bioinform.* **2012**, *7*, 96–108. [CrossRef] [PubMed]
41. Sugimori, N.; Espinoza, J.L.; Trung, L.Q.; Takami, A.; Kondo, Y.; An, D.T.; Sasaki, M.; Wakayama, T.; Nakao, S. Paraptosis cell death induction by the thiamine analog benfotiamine in leukemia cells. *PLoS ONE* **2015**, *10*, e0120709. [CrossRef] [PubMed]
42. Koh, T.; Murakami, Y.; Tanaka, S.; Machino, M.; Sakagami, H. Re-evaluation of anti-inflammatory potential of eugenol in IL-1β-stimulated gingival fibroblast and pulp cells. *In Vivo* **2013**, *27*, 269–274. [PubMed]

43. Ma, Y.; Jiang, J.; Gao, Y.; Shi, T.; Zhu, X.; Zhang, K.; Lu, K.; Xue, B. Research progress of the relationship between pyroptosis and disease. *Am. J. Transl. Res.* **2018**, *10*, 2213–2219. [PubMed]
44. Guamán-Ortiz, L.M.; Orellana, M.I.; Ratovitski, E.A. Natural compounds as modulators of non-apoptotic cell death in cancer cells. *Curr. Genom.* **2017**, *18*, 132–155. [CrossRef] [PubMed]
45. Sakagami, H.; Okudaira, N.; Masuda, Y.; Amano, O.; Yokose, S.; Kanda, Y.; Suguro, M.; Natori, T.; Oizumi, H.; Oizumi, T. Induction of apoptosis in human oral keratinocyte by doxorubicin. *Anticancer Res.* **2017**, *37*, 1023–1029. [PubMed]

Permissions

All chapters in this book were first published by MDPI; hereby published with permission under the Creative Commons Attribution License or equivalent. Every chapter published in this book has been scrutinized by our experts. Their significance has been extensively debated. The topics covered herein carry significant findings which will fuel the growth of the discipline. They may even be implemented as practical applications or may be referred to as a beginning point for another development.

The contributors of this book come from diverse backgrounds, making this book a truly international effort. This book will bring forth new frontiers with its revolutionizing research information and detailed analysis of the nascent developments around the world.

We would like to thank all the contributing authors for lending their expertise to make the book truly unique. They have played a crucial role in the development of this book. Without their invaluable contributions this book wouldn't have been possible. They have made vital efforts to compile up to date information on the varied aspects of this subject to make this book a valuable addition to the collection of many professionals and students.

This book was conceptualized with the vision of imparting up-to-date information and advanced data in this field. To ensure the same, a matchless editorial board was set up. Every individual on the board went through rigorous rounds of assessment to prove their worth. After which they invested a large part of their time researching and compiling the most relevant data for our readers.

The editorial board has been involved in producing this book since its inception. They have spent rigorous hours researching and exploring the diverse topics which have resulted in the successful publishing of this book. They have passed on their knowledge of decades through this book. To expedite this challenging task, the publisher supported the team at every step. A small team of assistant editors was also appointed to further simplify the editing procedure and attain best results for the readers.

Apart from the editorial board, the designing team has also invested a significant amount of their time in understanding the subject and creating the most relevant covers. They scrutinized every image to scout for the most suitable representation of the subject and create an appropriate cover for the book.

The publishing team has been an ardent support to the editorial, designing and production team. Their endless efforts to recruit the best for this project, has resulted in the accomplishment of this book. They are a veteran in the field of academics and their pool of knowledge is as vast as their experience in printing. Their expertise and guidance has proved useful at every step. Their uncompromising quality standards have made this book an exceptional effort. Their encouragement from time to time has been an inspiration for everyone.

The publisher and the editorial board hope that this book will prove to be a valuable piece of knowledge for researchers, students, practitioners and scholars across the globe.

List of Contributors

Corinna L. Seidel, Patrick Wiedemann, Matthias Weider, Gabriele Rodrian and Lina Gölz
Department of Orthodontics and Orofacial Orthopedics, Universitätsklinikum Erlangen and Friedrich-Alexander Universität (FAU) Erlangen-Nürnberg, Glückstr. 11, 91054 Erlangen, Germany

Roman G. Gerlach
Mikrobiologisches Institut-KlinischeMikrobiologie, Immunologie und Hygiene, Universitätsklinikum Erlangen and Friedrich-Alexander-Universität (FAU) Erlangen-Nürnberg, Wasserturmstraße 3/5, 91054 Erlangen, Germany

Michael Hader
Department of Radiation Oncology, Universitätsklinikum Erlangen and Friedrich- Alexander-Universität (FAU) Erlangen-Nürnberg, Universitätsstr. 27, 91054 Erlangen, Germany

Benjamin Frey and Udo S. Gaipl
Department of Radiation Oncology, Universitätsklinikum Erlangen and Friedrich- Alexander-Universität (FAU) Erlangen-Nürnberg, Universitätsstr. 27, 91054 Erlangen, Germany
Medical Immunology Campus Erlangen, FAU Erlangen-Nürnberg, 91054 Erlangen, Germany

Christian Bogdan
Mikrobiologisches Institut-KlinischeMikrobiologie, Immunologie und Hygiene, Universitätsklinikum Erlangen and Friedrich-Alexander-Universität (FAU) Erlangen-Nürnberg, Wasserturmstraße 3/5, 91054 Erlangen, Germany
Medical Immunology Campus Erlangen, FAU Erlangen-Nürnberg, 91054 Erlangen, Germany

Aline Bozec
Medical Immunology Campus Erlangen, FAU Erlangen-Nürnberg, 91054 Erlangen, Germany
Department of Medicine 3, Rheumatology and Immunology, Universitätsklinikum Erlangen and Friedrich-Alexander-Universität (FAU) Erlangen-Nürnberg, Glückstr. 6, 91054 Erlangen, Germany

Fabian Cieplik
Department of Conservative Dentistry and Periodontology, University Hospital Regensburg, Franz-Josef-Strauß-Allee 11, 93053 Regensburg, Germany

Christian Kirschneck
Department of Orthodontics, University Hospital Regensburg, Franz-Josef-Strauß-Allee 11, 93053 Regensburg, Germany

Hannah M. Herzog, Michelle G. James and Giancarlo A. Cuadra
Department of Biology, Muhlenberg College, 2400 W. Chew Street, Allentown, PA 18104, USA

Alyssa N. Hanel
Department of Biology, Muhlenberg College, 2400 W. Chew Street, Allentown, PA 18104, USA
College of Dental Medicine, Columbia University, 622 W 168th St, New York, NY 10032, USA

Nicole B. Arweiler and Thorsten M. Auschill
Department of Periodontology and Peri-Implant Diseases, Philipps-University, 35039 Marburg, Germany

Christian Heumann
Department of Statistics, Ludwig-Maximilians University, 80539 Munich, Germany

Elmar Hellwig and Ali Al-Ahmad
Department of Operative Dentistry & Periodontology, Center for Dental Medicine, Faculty of Medicine, University of Freiburg, 79106 Freiburg, Germany

Kübra Bunte and Thomas Beikler
Department of Periodontics, Preventive and Restorative Dentistry, University Medical Centre Hamburg-Eppendorf, 20246 Hamburg, Germany

Taihei Watanabe and Tomonori Hoshino
Division of Pediatric Dentistry, Meikai University School of Dentistry, 1-1 Keyakidai, Sakado, Saitama 350-0283, Japan

Naoto Suda
Division of Orthodontics, Meikai University School of Dentistry, 1-1 Keyakidai, Sakado, Saitama 350-0283, Japan

Kazumasa Mori
Division of First Oral and Maxillofacial Surgery, Meikai University School of Dentistry, 1-1 Keyakidai, Sakado, Saitama 350-0283, Japan

Toshikazu Yasui
Division of Oral Health, Meikai University School of Dentistry, 1-1 Keyakidai, Sakado, Saitama 350-0283, Japan

Naoki Yamauchi
Masuko Memorial Hospital, 35-28 Takehashi-cho, Nakamura-ku, Nagoya 453-8566, Japan

Harutsugu Kashiwagi
Ecopale Co., Ltd., 885 Minamiisshiki, Nagaizumi-cho, Suntou-gun, Shizuoka 411-0932, Japan

Tsuneaki Gomi
Gomi clinic, 1-10-12 Hyakunin-cho, Shinjuku-ku, Tokyo 169-0073, Japan

Takaaki Oizumi
Daiwa Biological Research Institute Co., Ltd., 3-2-1 Sakado, Takatsu-ku, Kawasaki, Kanagawa 213-0012, Japan

Koichi Takao and Yoshiaki Sugita
Department of Pharmaceutical Sciences, Faculty of Pharmacy and Pharmaceutical Sciences, Josai University, Sakado, Saitama 350-0295, Japan

R.M. Love
School of Dentistry and Oral Health, Griffith University, Queensland 4222, Australia

C.M. Figueredo
School of Dentistry and Oral Health, Griffith University, Queensland 4222, Australia
Menzies Health Institute Queensland, Griffith University, Gold Coast, QLD 4222, Australia

R. Lira-Junior
Division of Oral Diseases, Department of Dental Medicine, Karolinska Institutet, 141 04 Stockholm, Sweden

Sadayuki Hashioka, Tsuyoshi Miyaoka, Maiko Hayashida, Rei Wake, Arata Oh-Nishi and Masatoshi Inagaki
Department of Psychiatry, Shimane University, 89-1 Enya-cho, Izumo 693-8501, Japan

Ken Inoue
Health Service Center, Kochi University, 2-5-1 Akebono-cho, Kochi 780-8520, Japan

Siddharth Garde, Rahena Akhter, Mai Anh Nguyen and Joerg Eberhard
The University of Sydney School of Dentistry, Faculty of Medicine and Health, The University of Sydney, Camperdown 2006, Australia

Clara K. Chow
Westmead Applied Research Centre, Sydney Medical School, Westmead 2145, Australia

Norifumi H. Moritani
Department of Oral and Maxillofacial Reconstructive Surgery, Okayama University Graduate School of Medicine, Dentistry and Pharmaceutical Sciences, Okayama 700-8558, Japan

Emilio Satoshi Hara
Department of Biomaterials, Okayama University Graduate School of Medicine, Dentistry and Pharmaceutical Sciences, Okayama 700-8558, Japan

Satoshi Kubota
Department of Biochemistry and Molecular Dentistry, Okayama University Graduate School of Medicine, Dentistry and Pharmaceutical Sciences, Okayama 700-8558, Japan

Junko Nagai, Mai Imamura and Yoshihiro Uesawa
Department of Medical Molecular Informatics, Meiji Pharmaceutical University, 2-522-1 Noshio, Kiyose, Tokyo 204-8588, Japan

Yasuyoshi Miyata, Kensuke Mitsunari and Tomohiro Matsuo
Department of Urology, Nagasaki University Graduate School of Biomedical Sciences, Nagasaki 852-8501, Japan

Yasushi Mochizuki and Hideki Sakai
Department of Urology, Nagasaki University Graduate School of Biomedical Sciences, Nagasaki 852-8501, Japan
Division of Blood Purification, Nagasaki University Hospital, Nagasaki 852-8501, Japan

Hiroshi Mukae
Department of Respiratory Medicine, Unit of Basic Medical Sciences, Nagasaki University Graduate School of Biomedical Sciences, Nagasaki 852-8591, Japan

Yoko Obata and Tomoya Nishino
Department of Nephrology, Nagasaki University Hospital, Nagasaki 852-8501, Japan

Mineaki Kitamura
Department of Nephrology, Nagasaki University Hospital, Nagasaki 852-8501, Japan
Division of Blood Purification, Nagasaki University Hospital, Nagasaki 852-8501, Japan

Hiroshi Mukae
Department of Respiratory Medicine, Unit of Basic Medical Sciences, Nagasaki University Graduate School of Biomedical Sciences, Nagasaki 852-8501, Japan

Kojiro Ohba
Department of Respiratory Medicine, Unit of Basic Medical Sciences, Nagasaki University Graduate School of Biomedical Sciences, Nagasaki 852-8501, Japan
Department of Urology, Nagasaki University Graduate School of Biomedical Sciences, Nagasaki 852-8501, Japan

Atsutoshi Yoshimura
Department of Periodontology and Endodontology, Nagasaki University Graduate School of Biomedical Sciences, Nagasaki 852-8501, Japan

Hiroshi Sakagami
Meikai University Research Institute of Odontology (M-RIO), 1-1 Keyakidai, Sakado, Saitama 350-0283, Japan

Masahiro Sugimoto
Institute for Advanced Biosciences, Keio University, Tsuruoka 997-0052, Japan
Health Promotion and Preemptive Medicine, Research and Development Center for Minimally Invasive Therapies, Tokyo Medical University, Shinjuku, Tokyo 160-0022, Japan
Research and Development Center for Precision Medicine, University of Tsukuba, Tukuba, Ibaraki 305-8550, Japan

Yumiko Kanda
Department of Microscope, Meikai University School of Dentistry, 1-1 Keyakidai, Sakado, Saitama 350-0283, Japan

Yukio Murakami
Division of Oral Diagnosis and General Dentistry, Meikai University School of Dentistry, 1-1 Keyakidai, Sakado, Saitama 350-0283, Japan

Osamu Amano
Division of Anatomy, Meikai University School of Dentistry, 1-1 Keyakidai, Sakado, Saitama 350-0283, Japan

Junko Saitoh and Atsuko Kochi
Ichijokai Hospital, 4-26-1 Kitakokubu, Ichikawa, Chiba 272-0836, Japan

Index